The Cancer Clock

The Cancer Clock

Edited by

Sotiris Missailidis

The Open University, UK

John Wiley & Sons, Ltd

Other Wiley Editorial Offices

John Wiley & Sons Inc., 111 River Street, Hoboken, NJ 07030, USA

Jossey-Bass, 989 Market Street, San Francisco, CA 94103-1741, USA

Wiley-VCH Verlag GmbH, Boschstr. 12, D-69469 Weinheim, Germany

John Wiley & Sons Australia Ltd, 42 McDougall Street, Milton, Queensland 4064, Australia

John Wiley & Sons (Asia) Pte Ltd, 2 Clementi Loop #02-01, Jin Xing Distripark, Singapore 129809

John Wiley & Sons Canada Ltd, 6045 Freemont Blvd, Mississauga, Ontario, L5R 4J3, Canada

Wiley also publishes its books in a variety of electronic
available in electronic books.

Anniversary Logo Design: Richard J. Pacifico

Library of Congress Cataloging-in-Publication Data

The cancer clock / [edited by] Sotiris Missailidis.
   p. ; cm.
 Includes bibliographical references.
 ISBN 978-0-470-06151-0 (cloth : alk. paper)
1. Cancer. 2. Oncology. I. Missailidis, Sotiris.
 [DNLM: 1. Neoplasms. QZ 200 C2151227 2007]
 RC261.C2732 2007
 616.99′4–dc22

2007029109

British Library Cataloguing in Publication Data

A catalogue record for this book is available from the British Library

ISBN 9780470061510 (HB)
ISBN 9780470061527 (PB)

Typeset in 10/12 pt Times by Thomson Digital, Noida, India
Printed and bound by Printer Trento Srl., Trento, Italy
This book is printed on acid-free paper responsibly manufactured from sustainable forestry
in which at least two trees are planted for each one used for paper production.

Contents

5. Inflammation and cancer

Nigel Courtenay-Luck

6. Cancer diagnosis

Anna Batistatou and Konstantinos Charalabopoulos

9. Anticancer therapeutics   173

Teni Boulikas, Nassos Alevizopoulos, Angela Ladopoulou, Maria Belimezi, Alexandros Pantos, Petros Christofis and Michael Roberts

10. Palliative care in oncology 221

*Silvana dos Santos Barreto, Mariângela Freitas Lavor, Maria da Glória
Nunes dos Santos, Marcelle Miranda da Silva, Benedita Maria Rego
Deusdará Rodrigues and Maria Therezinha Nóbrega da Silva*

11. Physiotherapy in cancer patients 245

Mario Bernardo-Filho, Anke Bergmann and Ângela Tavares

Preface

Cancer, like most processes in life, resembles a clock, or perhaps a stop-watch in it's development. It has a beginning, a stage where the process is initiated, still imperceptible, inside our body. As the process moves along, it is discovered, either by the patient themselves as a suspicious lump or an ill feeling, or, more often nowadays, by the medical examiner in a diagnostic test, an examination, a standard screening like mammography or smear test (in women after a certain age). This discovery initiates a series of events such as further tests, biopsies, perhaps surgery, chemotherapy, radiotherapy, or all of the above, and these elicit feelings that vary from person to person and manifest themselves in all sorts of ways. But, like a clock that is ticking, the process continues onwords. Perhaps the clock ticks along and the patient runs out of time, sooner or later, and all that is left is to care for the individual and make this process as painless as possible, reduce suffering and help them to keep their dignity. However, it is equally possible, and more and more common nowadays, with early diagnosis, modern medical care and novel therapies available, that the clock is can be stopped. The stop-watch is reset and the individual moves back to the pool of the healthy, to live happily ever after, or to face other difficulties as they may come. Yet again, there is a further possibility. The clock neither runs out of time, nor, unfortunately, is it stopped and reset, but it is slowed down. That slowing down varies very much, ranging from a few months to years of healthy life, before eventually time runs out. Or it can be prolonged so much that the individual does not actually die of cancer, but lives their life to its natural conclusion, having passed through the realm of the chronic disorder patients. Appropriate medicines can control the disease indefinitely, allowing life to progress. Cancer is a disease that, in the vast majority, affects older people. Learning about ways to prevent or delay the onset of the disease and control its progression may just about give us enough time to push the disease outside the limit of our lives. As a colleague told me recently, if cancer was to develop when we are 90 or 100 years old. . . well, it wouldn't really matter that much.

So far, books about cancer are mostly addressed to experts, or students of specific disciplines, describing individual, specific aspects of the disease, epidemiology, cancer biology, surgery, nuclear medicine, or medicinal chemistry. But such volumes are not approachable by the general audience, people who suffer or have suffered from the disease, their families, people who are interested in learning about the disease, or new students that have not yet made up their minds as to what they will focus on during their studies. Information is only available from websites and support groups and charities. Thus, this book aims to provide the reader with information on the various issues involved in this cancer process, the cancer clock, as the title describes.

We see often enough advertisements about tobacco smoking and cancer and cigarette packs have logos or pictures (depending on the country) of the possible harmful effects. But why is it that tobacco can cause cancer? Why can alcohol, or its abuse, cause cancer? What about UV radiation from the sun? And then of course, we have all been witnesses to comments and questions such as the following 'My grandmother was smoking a pack of cigarettes a day and lived to a hundred and twenty years old'. Well. . . that may be so, but what other factors influenced her life? Perhaps she lived in a mountain village, breathing fresh, clean air; eating fresh, healthy food; exercising, even if by walking up the mountain slope to tend the goats, and so on. Tobacco may have increased her risk of getting cancer, but many other factors are involved in the process. There are also various environmental factors that can affect the onset of the disease. 'But no' goes no the argument', such and such both lived in the big city, even close to each other'. Well, what about diet? One perhaps cooked fresh food every day, when another, with a fast lifestyle and increased time pressures, often resorted to fast-food, pre-cooked and pre-packaged food, microwavable dishes and quickly fried meat. Could this be a reason? Evidence suggests that it often is. But what about people who enjoy similar diets? That may be so, but there are also genetic factors at hand.

Parts of our genome, the genetic code inside every one of our cells, may, in some people, contain mutations in what are called oncogenes, or even proto-oncogenes or tumour suppressor genes that increase the risk of cancer. Genes are parts of our DNA. As for the term 'onco', it comes from the Greek word *oncos*, which means tumour, and 'proto' also comes from a Greek word and means pre. So. . . a protooncogene would in lay English refer to a pre-tumour gene, and these are often responsible for the initiation of cancer. There are also genes that are responsible for correcting damage and preventing cancer, known as tumour suppressor genes. These would need to be knocked out within the cell, in order to remove the various controls they impose, which can prevent cancer. Thus, genetics, is another factor that plays a crucial role in the development of the disease and can account for the difference between one person getting cancer when another one does not, even if they live in a similar place and enjoy a similar lifestyle. Then again it may be a chronic inflammation, or an infection that was left unattended that caused the onset of the disease. I will not refer to serendipity, as this is not a factor we can control and plan, although it is always there. This can be covered by beliefs in some higher power, penance or simply bad luck. But a lot of other factors, crucial for the development of the disease, can be controlled and it is within our power, if not our responsibility, to control them.

The book will also look briefly at how the disease develops and establish the necessary steps for the generation and spread of a tumour. The various processes of the disease are examined and we see what a tumour needs in order to progress from that single first cell that went wrong to becoming a life threatening disease.

What are the options we have in identifying the possibility of having cancer, or, even before that, a propensity for developing the disease? There are often chemicals secreted in the blood stream or in the urine as a result of biological processes that may potentially lead to the formation of a tumour, or as a result of the formation and growth of the tumour itself. These are known as tumour markers and there are sensitive assays that can diagnose some of them early on. However, tumour markers can often give false alarms, and though they are valuable tools for diagnosing and monitoring the disease, at early stages they may not be as accurate as we would like. Imaging then becomes an option, as we can successfully image a small tumour in the body using various imaging techniques. If such a mass is identified through an imaging technique, such as mammography for example, then further measures can be taken to identify this mass and find out whether it is malignant or not. If it is, then the scenario changes and the fight against the disease begins.

Surgery is one of the various weapons in our arsenal for the fight against cancer. The tumour can be removed from the body entirely, or at least in part to reduce the burden and assist other therapies. Another procedure is cancer therapy, where a drug is given to the patient with the aim of killing the cancer cells without damaging the healthy ones. This often relies simply on the ability of cancer cells to multiply faster than the normal cells, but newer medicines rely increasingly on specific differences between the cancer cell and the healthy one. Different proteins are present in the cancer cell, or even different, mutated, forms of proteins that exist in normal tissue. These perform a particular function in the development of the cancer, and their blocking by a drug could cause malfunction to the cancer cell and kill it or lead it to self-destruction, as often is the case. Many modern therapeutic regimes aim at that effect, both using the so called small chemotherapy agents and the new series of biologics, drugs based on biological macro-molecules, such as antibodies and nucleic acids.

Delivery of old drugs to the cancer cell, using specific delivery methods also play an important role in the development of current and future therapeutics. The reader will have the opportunity to find out some of the scientific discoveries that drive the development of new anticancer agents that hit the market every so often.

But care of the patient does not stop with the prescription of a drug, for cancer patients often need to spend a significant amount of time in a hospital, and nursing of these patients, as well as palliative care is another important factor on their way through this fight, whether attempting to re-integrate patient into normal life or ease their passing. Every step of the way comes with various psychological effects, fear, anxiety and often despair at the prospect of having the disease, various ups and downs during treatment, coping with the pain that is often associated with the disease, dealing with the side effects of therapies, the loss of hair and stomach problems often associated with chemotherapy, the loss of taste and smell associated with radiotherapy.

These feelings are an important part of the process and can help patients on their way to full recovery or the enjoyment of their last moments with their loved ones, or pull them into despair and heighten the sense of loss and death. These aspects, too, will be considered in this volume. I realised that I wanted to provide the reader with a full view of this complicated disease, or series of diseases (as cancer is not really one disease), and provide them with an overview of the processes associated, I discovered that after 15 years of working in cancer research, University Departments and Hospitals, I still only had a brief glimpse of these areas and only knew in great depth my own narrow field of research on drug design. But whilst I wanted to provide the reader with a broad view of the disease, I wanted this to be an authoritative view, one with the clarity and accuracy of an expert in the area. To this end, a series of experts in the individual areas of cancer research have been asked and agreed to contribute to this volume, bringing an accurate and up to date picture of the research on the field of cancer, together with their view of the future, making this volume a valuable companion to anyone who wishes to learn more, either as a student or as somebody who wishes to be informed, for themselves or for somebody they know or care for.

This book is by no means comprehensive or exhaustive. However, it is my hope that the reader will find it useful and can use this book both as a source of background information on cancer and as a first reference for seeking additional information through the hundreds of references and websites that have been used in the compilation of this work.

Sotiris Missailidis
February 2007

Acknowledgements

There are a number of people that I would like to acknowledge for their contribution in the completion of this volume. First of all, I would like to acknowledge my wife Giselle for being the inspiration of this work and for her constructive comments on the outline and material. Furthermore, I would like to thank her and our daughter Ananda for their patience and support during the frantic time of putting this volume together. I could not have done it without their support and encouragement.

An edited volume is only as good as its contributions. For that, I would like to thank all the authors of the various chapters for preparing very interesting pieces of work, working meticulously and with good timing to see this effort completed within the time plan that was originally agreed and at the highest standard. It was very daring to name the book *The Cancer Clock* as this necessarily dictated the number of chapters, which could not be more or less than what they actually are. But, even in the rare occasion where an author was unable to deliver, somebody else always stepped in and completed the task in time. I thank all the authors for their chapter contributions. They made the volume what I hope to be a very interesting and informative reading.

Such a piece of work takes a lot of time to be completed. There is no amount of late nights that can account for it. Thus, I would like to thank the Open University for their support in preparing this work. The Chemistry Department and Faculty of Science, apart from providing me with all the necessary facilities, has allowed me to utilise my study leave time to devote all my efforts in the compilation of this work, which has made a critical difference in completing the volume in time.

The photographs in the volume were taken using a Nikon digital camera of our good friends Dr Jon Hall and Dr Lucia Rapanoti. They have always been there to offer a helping hand or let some steam off, over a big meal, when the going got tough.

Dr David Ray is acknowledged for his offer to further proof-read the material, in case I got too close to the manuscript and missed anything. I am very grateful for that.

Finally, I would like to thank the team at Wiley, Rachael Ballard, Liz Renwick, Fiona Woods and Robert Hambrook, as well as our editor, Alison Woodhouse, who guided me through the various stages of the publishing process and with whom I have worked so well in the preparation of this volume and are already preparing the next.

List of Contributors

Dr. Toni Aebischer
Marie Curie Excellence Team Pathogen
Habitats
Institute of Immunology and Infection
Research
University of Edinburgh
King's Buildings
Ashworth Laboratories
West Mains Road
Edinburgh EH9 3JT, UK

Dr Nassos Alevizopoulos
Regulon Inc. (USA)
Afxentiou 7, Alimos
Athens 17455, Greece

Professor Jane Anastassopoulou
National Technical University of Athens
Chemical Engineering Department
Radiation Chemistry and
Biospectroscopy
Zografou Campus
15780 Zografou
Athens, Greece.

Ass Professor Anna Batistatou
Department of Pathology
Ioannina University Medical School
5A Daidalou Str.
453 33, Ioannina, Greece

Dr Maria Belimezi
Regulon Inc. (USA)
Afxentiou 7, Alimos,
Athens 17455, Greece

Professor Anke Bergmann
Physiotherapist, Head of Department
Physioterapy Department
Hospital do Câncer III

Instituto Nacional de Câncer
Rio de Janeiro, RJ
Brasil

Professor Mario Bernardo-Filho
Physiotherapist, Full Professor
Universidade do Estado do Rio de
Janeiro and Researcher, Instituto
Nacional de Câncer,
Boulevard Vinte e Oito de Setembro 257
Vila Isabel
Rio de Janeiro, RJ
Brasil

Teni Boulikas, Ph.D.
Chairman of the Board, Regulon Inc.
(USA)
Afxentiou 7, Alimos,
Athens 17455, Greece

**Professor Konstantinos
Charalabopoulos**
Department of Physiology, Clinical Unit
Ioannina University Medical School
Ioannina, Greece
Address: 13 Solomou Str., 452 21,
Ioannina, Greece

Dr Nigel Courtenay-Luck
Chief Scientific Officer
Antisoma Research Ltd
Antisoma plc
West Africa House, Hanger Lane
Ealing
London W5 3QR, UK

Dr Petros Christofis
Regulon Inc. (USA)
Afxentiou 7, Alimos,
Athens 17455, Greece

Dr Athanasios Dovas
Albert Einstein Medical College
New York, USA

Dr Angela Ladopoulou
Regulon Inc. (USA)
Afxentiou 7, Alimos,
Athens 17455, Greece

Mariângela Freitas Lavor RN, M.Sc.
Former President of Brazilian
Oncology Nursing Society;
Former President of Oncology
Supportive Therapeutic Group
of National Cancer Institute;
Ex-director of Palliative Care
Hospital of National Cancer Institute,
Rio de Janeiro, Brazil;
Chief Cabinet of Rio de Janeiro Action
and Health Service Secretariat, Brazil.
Contact: R Afonso Pena, 71/302 Tijuca
Rio de Janeiro-RJ, Zip Code 20270-240
Brazil

Dr Sotiris Missailidis
Chemistry Department
Robert Hooke Building
The Open University
Walton Hall
Milton Keynes, MK7 6AA, UK

Marcelle Miranda da Silva, RN, M.Sc.,
Specialist Oncology Nursing
Contact: R. Rodrigues da Fonseca.
661/ bl 4 204 - Ze Garoto, - São Gonçalo
Rio de Janeiro RJ, Zip Code: 24440-110,
Brazil

Dr Ian McCubbin
NHS Ayrshire and Arran
Pavilion 7
Ayrshire Central Hospital
Kilwinning Road
Irvine, KA12 8SS, UK

**Professora Maria Therezinha Nóbrega
da Silva**
Faculdade de Enfermagem da UERJ
Universidade do Estado do Rio de
Janeiro
Boulevard Vinte e Oito de Setembro 257
Vila Isabel
Rio de Janeiro, RJ, CEP 20551-030
Brasil

Maria da Glória dos Santos Nunes RN,
Specialist Oncology Nursing, Palliative
Care Hospital of National Cancer
Institute, Rio de Janeiro, Brazil
Contact: R. Ferreira de Andrade, 616 Bl
1 apto 503 – Cachambi
Rio de Janeiro-RJ, Zip Code 20780-200
Brazil

Dr Alexandros Pantos
Regulon Inc. (USA)
Afxentiou 7, Alimos,
Athens 17455, Greece

Prof. Alan Perkins
Professor of Medical Physics
School of Human Development
Department of Medical Physics
Medical School, Queen's Medical Centre
Nottingham, NG7 2UH

Dr Michael Roberts
Regulon Inc. (USA)
Afxentiou 7, Alimos,
Athens 17455, Greece

**Benedita Maria Rego Deusdará
Rodrigues, RN, Ph.D.**
Full Professor, Director of Rio de
Janeiro State University School of
Nursing, Brazil.
Contact: R. Mariz e Barros, 856/203
Rio de Janeiro-RJ, Postal Zip Code
20270-002, Brazil

Rio de Janeiro State University School
of Nursing
Boulevard Vinte e Oito de Setembro,
157/706
Rio de Janeiro-RJ, Zip Code Cep
20551-030, Brazil

Priv. Doz. Dr. Thomas Rudel
Max-Planck-Institute for Infection
Biology
Dept. of Molecular Biology
Charitéplatz 1
D-10117 Berlin
Germany

Silvana dos Santos Barreto, RN, M.Sc.
Specialist Oncology Nursing,
Member of Brazilian Oncology
Nursing Society, Oncology Nursing
Society (US), International Association
for Hospice and Palliative Care (US)
R. Jose Higino, 136/202 – Tijuca
Rio de Janeiro-RJ, CEP 20520-202
Brazil

Prof. David E.G. Shuker
Chemistry Department
Robert Hooke Building
The Open University
Walton Hall
Milton Keynes, MK7 6AA, UK

Professor Ângela Tavares
Physiotherapist, Professor
Faculdade de Fisioterapia
Fundação Oswaldo Aranha
Volta Redonda, RJ, Brasil

Professor Craig A White
NHS Ayrshire and Arran
Pavilion 7
Ayrshire Central Hospital
Kilwinning Road
Irvine, KA12 8SS, UK

Dr Bassam Zeina
Dermatology Department
Milton Keynes Hospital
Milton Keynes MK6 5LD, UK

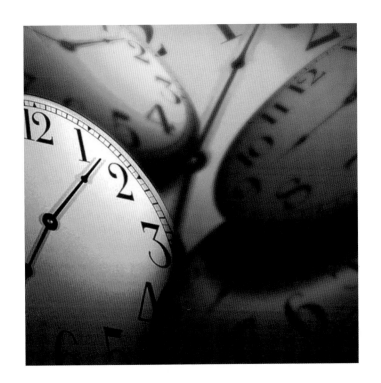

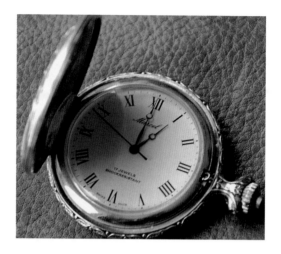

This first chapter of the book aims to set the scene on issues pertaining to cancer epidemiology, as well as the socioeconomic and molecular basis of the disease. It will clearly demonstrate various aspects of cancer initiation. Cancer, as a disease, is often different from other diseases in that it has various reasons why it can be initiated. It has often been thought off as a genetic disease, as an infectious disease, even as an inflammatory disorder, and has shared many similarities with all of them. However, cancer is a very complex disorder, or group of disorders in fact, that are very much dependent on all of the above as we will see later on. However, it is also very much related to our environment, the cultural and socioeconomic aspects of our life, even the *place* where we live and the *time* of our lives. As you will see in this chapter, contrary to popular belief, cancer is a disease that takes a very long time to develop. So, if we can only extend this process a bit further, we will all be suffering from old age before we have to encounter cancer. And though it may be frightening to know that in many of us cancer has started years before we ever find out, it is always reassuring to discover that there are things we can do to slow this process or even avoid it in our lifetime. It is reassuring to know that by changing our habits, our diet and behaviour, we can, more often than not, postpone this disease perhaps indefinitely. The socioeconomic and molecular basis of cancer will be discussed in this first chapter, together with some indication of the world cancer incidence and the 'time' and 'place' distribution of the disease, also hoping to shed light on some of the differences between parts of the population.

1

Socioeconomic and molecular basis of cancer

David E. G. Shuker

Department of Chemistry, The Open University, UK

1.1 Introduction

Cancer is a disease that is characterized by the slow rate at which it develops. This might seem at odds with our experience of seeing people diagnosed with a cancer seeming, for the most part, to have a short life expectancy. However, the clinical stage of most cancers is literally the 'tip of the iceberg', because the cancer will have been growing undetected for many years in the early stages of its natural history.

As we have come to understand more about the phenomenon of cancer at both the biological and epidemiological level it has become apparent that there are two main factors that influence the risk of developing cancer – *time* and *place*.

The importance of *time* can be seen by looking at the age-specific mortality of cancer at all sites in men and women (Figure 1.1). The age-specific rates of different cancers display similar patterns (with the notable exception of some childhood cancers such as neuroblastoma), namely, the incidence is very low until about 40 years of age and then displays a dramatic rise thereafter. This overall pattern is driven by the profiles of some of the major cancers – the age-specific incidence of colorectal cancer rises relentlessly with age (Figure 1.2). However, within this overall pattern there are some significant differences for particular cancer sites. For example, the incidence of ovarian cancer in women shows a peak at age 70–80 with a noticeable decline thereafter (Figure 1.3). Somewhat more spectacularly, the peak incidence of testicular cancer is seen in men at around age 40 with

The Cancer Clock Edited by Sotiris Missailidis
© 2007 John Wiley & Sons Ltd

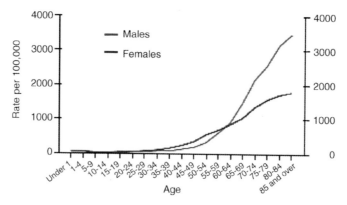

Figure 1.1 Age-specific mortality from all cancers (excluding non-melanoma skin cancer), England and Wales, 1997. Data from *Cancer trends in England and Wales 1950–1999 (Studies on Medical and Population Subjects No. 66)* Stationery Office, 2001. Reproduced under the terms of the click-use licence

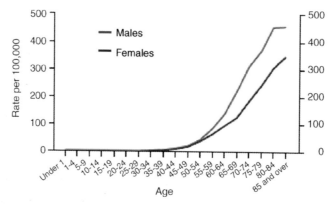

Figure 1.2 Age-specific incidence of colorectal cancer, England and Wales, 1997. Data from *Cancer trends in England and Wales 1950–1999 (Studies on Medical and Population Subjects No. 66)* Stationery Office, 2001. Reproduced under the terms of the click-use licence

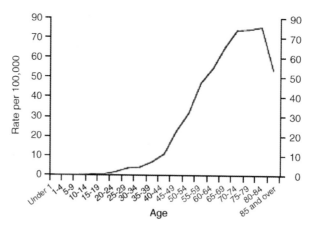

Figure 1.3 Age-specific incidence of ovarian cancer in women, England and Wales, 1997. Data from *Cancer trends in England and Wales 1950–1999 (Studies on Medical and Population Subjects No. 66)* Stationery Office, 2001. Reproduced under the terms of the click-use licence

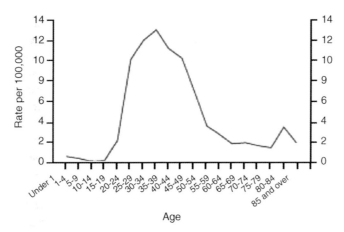

Figure 1.4   Age-specific incidence of cancer of the testis in men, England and Wales, 1997. Data from *Cancer trends in England and Wales 1950–1999 (Studies on Medical and Population Subjects No. 66)* Stationery Office, 2001. Reproduced under the terms of the click-use licence

the incidence at age 70 being not much more than that for young men (Figure 1.4). These exceptions are probably linked to hormonal effects that change throughout lifetime. Note also that the incidence rates (as incident cases per 100 000 individuals of the population, shown on the vertical axes) vary greatly between the different cancers.

So far we have discussed *time* as it is measured in epidemiological studies. There is another way in which time is important in the cancer process and that is at the molecular and biological level. One of the best characterized cancer progressions is that of color-ectal cancer, for which the key molecular steps have been identified. Vogelstein and colleagues at Johns Hopkins University in Baltimore have built up a picture of the natural history of colorectal cancer that can be summarized in a diagram that has become affectionately known as a 'Vogelgram' (Figure 1.5). Colorectal cancers are believed to develop over the course of 20–40 years as a consequence of the episodic accrual of specific mutations in oncogenes such as *KRAS* (*Kirsten Ras*) and tumour suppressor genes such as *APC* (a gene first identified in the hereditary susceptibility to adenomatous polyposis coli) and *TP53* (a gene encoding for the p53 tumour suppressor

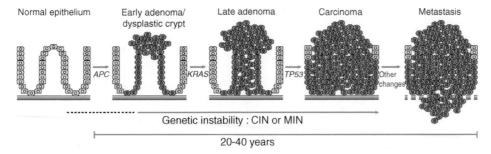

Figure 1.5   A step-wise model of colorectal tumorigenesis developed by Vogelstein and colleagues. Reprinted by permission from Macmillan Publishers Ltd: Nature Reviews Cancer *3*, 695–700 © 2003

protein). These mutations arise within the tumour in a characteristic sequence. A single cell acquires a mutation in one such gene, and this mutation soon reaches fixation because of the growth advantage it provides to the cell. Genetic instability is thought to occur somewhere during the process of colorectal tumorigenesis to accelerate the rate of mutations in dividing cancer cells. Each of the individual mutations is itself a rare event. For a cancer to progress to the clinical stage, a progenitor cell, or clone of cells, would have to accumulate three or more of these mutations. It is the time that it takes for such a 'jackpot' of rare mutations to occur in sporadic cancers that probably explains why it can take up to 40 years for a cancer to develop. Some evidence for this comes from studies of rare inherited genetic disorders such as the Li–Fraumeni and Lynch syndromes that predispose to the virtually certain development of cancers in early life. In such syndromes mutations in key genes are inherited in the germline so that every cell in the body contains mutated *APC* or *TP53*. This circumstance vastly increases the likelihood that a subsequent rare somatic mutation will occur in an already mutated cell.

We now turn our attention to the role of *place* in influencing cancer risk. The incidence of many cancers varies greatly from country to country and from region to region (Figure 1.6). One possible explanation of this could be that variations in the genetic make-up of different populations would lead to differing susceptibilities to cancer. Alternatively, variations in exposure to environmental carcinogens, or

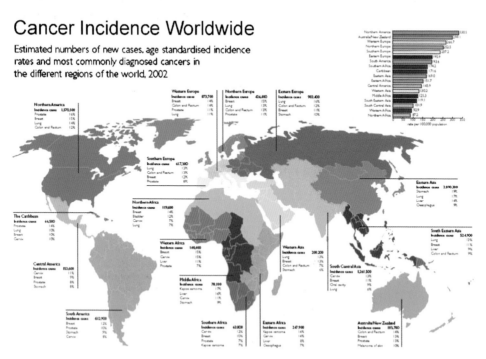

Figure 1.6   The variation in incidence of cancers at major sites around the world. (Figure reproduced from http://info.cancerresearchuk.org/cancerstats/geographic/world/?a=5441; accessed 20 April 2007) used with permission

differences in lifestyle because of the range of cultural profiles around the world, might lead to differences in cancer risk. Studies of migrant populations offer the possibility to examine the contributions of these alternative explanations. The genetic profile of individuals within a migrant population will not change within one generation, or within several generations for that matter. In contrast, exposures to environmental carcinogens will change immediately upon arrival and lifestyle changes will follow as assimilation of migrants into a new culture occurs. Thus, cancer risks driven predominantly by genetic factors would show little if any change in migrant populations, whereas those influenced by environmental or lifestyle factors would reflect the changes in the profile of exposures. The available evidence suggests that most cancer risks fit the environmental/lifestyle model of causation rather than the genetic model.

Migrant studies provide compelling evidence that cancer risk is principally determined by environmental factors, including diet. Patterns of cancer among migrant groups, as they move from country to country, often change faster than those within any country. Patterns of diet also change over time as a result of migration, sometimes dramatically.

A classic example of changes in cancer risk, in both directions, for different cancers is found in Japanese migrants to Hawaii (Figure 1.7). Japanese women living in Japan typically have a high risk of stomach cancer and an almost three times lower risk of breast cancer. The first generation of Japanese migrants in Hawaii showed a halving of their stomach cancer risk and an almost trebling of their breast cancer risk. By the second generation the Japanese–Hawaiians had a stomach cancer risk one-third that of women in Japan but a breast cancer risk that was four times higher. In a number of migrant studies a similar pattern has been seen with incoming migrants 'adopting' the profile of

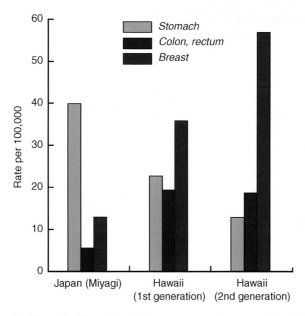

Figure 1.7 Cancer incidence for three sites in Japanese women by generation in Hawaii and Japan, 1968–1977. *WCRF/AICR Report 'Food, Nutrition and the Prevention of Cancer: A Global Perspective'* 1997. Fig. 1.1.20 Washington DC: American Institute for Cancer Research (Source: used with permission)

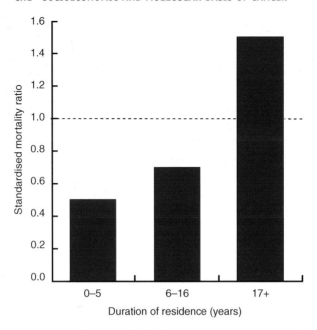

Figure 1.8 Breast cancer mortality ratios for Italian women migrants by duration of residence in Australia, 1962–1971. *WCRF/AICR Report 'Food, Nutrition and the Prevention of Cancer: A Global Perspective'* 1997. Fig. 1.2.21. Washington DC: American Institute for Cancer Research (Source: used with permission)

cancer risks of the indigenous populations. The rapidity with which cancer risks change is illustrated by a study of breast cancer mortality in Italian women migrants in Australia. Changes in rates of cancer mortality could be seen as soon as 5 years after the arrival of migrants in the host country (Figure 1.8).

In the discussion so far of the effects of *time* and *place* on cancer risk we have hinted at a number of environmental, lifestyle and dietary factors as causative, or aetiological agents. We will now turn our attention to a more detailed discussion of the role of certain factors in the determination of cancer risk.

1.2   Diet and cancer

Human beings need to consume a certain amount of food and water each day in order to acquire the basic energy required to keep the system going, as well as obtain the raw materials essential for building and repairing cellular components. The sheer quantity of food consumed by an average British family during a year in the late 1980s is rather impressive (Figure 1.9).

Until quite recently, the 'normal' diet was assumed to be either largely neutral in its effects on cancer risk or, for the most part, beneficial or protective. The role of diet in some other chronic diseases, such as diabetes and coeliac disease, had been long recognized as being linked to the presence of particular food components interacting with a defective metabolic function. In the case of cancer, the available evidence suggested that some cancers were linked to the presence of contaminants of man-made or natural origin. However, despite the public concern about cancer risk from pesticides, arising in

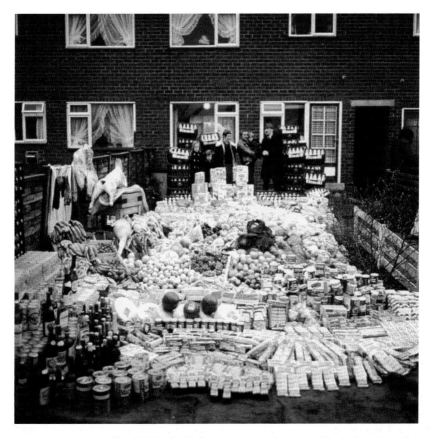

Figure 1.9 Food consumed by a British family in the 1980s during a year (image from Open University ST240 Our Chemical Environment, course book 3. Copyright © The Open University)

large part from the publication of Rachel Carson's book *Silent Spring* in the 1960s, there is little, if any, evidence that the use of pesticides raises the risk of cancer. This is not to say that pesticides are not toxic or carcinogenic, for many of them are, but the reality of the situation is that the levels of pesticide residues in foods are so low that, for all practical purposes, these exposures do not add perceptibly to the burden of cancer. It is important to note that this conclusion is not based on the extrapolation of data obtained in experimental animals to the human situation but on large epidemiological studies where pesticide exposures were assessed and for which data on cancer outcome were available. Notwithstanding, there is evidence that occupational exposure to pesticides in agricultural workers working with high volumes of concentrated pesticide solutions does lead to a somewhat increased risk of developing non-Hodgkin's lymphoma. Perhaps this is as good an example as any of the well-known aphorism – 'it is the dose that makes the poison' – attributed to the wonderfully named 16th century physician Philippus Aureolus Theophrastus Bombastus von Hohenheim (aka Paracelsus, 1493–1541).

In contrast, there is evidence that exposure to certain naturally occurring toxins, at levels consumed in the diet, does lead to a significantly increased risk of cancer. The aflatoxins, for example, are a group of fungal metabolites that are found in foodstuffs contaminated with *Aspergillus* fungi. The fungal contamination occurs when the susceptible foodstuffs (maize and groundnuts) are stored in warm and humid climates. There has been concern for a long time that human exposure to aflatoxins is a major risk factor for liver cancer but the epidemiology has been confounded by the risks of the same disease due to hepatitis infections. The distinctive chemical structure of aflatoxins has enabled the development of various assays capable of measuring human exposure to these carcinogens. The assays are based on the measurement of urinary metabolites as well as products of the interactions between aflatoxin and proteins or DNA (protein or DNA adducts; Box 1.1).

Box 1.1 **Metabolic activation of aflatoxin B$_1$ (AFB$_1$) to a reactive epoxide that binds to DNA, giving rise to a major DNA adduct (aflatoxin B$_1$-guanine) that is repaired and excreted in urine**

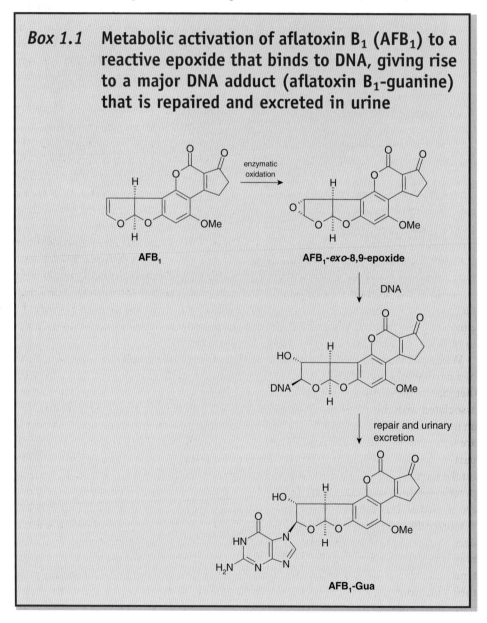

The demonstration that DNA adducts and other measures of aflatoxin exposure could really contribute to human risk assessment came with the results of a large prospective cohort study in south-east Asia. Between 1986 and 1989, 18 244 men (aged 45–64 years) were recruited into a cohort which was followed up with respect to the occurrence of hepatocellular carcinoma. At recruitment into the study each subject was interviewed, using a questionnaire, for details of dietary and other past exposures. Samples of blood and urine were also collected and stored for future analysis for a number of markers. Over the following years, 55 cases of liver cancer and 267 matched controls were collected and analysed as a nested case-control study. The presence of any urinary biomarker of aflatoxin exposure indicated a four-fold elevated risk of liver cancer. The presence of urinary aflatoxin B1-guanine (AFB1-Gua), derived from the breakdown of specific liver DNA adducts, was linked to an almost eight-fold increase in risk. The combination of urinary AFB1-Gua and specific urinary metabolites of aflatoxins indicated a ten-fold increase in risk. The study also allowed an analysis of the effect of hepatitis. Previous exposure to hepatitis B results in the presence of antibodies to a surface antigen (HBsAg) that can be detected many years after the infection and this antibody is, therefore, a biomarker of the past infection. The simultaneous presence of markers of exposure to aflatoxin and hepatitis indicated an almost 60-fold increase in the risk of developing liver cancer. Interestingly, a classic epidemiological analysis of the questionnaire data for the cases and controls failed to reveal the same effects.

This study dramatically demonstrated the value of using biomarkers of exposure to an environmental carcinogen as means to identify risk factors for a disease outcome with much greater sensitivity than traditional methods of epidemiological enquiry. Having established that certain biomarkers of aflatoxin exposure did indeed have good predictive value for the disease outcome, there are now efforts to use them to evaluate the effect of intervention studies using a drug, oltipraz, which is known from animal studies to reduce the risk of liver cancer caused by aflatoxins.

Whilst the story of aflatoxins and liver cancer is a good example of the identification of a particularly potent foodborne carcinogen, much of the cancer risk associated with diet has proved much more difficult to characterise. There are several problems associated with the study of diet and cancer. First, establishing exactly what constitutes an individual's diet is not as easy to determine as might be thought. Surprisingly, people are very unreliable in their recollection, even within the past 24 hours, of what they ate, particularly with respect to portion size. Studies using biomarkers of protein and salt intake have shown how inaccurate a 24-h dietary recall questionnaire can be. From a practical standpoint, a diet diary, in which all types of food and the quantities consumed are recorded, has been shown to provide an acceptably complete account of what a person really has eaten. Moreover, the use of photographic prompts for portion size has been shown to provide a quantitatively accurate measure of the amount consumed. You may not, however, be surprised to hear that, in the absence of such approaches, people tend to overestimate how much fruit and vegetables they have eaten and underestimate their consumption of meat. Second, it is not particularly obvious what it is about a particularly dietary component that is important for its effect on cancer risk. For example, with respect to meat consumption, is it important to know how the meat was prepared? – was it processed with the addition of additives such as nitrite, leading to the formation of nitrosamines? – was it cooked at a high temperature, leading to the production of mutagenic pyrolysis products? – or is the protein content an important source of precursors for endogenous processes that lead to mutagen formation? Similarly, for fruit and vegetables – is it the frequency and type of fruit/vegetable that is important? – is it the vitamin C/E content? – or, is it the amount of fibre that is important? Third, the level of cancer risk associated with dietary components is usually not very large. This is perhaps not surprising. If a food was strongly associated with cancer, this would have been recognized long ago and its use would have been avoided. This is certainly the case with other chronic and acute diseases – particularly if the cause of the problem is related to food being mouldy or tainted. Thus, the study of links between diet and cancer require large groups of people to be followed over many years (10–20 or more years). Such studies are expensive and do not yield many results in the early stages. However, several large studies were set up in the late 1980s – the Nurses' Health Study in the US and the European Prospective Investigation on Diet and Cancer (EPIC) – and are now beginning to yield important results. The scale of these studies is truly vast – in the second stage of the US Nurses' Health Study there were over 110 000 volunteers and in the entire EPIC cohort there were over 500 000 people recruited. The size of these prospective studies means that nested case–control studies with high statistical power for particular endpoints can be carried out within the cohort. The use of stored biological samples (notably blood and urine) adds further power to these studies, as biomarkers provide objective measures of dietary components. Furthermore, because the studies are prospective, the dietary questionnaires and biological samples were collected when the volunteers were healthy. If such markers are predictive of subsequent cancer risk they have the potential to be used in future studies where dietary interventions designed to reduce cancer risk can be tested.

Examples of the kind of results that can be obtained using the large cohort studies include the links between meat and colorectal cancer, and, saturated fat and breast cancer.

There has been much controversy as to whether high meat intake increases risk of bowel cancer. In the EPIC study, it has been found that high dietary fibre intake lowers and high meat intake increases risk of bowel cancer. However, there is an interaction between the different foods. Meat intake increases cancer risk only in those people with low intakes of dietary fibre; high dietary fibre or high fish intake appear to protect against the effects of meat intake and risk of bowel cancer.

In a study based on 13 000 women participants in EPIC, it was found that those who ate the most saturated fat were almost twice as likely to develop breast cancer as those who ate the least. Saturated fats are found mainly in full-fat milk, meat, and products such as biscuits and cakes. In the past, many large studies have failed to find a link between fat intake and breast cancer, possibly due to imprecise methods. The EPIC participants were asked to complete a detailed food diary over the course of 7 days. Even the brand of food was recorded so that the nutritional content could be worked out more precisely. It was found that women who ate more than 90 g of fat per day have twice the risk of developing breast cancer as women who ate less than 40 g of fat per day. Two-thirds of a pint of full-fat milk contains 16 g of fat, whereas the same volume of semi-skimmed milk contains 7 g of fat.

In 1997 the World Cancer Research Fund (WCRF) and the American Institute for Cancer Research (AICR) published an influential report entitled *Food, Nutrition and the Prevention of Cancer: A Global Perspective*. The WCRF/AICR report summarized the large amount of data on diet and cancer and drew conclusions on which six main dietary recommendations are based. These can be summarized as follows:

1. Choose a diet rich in a variety of plant-based foods.

2. Eat plenty of vegetables and fruits.

3. Maintain a healthy weight and be physically active.

4. Drink alcohol in moderation, if at all.

5. Select foods low in fat and salt.

6. Prepare and store foods safely.

These recommendations are broadly similar to those that have been made by the World Health Organization, the US National Cancer Institute and a number of cancer research organizations worldwide.

The decade following the 1997 WCRF/AICR report there has been much further work on the links between diet and cancer. Body mass and physical activity are things that are likely to emerge as important factors for cancer risk and some of the earlier conclusions about fruit and vegetables may be revised in the light of new information, particularly from recently concluded prospective studies of large cohorts.

We began this section by noting that human beings need to eat food and drink water regularly to maintain good health. Although we can try and optimize our diet so that it is compatible with acceptable nutritional requirements, as well as carrying the minimum attainable risk of cancer, there really is no practical alternative to eating food in order to obtain the main macro- and micro-nutrients. There are however a number of 'optional extras' that we consume which affect cancer risk in a substantial way and which would be possible, in principle, to substantially reduce or completely eliminate from our lives: alcohol and tobacco.

1.3 Alcohol and cancer

The consumption of alcoholic beverages is something that almost all societies have indulged in, from the earliest recorded times. It is likely that the production of alcoholic beverages was an accidental discovery made in several parts of the world at different times. Once the pleasurable and potent effects of alcoholic drinks were discovered, their consumption became a regular feature of social gatherings. Drinking patterns – overall level of alcohol consumption, choice of alcoholic beverages, differences by sex and age and temporal variations – differ among and within societies. Recorded consumption tends to be higher in societies with populations of European origin and lower in Muslim societies. In most of the developed countries, the majority of adults consume alcoholic beverages, at least occasionally.

Alcoholic beverages are produced from raw materials by fermentation. The predominant types of commercially produced alcoholic beverages are beer, wine and spirits. The main components of all alcoholic beverages are ethanol and water; beers also contain substantial amounts of carbohydrates. Furthermore, many compounds have been identified as common to all alcoholic beverages and are present in different quantities, depending on the beverage. Some components and occasional contaminants include known and suspected carcinogens. Beers and wines, however, also contain vitamins and other nutrients which are usually absent from distilled spirits. Despite the differences in concentration, the average intake of ethanol per drink is approximately constant across beverage types.

Alcohol is rapidly converted in the liver to acetaldehyde and then to acetate, in which form it is excreted in urine. These metabolic steps are carried out by specific enzymes (protein-based molecules with the ability to act as biological catalysts and facilitate reactions in the body), namely alcohol dehydrogenase (ADH) and aldehyde dehydrogenase (ALDH). Acetaldehyde is not a complete carcinogen in experimental animals, but it exhibits potent co-carcinogenic effects when administered with other chemicals such as nitrosamines. Furthermore, acetaldehyde is a very reactive molecule and binds covalently to proteins and DNA (Figure 1.10, Box 1.2). People who lack the enzyme ALDH, or express it at low levels or inactive forms, exhibit symptoms of acute toxicity to acetaldehyde, such as flushing, following consumption of alcoholic beverages. There is considerable variation between various populations in the expression of ALDH and this may contribute to differences in the risk of cancer linked to alcohol.

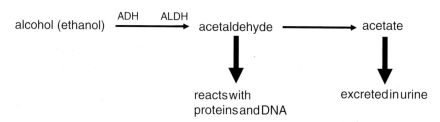

Figure 1.10 Summary of the metabolic and biochemical pathways of alcohol (ethanol)

Box 1.2 Alcohol metabolism in the body

The metabolism of ethanol in the presence of nicotinamide adenine dinucleotide (NAD) takes place with the assistance of the enzyme alcohol dehydrogenase (ADH) as shown in the following reaction:

$$CH_3CH_2OH \ + \ NAD^+ \ \underset{}{\overset{ADH}{\rightleftharpoons}} \ CH_3C\overset{O}{\underset{H}{\big\langle}} \ + \ NADH \ + \ H^+$$

$$\text{ethanol} \qquad\qquad\qquad\qquad \text{acetaldehyde}$$

Acetaldehyde, a substance even more toxic than ethanol, is quickly converted by another liver enzyme, called aldehyde dehydrogenase (ALDH), to acetate, a normal, non-toxic metabolite in humans. Non-metabolized acetaldehyde can interact with proteins and DNA and form adducts. It is also responsible for some of the obvious effects of alcohol, such as blushing. The metabolic reaction of acetaldehyde to acetate also needs NAD for its completion:

$$CH_3C\overset{O}{\underset{H}{\big\langle}} \ + \ NAD^+ \ \underset{}{\overset{ADH}{\rightleftharpoons}} \ CH_3C\overset{O}{\underset{O^-}{\big\langle}} \ + \ NADH \ + \ H^+$$

$$\text{acetaldehyde} \qquad\qquad\qquad\qquad \text{acetate}$$

Acetate is finally broken down into carbon dioxide and water and is eliminated, mainly through the kidneys in the urine but also through the lungs.

Epidemiological studies clearly indicate that drinking of alcoholic beverages is causally related to cancers of the oral cavity and pharynx (excluding the nasopharynx), larynx and oesophagus. Alcoholic beverages are also causally linked to liver cancer, with the relationship being most evident in cirrhosis. There is no indication that these effects are dependent on type of beverage. The available evidence indicates an increased risk for cancers of the breast, colon and rectum, whereas there is little evidence to suggest a causal role for drinking of alcoholic beverages in stomach and pancreatic cancer.

The link between alcohol consumption and breast cancer in women has been a subject of controversy for a number of years. This is because many studies have failed to give conclusive results, although there has been evidence of small but consistent increases in risk of cancer. There have been several attempts to merge the available epidemiological results into one large dataset – this is the technique of meta-analysis. By and large, such meta-analyses have reached the same conclusion that there is a dose-dependent increase in risk of breast cancer that does not show a threshold. On average, consumption of each additional 10 g ethanol/day was associated with risk higher by 10 per cent. Risk did not differ significantly by beverage type or menopausal status. Because of the widespread consumption of alcohol, even at modest levels, this low risk contributes to a large number of breast cancer cases at the population level.

Red wine and cancer prevention

Alcohol, itself, has been shown in various studies to increase cancer risk. However, there has also been good news for moderate consumers of alcohol. Drinking a glass of an alcoholic drink a day has been shown to have a beneficial effect on cardiovascular disease and decrease the risk for Alzheimer's and dementia at old age. Besides that, alcohol, even though only in particular form and indirectly, has been shown to have protective properties against cancer.

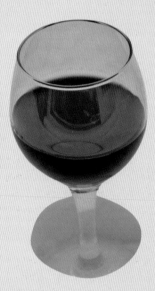

Red wine has been found to be a rich source of antioxidants (compounds that protect the cells from oxidative damage caused by free radicals) in the form of polyphenols. These are compounds that are in the skin and seeds of the grapes. However, during the wine-making process, the alcohol dissolves the polyphenols from the skin and seeds of the fruit and into the wine. Red wine is much richer in polyphenols than white wine, due to the making process that requires the removal of the skins after the grapes are crushed in the white wine. One particular type of polyphenol compound, resveratrol, is present in red wine, as is in grapes, raspberries and other plants. This compound has shown significant antitumour and cancer preventive activity in experimental animals and human tumour cell cultures. Furthermore, resveratrol has been found to reduce inflammation, which often increases the risk of cancer or is used by cancer for growth and metastasis (see Chapter 5). Thus, resveratrol has been shown to have both preventative properties against the initiation of the disease, but it can also inhibit cancer promotion and progression.

Research has shown that drinking a glass of red wine a day reduces the risk of prostate cancer by half, with even stronger effects against the most aggressive forms of the disease. Consumption of four glasses of wine per week can reduce the cancer risk of aggressive forms of prostate cancer by 60 per cent. Furthermore, epidemiological studies in regions of France, where the consumption of red wine is higher, have confirmed a reduced cancer incidence associated with red wine drinking.

Thus, although alcohol itself can increase the risk of cancer, and any cancer prophylactic properties are related to non-alcoholic substances, a glass of red wine a day can not only be an enjoyable experience and help one relax at the end of a longday, but it can ultimately assist in the control of some of the major disease of our time, such as cardiovascular and mental illnesses, and confer protection against cancer initiation and progression.

1.4 Tobacco and cancer

Smoking of tobacco is practised worldwide by over one thousand million people. However, while smoking prevalence has declined in many developed countries, it remains high in others and is increasing among women and in developing countries. Between one-fifth and two-thirds of men in most populations smoke. Women's smoking rates vary more widely, but rarely equal male rates. Tobacco is most commonly smoked as cigarettes, both manufactured – which are a highly sophisticated nicotine delivery system – and hand-rolled. Pipes, cigars, bidis and other products are used to a lesser extent or predominantly in particular regions. Cigarettes are made from fine-cut tobaccos that are wrapped in paper or a maize leaf. Cigars consist of cut tobacco filler formed in a binder leaf and with a wrapper leaf rolled spirally around the bunch. Bidis (smoked in India) contain shredded tobacco wrapped in non-tobacco leaves.

The peak of tobacco consumption in the USA occurred around 1960, but the peak of lung cancer deaths followed some 20 years later in men and is just becoming apparent in women. The 20-year lag between the consumption peak and cancer peak in men is characteristic of the time it takes for cancer to manifest itself as a clinical disease (see above). The difference between the peak cancer death rates for men and women is due to the fact that women began smoking cigarettes in the USA somewhat later than men (Figure 1.11). One of the most remarkable trends in disease over the 20th century was that in 1900 stomach cancer was the leading cause of cancer deaths in men and lung cancer was a comparatively rare condition (Figure 1.12). The gradual decline of stomach cancer over the past century has been called 'the great unplanned triumph of cancer epidemiology' because it is still not quite clear why it occurred. Unfortunately, it has been supplanted by 'the great unplanned disaster in cancer epidemiology' which is the lung cancer epidemic of the 20th and 21st centuries. In women, lung cancer took over from breast cancer as the leading cause

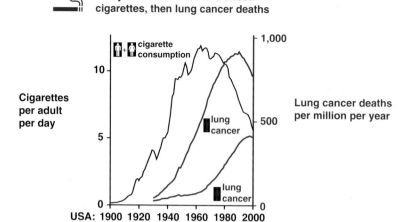

Figure 1.11 The relationship between cigarette smoking and lung cancer in US men and women over time (*Source*: www.deathsfromsmoking.net)

of cancer in 1990 – perhaps 'a great unplanned triumph of equal opportunity in disease provision' (Figure 1.13).

The link between tobacco and cancer was first identified in the 1930s in Germany and then studied in detail by Ernst Wynder in the US and Richard Doll in the UK in the late 1940s. Wynder asked a few simple questions to lung cancer patients and discovered that most of them were smokers. Many subsequent epidemiological studies have confirmed that 95 per cent of lung cancer deaths occur in smokers.

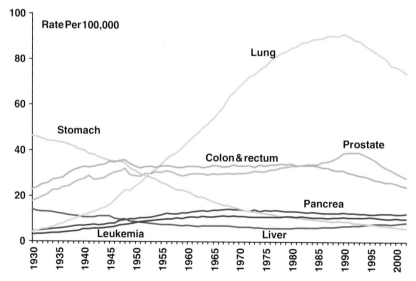

Figure 1.12 Cancer death rates, for men, US, 1930–2002 (*Source*: American Cancer Society. *Cancer Facts and Figures 2007* Atlanta: American Cancer Society, Inc.)

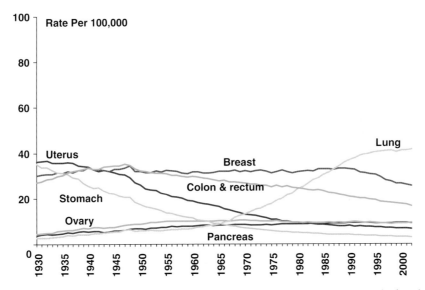

Figure 1.13 Cancer death rates, for women, US, 1930–2002 (*Source*: American Cancer Society *Cancer Facts and Figures 2007* Atlanta: American Cancer Society, Inc.)

Yet, most smokers do not die of lung cancer. This apparent paradox is due to such factors such as individual susceptibility to the development of cancer and death from other common, non-cancer, causes. Much of the detail of what we know about the links between tobacco and cancer has come from a study in a cohort of British doctors begun in 1951 by Richard Doll and colleagues. Doll recruited 34 439 male British doctors in a prospective study. Information about their smoking habits was obtained in 1951, and periodically thereafter; cause-specific mortality was monitored for 50 years. As more than 80 per cent of the doctors smoked at the time of recruitment, it took only a few years of follow-up to confirm the link between tobacco use and lung cancer. In the subsequent decades of follow-up more cancers were shown to be linked to tobacco use, including bladder cancer. The prospective design of the British doctors' study also revealed the sustained difference in numbers of years of life lost between lifelong non-smokers and continuing smokers (Figure 1.14). However, it was also possible to show that the benefits of stopping smoking could even be seen at age 55–64 in lifelong smokers. There are even larger benefits to be gained from stopping smoking at earlier ages.

By reviewing a large number of epidemiological studies carried out in many parts of the world, a World Health Organization expert working group came to the conclusion that tobacco use is causally associated with cancers at many sites in addition to lung, including oral cavity, pharynx, larynx, oesophagus (squamous-cell carcinoma and adenocarcinoma), pancreas, urinary bladder, renal pelvis nasal cavities and nasal sinuses, stomach, liver, kidney (renal-cell carcinoma), uterine cervix and myeloid leukaemia.

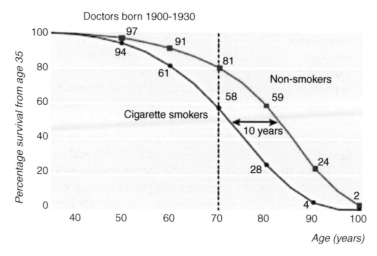

Figure 1.14 Survival from age 35 for continuing cigarette smokers and lifelong non-smokers among UK male doctors born 1900–1930, with percentages alive at each decade of age (*Source*: Doll *et al.* BMJ, 2004 *328*, 1519–1528. Reproduced with permission from BMJ Publishing Group)

The chemical composition of tobacco smoke, although influenced by the specific manner in which individuals smoke, is primarily determined by the type of tobacco. It is also influenced by the design of the smoking device or product and, for cigarettes, by the presence or absence of filters, and by other factors including ventilation, paper porosity and types of additives. As a result, concentrations of individual chemicals in smoke vary. Analysis of the ways in which people smoke modern cigarettes shows that the actual doses of nicotine, carcinogens and toxins depend on the intensity and method of smoking and have little relation to the stated tar yields. The total volume of smoke drawn from cigarettes as a result of specific smoking patterns is the principal determinant of dose to the smoker. All presently available tobacco products that are smoked, deliver substantial amounts of established carcinogens to their users. More than 60 known carcinogens are present in tobacco smoke, including polyaromatic hydrocarbons such as benzo[a]pyrene and formaldehyde and the radioactive isotope polonium 210.

Active smoking raises the concentrations of carbon monoxide, benzene and volatile organic compounds in exhaled air. The concentrations of urinary metabolites of some important tobacco smoke carcinogens and related compounds are consistently higher in smokers than in non-smokers. These include metabolites of benzene, a known carcinogen in humans, as well as metabolites of several carcinogens that cause lung tumours in rodents. Binding to blood proteins by carcinogens present in tobacco smoke has been demonstrated to occur at significantly higher levels in smokers than in non-smokers. This binding results in the formation of adducts, which are derived from various compounds including aromatic amines (e.g. 4-aminobiphenyl), polycyclic aromatic hydrocarbons (e.g. benzo[a]pyrene), tobacco-specific nitrosamines (e.g. 4-(methylnitrosamino)-1-(3-pyridyl)-1-butanone), benzene, acrylamide and acrylonitrile.

Much early work on tobacco carcinogenesis concentrated on carcinogens that had been identified in occupational or environmental situations. It appeared to be the case that the various nicotine delivery systems that characterized tobacco use were perhaps a more efficient way of delivering such carcinogens to the lung. However, it has recently become apparent that derivatives of the main tobacco alkaloids themselves may be responsible for the particular carcinogenesis of tobacco. Nicotine is probably responsible for the addictive properties of tobacco but does not cause cancer itself. However, during the tobacco curing process, as well as during the process of smoking and chewing of tobacco, nicotine is converted to derivatives such as N-nitrosonornicotine (NNN) and a related compound known as NNK. Once in the body, NNK is further metabolized to an unstable metabolite (α-hydroxy) that spontaneously decomposes to a highly reactive species (diazonium ion) that binds covalently to DNA to give characteristic DNA adducts (Box 1.3).

Box 1.3   The connection between nicotine and DNA damage related to tobacco use

Smoking-related DNA adducts have been detected by a variety of analytical methods in the respiratory tract, urinary bladder, cervix and other tissues. In many studies, the levels of carcinogen-DNA adducts have been shown to be higher in tissues of smokers than in tissues of non-smokers. Some, but not all, studies have demonstrated elevated levels of these adducts in the peripheral blood and in full-term placenta. Smoking-related adducts have also been detected in cardiovascular tissues. Collectively, the available biomarker data provide convincing evidence that carcinogen uptake, activation and binding to cellular macromolecules, including DNA, are higher in smokers than in non-smokers.

1.5 Conclusions

We began this chapter by a consideration that *time* and *place* are two factors that have a great influence on cancer risk. The slow pace of the development of cancer means that the longer that you live the greater your chance of developing cancer. If the process of cancer can be slowed down or reversed, it probably will not matter how many deleterious mutations have been acquired in various genes because the clinical stage of the disease will be delayed and some other, more acute, form of death will intervene. Overall, much of the available evidence suggests that most cancers are preventable. As Doll and Peto have observed: 'Death in old age is inevitable, but death before old age is not'. The notion of *place* being important in the development of cancer is not to suggest that one's physical location on the planet has perforce an influence on cancer risk, except perhaps in the special case of ultraviolet light and sun exposure-related skin cancer, where latitude of habitation is a risk factor. Rather, the place of habitation has an important impact on the cultural and environmental milieu, which manifests itself in diet and lifestyles that do impact directly on cancer risk.

Despite public concern over environmental pollutants and contaminants as causes of cancer, there is little evidence that they are responsible for much of the burden of cancer. One of largest preventable causes of cancer is tobacco. The link between tobacco use and lung cancer is now so well defined that it is possible to predict that tens of millions of smokers and other tobacco users worldwide will die of cancer over the next 40 years. This epidemic would be entirely preventable if it were not for two addictions. The first is the now well-established nicotine addiction that keeps tobacco users hooked and the second is that large income flows into national treasuries from tobacco excise duties. The consumption of alcohol in its various forms is now so well integrated into many societies that it will be difficult to eliminate. The experience of the US during the prohibition era highlights the difficulties of separating drinkers from their source of alcohol. The widespread consumption of alcohol and use of tobacco are two 'natural experiments' that show that human beings are not resistant to the carcinogenic affects of these two exposures.

Diet is also a major source of cancer risk – but, unlike tobacco and alcohol, also has the potential to lower cancer risk providing that the balance between nutritional requirements and the unavoidable intrinsic risks of dietary components can be found. Because all of us need to eat on daily basis, the reduction of even very small cancer risks, and the enhancement of small benefits, associated with food will have a significant effect on cancer risks for many people. However, unlike the situation with cardiovascular disease, where readily measurable risk markers such as blood pressure and serum cholesterol are available, there are currently no widely usable markers of diet-related cancer risk. For the foreseeable future, governments and other organizations will have to continue to give the best possible advice to the public on lowering cancer risk without any measure, at the individual level, of the efficacy of any intervention.

1.6 Self-assessment questions

Question	'Cancer is a disease of old age'. In what ways is this statement *not* true?
Answer	(i) for most cancers the incidence rate begins to increase from about 40 years of age
	(ii) there are a number of cancers that occur in children
	(iii) the of rate testicular cancer peaks in young adult men
Question	What are the two major risk factors for liver cancer in south-east Asia?
Answer	Exposure to dietary aflatoxins and infection with hepatitis viruses.
Question	What is the major difference between approaches to managing possible cancer risks related to pesticides and diet?
Answer	Pesticides can, at least in principle, be removed from our environment whereas dietary patterns can only be altered.
Question	If smoking causes cancer why don't all smokers get cancer?
Answer	Individual variations in susceptibility to the development of cancer and variations in metabolic profiles mean that a proportion of smokers will not develop cancer during their lifetime
Question	Why did the rate of lung cancer peak in women 20 years after that of men?
Answer	Women began to smoke at a comparable rate to men after a delay of about 20 years

1.7 Further reading and resources

Note: Wherever possible, in addition to the literature citations, the URLs for appropriate websites are given. As the homepages for the various organizations are likely to be more stable than individual pages this is what is provided. Details correct as of January 2007.

American Cancer Society, *Cancer Facts and Figures 2007*; Atlanta, American Cancer Society; 2006 (http://www.cancer.org/docroot/home/index.asp)

Cancer Research UK. *Cancer Incidence Worldwide*. Wall chart. CRUK, 2006. (http://www.cancerresearchuk.org/)

Doll R, Peto R, Boreham J and Sutherland I. Mortality in relation to smoking: 50 years' observations on male British doctors. *BMJ* 2004, **328**, 1519–1528.

European Prospective Investigation on Cancer (EPIC). (http://www.srl.cam.ac.uk/epic/international/)

Hecht, S.S. Biochemistry, biology, and carcinogenicity of tobacco-specific N-nitrosamines. *Chem Res Toxicol* 1998, **11**, 559–603.

International Union Against Cancer (UICC). *Deaths from smoking*. CD-ROM. UICC, Geneva, 2006 (http://www.deathsfromsmoking.net/)

IARC Monographs on the Evaluation of Carcinogenic Risks to Humans. Volume 44. *Alcohol drinking*. International Agency for Research on Cancer, Lyon, France, 1988. (http://monographs.iarc.fr/index.php)

IARC Monographs on the Evaluation of Carcinogenic Risks to Humans. Volume 83. *Tobacco Smoke and Involuntary Smoking*. International Agency for Research on Cancer, Lyon, France, 2004. (http://monographs.iarc.fr/index.php)

Rajagopalan H, Nowak MA, Vogelstein B and Lengauer C. The significance of unstable chromosomes in colorectal cancer. *Nat Rev Cancer* 2003, **3**, 695–700.

UK National Statistics. *Cancer trends in England and Wales 1950–1999. (Studies on Medical and Population Subjects No. 66)*. The Stationery Office, London, 2001. (http://www.statistics.gov.uk/)

US National Cancer Institute (http://www.cancer.gov/)

World Cancer Research Fund/American Institute for Cancer Research. *Food, Nutrition and Cancer and the Prevention of Cancer; A Global Perspective*. WCRF/AICR, London and Washington, 1997 (http://www.wcrf.org)

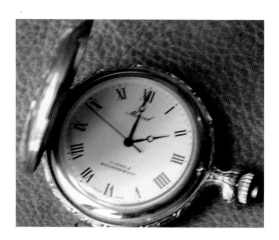

We have seen in the previous chapter the effect of *time* and *place* in the initiation of cancer. More specifically, we have discussed how dietary factors as well as socioeconomic, cultural and lifestyle factors can have a significant effect on the risk we are exposed with regards to cancer. Smoking and drinking can have a detrimental effect with regards to cancer risk. However, you may have noticed that for the cancer process to be initiated, a number of mutations are necessary. You may have also seen that the harmful effects of byproducts from fungal toxins, treated meat, tobacco smoking or alcohol consumption have ultimately been due to their interaction with DNA. Such interactions result in the so-called DNA adducts, which are subsequently removed and corrected by complicated DNA repair mechanisms within the cell, or can result in mutations after the division of the cell. Such mutations increase the possibility of oncogene activation or tumour suppressor gene suppression, thus assisting in the initiation of cancer. It can also lead to genetic instability, which allows faster accumulation of mutations, thus tipping the balance in favour of cancer formation.

In this chapter we will look at how elements, metals, widely present in our environment, can affect the formation of mutations through interactions with, or damaging of DNA. We will also have a brief discussion about other environmental factors, such as radiation, and their effect on promoting cancer initiation and growth.

2

Metal ions and cancer

J. Anastassopoulou[1] and A. Dovas[2]

1. Chemical Engineering Department, National Technical University of Athens, Greece
2. Albert Einstein Medical College, New York, USA

2.1 Introduction

The metals constitute 80 per cent of the elements of the Periodic Table (a table consisting of all known elements) and they are abundant in nature mostly in the form of metal oxides. At present, 13 metals are considered essential for life processes in both animals and plants. If you have ever taken multivitamin supplements, you will see that they often contain various metals, including for example iron, magnesium, zinc, manganese, copper and more rarely selenium, as the balance of such metals in the body is crucial for good health and growth. Furthermore, pregnant women are often prescribed extra iron in their diet. From the essential metals, sodium (Na^+), potassium (K^+), magnesium (Mg^{2+}) and calcium (Ca^{2+}) are known as the bulk metals, while vanadium (V^{2+}), chromium (Cr^{3+}), manganese (Mn^{2+}), iron (Fe^{2+}), cobalt (Co^{2+}), nickel (Ni^{3+}), copper (Cu^{2+}), zinc (Zn^{2+}) and molybdenum (Mo^{2+}) are the so-called trace metals. From the latter, iron, copper and zinc are at the top end of the scale while the other metals are present in extremely low concentrations (the *ultra-trace* elements). From the trace elements, vanadium, chromium, manganese, iron, cobalt and nickel are called transition elements, because of their particular chemical properties. Copper is also classified as a transition metal ion (TMI) but it has a different electronic configuration from the other metals. However, Cu^{2+} of d'configuration behaves as a transition metal.

Trace and ultra-trace metal ions control essential biological processes of living cells by catalysing biological reactions and controlling the activity of important biomolecules,

The Cancer Clock   Edited by Sotiris Missailidis
© 2007 John Wiley & Sons Ltd

for example protein kinases. The appearance of several diseases may be related to metal ion depletion. For instance, deficiency of iron, magnesium or calcium causes anaemia, cardiovascular diseases or osteoporosis, respectively. However, as with most things in nature, you can have 'too much of a good thing' and these metals become toxic to cells when their concentrations surpass certain optimal (natural) levels. When there is excess of metals, such as, copper and iron in Wilson's and thalassaemia diseases, correspondingly, then chelating agents may be used to reduce their concentration. There are also toxic metals, such as mercury, lead, nickel and chromium, which are difficult to detect immunotoxicologically and have been characterized as hazards in the work environment, particularly with their increasing industrial use. The metals beryllium, platinum and cobalt have been found to cause hypersensitivity and systemic allergy. Today we know that all metals are contact allergens and cause immediate allergic reactions, such as redness of the skin. Platinum (Pt) reacts violently with the skin and blood even at minute levels (10^{-11} g). Platinum salts represent a serious hazard causing asthma, rhinitis, urticaria and dermatitis. Whilst platinum can be a serious hazard, it is also one of the most potent chemotherapy drugs, as you will see later on in the book. A platinum-based compound, the neutral platinum coordination complex cis-Pt(NH$_3$)$_2$Cl$_2$, has been found to have significant antitumour activity and is used as a drug today for the treatment of various types of cancer. This drug exerts its anticancer action through selective interaction with cellular DNA.

On the other hand, the National Institute of Occupational Safety and Health has characterized seven metals as carcinogens. These are arsenic (As), beryllium (Be), cadmium (Cd), chromium (Cr), palladium (Pd), nickel (Ni) and thorium (Th). It is known that toxic metal ions such as cadmium (Cd^{2+}) and lead (Pb^{2+}) can antagonize and displace essential metal ions such as calcium (Ca^{2+}) and magnesium (Mg^{2+}) from their coordinating sites in cells, especially when these life metals are depleted and are in low concentrations. The coordination chemistry of the metals plays a specific role in their toxicity. The toxicity of heavy metal ions may depend partly on their binding to specific DNA sites.

The nature of metal–biomolecule binding is quite complex. This is because metal ions are normally surrounded by water molecules (hydrated) as salts. The approach, therefore, of a hydrated metal ion in order to come close to and interact with a biomolecule is through this hydration cell followed by substitution or not of a water molecule, as depicted in Figure 2.1.

You may have noticed that when metals are given above with their chemical symbol, they are accompanied by a positive charge. Thus, they often react with an electronegative

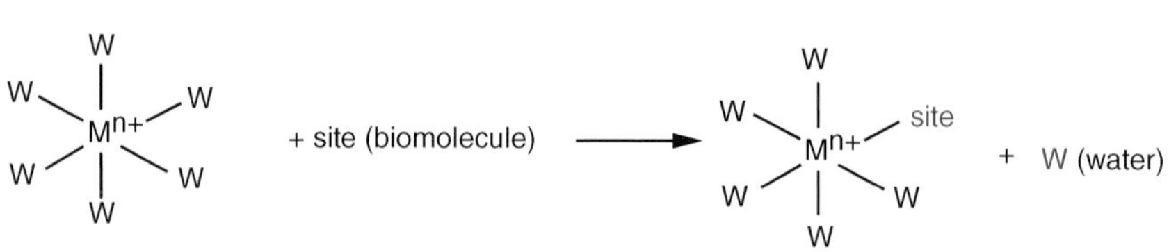

Figure 2.1 Hydrated metal–biological active site interactions

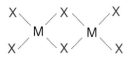

Figure 2.2 Metal–halogen bridges

atom of the biological molecule, such as nitrogen (N), oxygen (O) or sulfur (S). The DNA, for example is an overall negatively charged biomolecule, because of the phosphate groups in the backbone that holds the molecule together. That makes it an ideal target for interactions with metal ions, either through the waters of their hydration cell, or directly through the attraction of the positive charge of the metal to the negative charge of the DNA phosphate backbone. In the cases where the metal is linked to the halogens fluorine (F), chlorine (Cl), bromine (Br), or a hydroxyl group (OH) the metal can also form bridges (X=F, Cl, Br, OH) as shown in Figure 2.2.

2.2 Metal–DNA interactions

The binding of metal ions to nucleic acids has been subject of study for many years, but the mechanism of their action is still unknown. DNA is a supercoiled, negatively charged polymer of nucleotide units, characterized by its helical nature, the base pairs and the major and minor grove, formed by the supercoiling. The familiar structure of DNA is the right-handed helix (B-DNA), with the phosphate-sugar residues on the outside and the complimentary base pairs (adenine–thymine, guanine–cytosine) held together by hydrogen bonding in the interior. The positively charged metal ions interact directly or indirectly with sites characterized by an overall negative charge (high electron density) or particular negatively charged residues of the DNA. Such sites on DNA could be the negatively charged phosphates of the backbone of both strands and the nitrogen (N) or oxygen (O) atoms of the bases (electron donor atoms). Metal ions can bind tightly or weakly to DNA as partially dehydrated or fully hydrated 'free' ions respectively, or both (Figure 2.3).

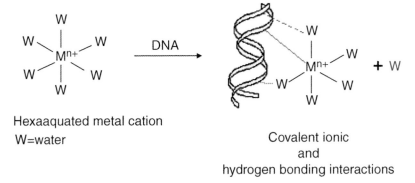

Figure 2.3 Schematic presentation of metal–DNA interaction

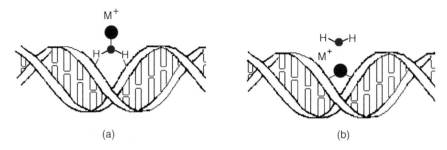

Figure 2.4   Monovalent cation in the minor groove of DNA

The sites that are most reactive of the bases are the nitrogen at position 7 of guanine and adenine, the nitrogen at position 3 of cytidine and the carbonyl oxygens of the bases. Monovalent metal ions, such as sodium (Na^+) and potassium (K^+) prefer to interact with AT rich regions of the minor groove. As everything inside the cell is surrounded by water, it is known that both metal ions and nucleic acids are specifically hydrated, encapsulated in a sphere of water molecules, and an overlapping of their hydration spheres and the release of water molecules accompany the interaction between them and the bulk state. Thus, metal ions, in order to enter in the groove as it is shown above (Figure 2.4), they should release their coordinated water and interact directly with the bases.

Various computation and experimental techniques, such as molecular dynamic (MD) simulations, solution nuclear magnetic resonance (NMR) and crystallographic results agree that the monovalent cations Na^+, K^+, Rb^+, Cs^+ and NH_4^+ prefer direct binding (inner sphere) at the AT step in the minor groove of DNA.

The divalent alkaline earth metals are rather more reactive than the alkali metals. They react as the alkali metals do and more. From alkaline earth metals magnesium is the major intracellular divalent ion and is present in all DNA and RNA activation processes. Mg^{2+} cations can act as bridge between specific enzymes and nucleotides, nucleosides and their derivatives. From the alkaline earth metals calcium (Ca^{2+}), strontium (Sr^{2+}) and barium (Ba^{2+} usually interact with DNA in an inner sphere manner, whereas magnesium (Mg^{2+}) is engaged in more outer-sphere complexes, because of its stability and higher energy of hydration.

Transition metals can act as free radicals[*]. Transition metals interact with more than two different sites and their interactions with DNA are more complicated. Transition metals lose their water molecules very easily and give inner sphere coordinated complexes. They usually bind directly to the bases and indirectly to the phosphate groups. The conformation of nucleic acids depends on the kind of metal ion that binds to DNA. Metal binding to the bases will usually disrupt base-pair hydrogen bonding and

---

[*]Free radicals are species or molecules, which contain one or more unpaired electrons. This causes the species to be paramagnetic (i.e. attracted slightly to a magnetic field) and sometimes makes the species highly reactive. They can be neutral, negatively or positively charged (radical ion, i.e. superoxide anion O_2^-.). HO. radicals and H atoms are more reactive species than OH^- and H^+, which are produced in the ionic dissociation of water, since they do not contain unpaired electrons.

destabilize the double helix. On the other hand, metal ions bound to the phosphates neutralize the excess negatively charged phosphate groups, an event that stabilizes the helix.

The binding of metals to nucleotides or polynucleotides also influences the conformation of the DNA, which is changed from the B-DNA (the standard DNA double helix) to other DNA forms such as A- or Z-DNA, which are characterized by the different orientation of the bases with respect to the axis of the DNA double helix. Furthermore, in the minor groove, cations localize preferentially at AT-rich sequences, while in the major groove the preferential site is the GC-rich sequences. The binding of metal ions to DNA is therefore sequence dependent.

In general, the metal properties of importance in their interaction with DNA are their size, polarity and ability to form hydrogen bonds as hydrated cations.

In the following sections we will examine the interactions of some metal ions with DNA.

2.3 Uranium–nucleotide interaction

Uranium is a natural radioactive element and the most important in the actinide series. All uranium isotopes are radioactive (U234, U235, U238) and they emit alpha particles. Lignites, like most materials found in nature, contain quantities of uranium and primordial radionuclides. The existence of uranium in coals is of considerable environmental interest, because the flying ash contains uranium pollutants. Furthermore, uranium is used as a fuel in nuclear power reactors and for the last two decades in the nuclear and conventional weapons field. The expanded use of this radioactive and toxic heavy metal in weapons influences the health of the general population and has lead to the known Gulf and Balkan syndromes. Large intakes of uranium lead to kidney damage and increase the risk of carcinogenesis because of its toxicity and radioactivity. As uranium tends to concentrate in specific locations in the body, risk of cancer of the bone, liver cancer, and blood (such as leukaemia) are increased. Inhaled uranium also increases the risk of lung cancer.

Special attention was paid to a particular form of uranium, its dioxouranium cation U_2^{O++} (μronyl), as this has the ability to react with polyfunctional ligands containing negative phosphate groups and other electronegative atoms, i.e. oxygen or nitrogen, as for example DNA. It was reported that uranyl ions induce necrosis of renal tubules. It was also found that the radioactivity of exposed Swiss-Albino mice increases in liver, kidney and brain. We found using Fourier transform infrared spectroscopy (FT-IR) in solid state, that uranium interacts strongly with the nucleotide 5′-guanosine monophosphate (5′-GMP) and produces a stable complex and that the major binding sites are the oxygens of the phosphate group and the N7 and O6 atoms of the base moiety, directly or indirectly through hydrogen bonding, as shown in Figure 2.5.

Accumulation of uranium and its daughter isotopes by plants grown on soils that contain uranium pollutants requires a better understanding. There is limited information on heavy-metal absorption by vegetables. The rate of release of uranium into soil

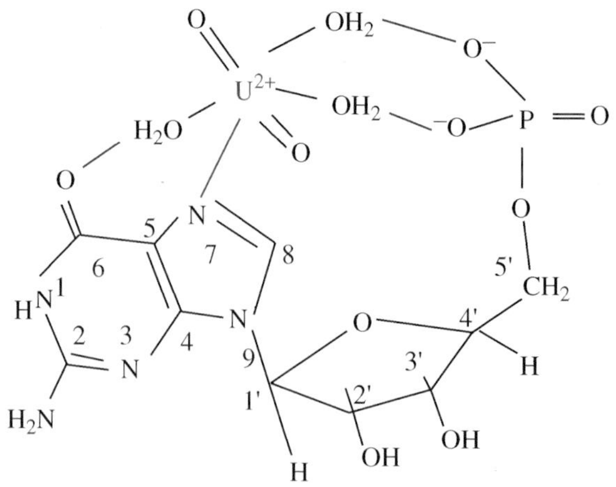

Figure 2.5 Proposed structure of uranium–guanosine-5′-monophosphate complex

and the subsequent uptake by plants could result in phytotoxicity. On the other hand, metal plant uptake is one of the main pathways through which metals enter the food chain. This pathway transfers the metals through higher trophic levels to humans.

The vegetables collected in polluted areas show significant absorption of radio-isotopes (Figure 2.6). From the Figure it is clearly seen that the wild herbs sampled in the contaminated area absorb uranium (Figure 2.6(a)). On the contrary, the same wild herbs from a non-contaminated region do not show any absorption of radioactive

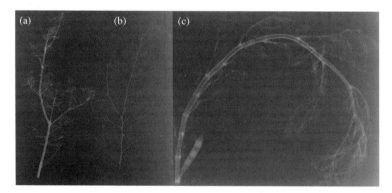

Figure 2.6 (a) Wild herb in a contaminated region; (b) wild herb in a non-contaminated region; (c) stems of beans containing potassium (^{40}K) radioisotope

elements (Figure 2.6(b)). It was also found that the steams of beans absorb potassium radioactive isotope (Figure 2.6(c)). The different absorption pattern of radioisotopes among the vegetables could be attributed to individual plant characteristics.

The use of special herbs could become a useful technique for trapping radioisotopes or heavy metals and could be used to reduce surface contamination. Thus, biosolids from different origins should be thoroughly investigated in the soil/water/plant ecosystem.

2.4 Toxicity and biological roles of copper

Copper is an essential trace element for life and participates in the transportation of oxygen, and the oxidation of iron (Fe^{2+}). The brain contains the highest cellular concentrations of copper in the body, next to the liver. Out of a total of 80–120 mg in a healthy human adult of 70 kg there are 8 mg in the liver and 15 mg in the heart, spleen, kidneys, brain and blood. Excess or deficiency of copper in the human body leads to diseases such as Wilson's disease, Mankes' syndrome and neurodegeneration. Wilson's disease (WD) is genetically determined as a metal storage disorder that leads to accumulation of copper ions in the liver. Recently, it has been reported that copper accumulation in the livers of WD patients, if not treated by chelation therapy, leads to liver injury and a 100-fold increase in the relative risk for primary liver cancer in patients with primary haemochromatosis. Also, in the cases of acute hemolytic anemia, which is associated with liver failure, WD must be considered.

The copper ion, the second most important ion that may participate in oxygen-dependent deleterious reactions *in vivo*, is tightly bound to proteins (mostly albumin), amino acids (mostly histidine) and to a specific plasma copper binding protein, caeruloplasmin. Copper compounds induce vomiting in humans. A 5 per cent copper sulfate solution can be used as an emetic for general poisoning. Copper(II) acetate, $[Cu(CH_3COO)_2 \cdot H_2O]$, is soluble in water and it is used as a mild caustic in medicine. Furthermore, copper(II) hydroxide, $Cu(OH)_2$, a light blue powder was formerly used as a pesticide and to treat seeds. On the other hand copper(I) oxide, Cu_2O, is a fungicide and $Cu(OH)_2$ or $CuCl_2$ are also used as fungicides. Copper in the form of bivalent ion, Cu^{2+} is very poisonous to lower organisms. Thus, bacteria and other decay microorganisms die in water contained in a copper vessel, and copper compounds in general prevent growth of algae. Oxygen toxicity is influenced by the presence in the diet of varying amounts of copper. Copper was found to bind DNA with high affinity, and facilitate the interaction of other molecules present in the diet (such as flavonoids) with DNA. A crystal structure of a complex formed between $CuCl_2$ and DNA demonstrated copper-binding to N7 of the guanine residue by forming a pseudo-octahedral geometry in which the other sites are occupied with water molecules. Copper(II)

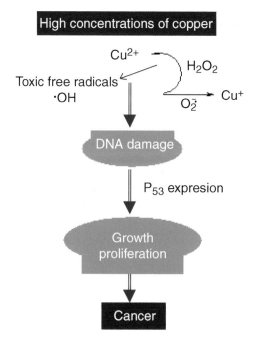

Figure 2.7   Schematic representation of the toxic role of copper

binds directly with a covalent bond to N7 of guanine and N3 of cytosine of DNA forming a more stable bond with DNA. The binding of copper ions to specific sites can modify the conformational structures of proteins, nucleic acids and biomembranes.

The formation of coordination complexes of copper with DNA may provide an advantageous active site for a reaction of highly reactive oxygen species (ROS), such as the free hydroxyl radicals, the hydroperoxyl anion (O_2^-) and the hydroperoxyl radical (HO_2·) or hydrogen peroxide (H_2O_2). The variation in the behaviour of the copper ions by its coordination sphere is considerable and accounts for the broad range of interactions with oxygen species that are observed in biological systems. Thus, if for any reason, a complex between a copper metal ion and an oxygen species is destabilized, then ROS may be liberated and cause oxidative damage leading to disease. Endogenous copper compounds catalyse ROS production from various organic carcinogens, resulting in oxidative DNA damage. This means that copper-mediated oxidative DNA damage plays an important role in chemical carcinogenesis.

The toxicity of copper depends on the concentration of the metal ion. Even though copper is essential as a life metal ion, it can become toxic for cells when its concentration is above normal levels and can induce growth proliferation and cancer by damaging DNA. Cu^{2+} ion, when acting as catalysts may also be toxic, through the generation of reactive oxygen species (ROS). Figure 2.7 demonstrates schematically the role of copper as toxic metal ion.

2.5   Formation of free radicals by metal ions

It is known that the superoxide anion radical (O_2^-) is the major reactive oxygen species generated in mitochondria, producing hydrogen peroxide (H_2O_2). Several biologically important molecules, such as glyceraldehydes, epinephrine (adrenaline) and norepinephrine (noradrenaline) are oxidized in the presence of molecular oxygen to produce superoxide anions. It is known that traces of soluble iron or copper could catalyse transfer electron reactions (Box 2.1).

Box 2.1   The Haber–Weiss reaction

In 1934, Haber and Weiss postulated the following reaction, which has become known as the Haber–Weiss reaction:

$$H_2O_2 + O_2^- \rightarrow O_2 + HO \cdot + OH^- \tag{2.1}$$

However, the rate constant for the reaction in aqueous solution is virtually zero. Therefore, it cannot take place unless it is catalysed by an oxidized transition metal, e.g. a copper ion, as proposed by Weiss and illustrated below:

$$Cu^{2+} + O_2^- \rightarrow Cu^+ + O_2$$

$$Cu^+ + H_2O_2 \rightarrow Cu^{2+} + HO \cdot + OH^-$$

$$Net : O_2^- + H_2O_2 \rightarrow HO \cdot + OH^- + O_2 \tag{2.2}$$

In this reaction the decomposition of H_2O_2 is independent of the presence of Cu(II) cations. It should be noted that in the original papers (Haber and Weiss, 1934) the initiation of the reaction (2.2) involves the hydroperoxyl radical (HO_2) and not the superoxide anion ($O_2^- \cdot$), as shown. This is only to simplify the steps of the reaction. The Haber–Weiss reaction may also be referred to as the 'superoxide-assisted Fenton reaction'.

These reactions are a prime example of a damaging free radical reaction catalysed by transition metals. A simple mixture of H_2O_2 and an iron Fe(II) salt can oxidize many different organic molecules, as was first observed by Fenton in 1894 (for a potential mechanism of this reaction see Box 2.2).

Box 2.2   A possible mechanism for the Fenton oxidation reaction of organic compounds

The exact mechanism of oxidation of organic compounds is still under debate, however, it probably involves several oxidizing species, the best characterized being $HO\cdot$:

$$O_2 \quad Fe^{2+} \quad Hys \quad \rightleftharpoons \quad O \quad Fe^{3+} \quad Hys \quad \longrightarrow \quad Fe^{3+} + HO^{\cdot} + OH^{-} \tag{2.3}$$

The mechanism of the reaction (2.3) is complex and involves $[FeO_2]^{2+}$ as intermediate. Even more reactions are possible in Fenton systems:

$$HO\cdot + H_2O_2 \rightarrow H_2O + H^+ + O_2^- \tag{2.4}$$

$$O_2^- + Fe^{3+} \rightarrow Fe^{2+} + O_2 \tag{2.5}$$

$$HO_2 + Fe^{2+} + H^+ \rightarrow Fe^{3+} + H_2O_2 \tag{2.6}$$

$$HO\cdot + Fe^{2+} \rightarrow Fe^{3+} + OH^- \tag{2.7}$$

$$HO_2 + Fe^{3+} \rightarrow Fe^{2+} + H^+ + O_2 \tag{2.8}$$

Various model systems for substrate oxidations and hydroxylations have been developed, in which iron and copper were replaced by chromium, nickel, cobalt, titanium, vanadium or tin. However, most attention has focused on iron and copper as potential mediators of $HO\cdot$ generation under normal physiological conditions, mostly due to their abundance in body tissues.

In cells, radicals are likely to be produced by bond homolysis, photolysis, radiolysis (see later) or redox reactions, processes in which radicals are produced in normal organic radical chemical reactions. There are many enzymes that produce free radicals, either as final products (e.g. xanthine oxidase, NADH oxidase) or as catalytic intermediates (e.g. prostaglandin synthase) and by-products (e.g. in the short circuit of the cytochrome P_{450}-dependent catalytic cycle; Figure 2.8). Moreover, exposure to highly reactive species such as NO or singlet oxygen can also initiate radical reactions.

Both one-electron oxidation and one-electron reduction reactions produce free radicals. Even though most biochemical oxidoreductions imply the exchange of two electrons, many oxidoreductases generate radicals as intermediates during their

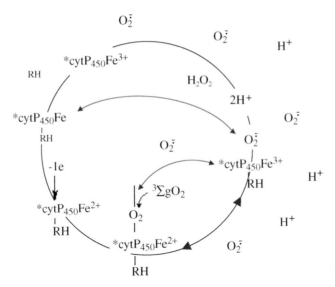

Figure 2.8 P_{450}-dependent catalytic cycle

catalytic cycle. Such radicals, formed during normal cell processes, may diffuse from the enzyme's catalytic site before their further oxidation or reduction to paired electron species.

Such an example is provided by the redox reactions of the mitochondrial electron transport chain. The mitochondrial electron transport chain not only is the cellular source of ATP (adenosine triphosphate and the body's energy store), generated by oxidative phosphorylation, but also the main source of cellular ROS. More specifically, the mitochondria produce both O_2^- and H_2O_2. This production, however, is a 'side reaction' as a result of 'leakage' of electrons directly onto oxygen rather than the next component of the electron transport chain. This effect depends on the partial oxygen pressure in the mitochondrial environment as well as in alterations in the efficiency of electron transport due to imbalances in the stoichiometry of functional electron transport proteins.

Redox reactions in which a complexed or a chelated transition metal ion (mainly iron but also copper, chromium and vanadium) act either as a binding site or as a catalyst, are also important for intracellular radical production. Indeed, the evidence is convincing that a redox reaction between a transition metal ion and a peroxide produces a radical *in vivo*.

The variable oxidation number of transition metals helps them to be effective catalysts of reactions involving oxidation and reduction. The single electron transfers promoted by metals can overcome the spin restriction on direct reaction of O_2 with non-radical species. The potential danger is that, unless their availability is carefully controlled, transition metals will catalyse unwanted free-radical reactions. For example, the human organism contains many auto-oxidizable compounds such as epinephrine (adrenaline), norepinephrine (noradrenaline), NADH, NADPH, etc., all of which are thermodynamically capable of reducing O_2 to O_2^-. However, the rates of these reactions are very low, but transition metals catalyse such autoxidations so that mixtures of these compounds with iron or copper ions will often result in free radical damage.

The reduction potentials of transition metal ions depend very much on the ligand and the metal. In this way different enzymes allow the same metal to catalyse different reactions. Similarly, different ligands confer a greater ability to their chelated metals to initiate free radical reactions.

2.6 Radiolysis

Radiolysis is the breaking of one or more interatomic bonds due to exposure to high energy radiation (ionizing radiation, α, β, γ, X, n), which follows random excitations and ionizations.

Exposure to radiation can occur both from natural sources and from industrial, medical or other man-made sources. We are constantly exposed to various forms of radiation. The highest energy radiation is X and γ radiation, which are rich in photon energy and can produce ionization (create positive and negative electrically charged atoms or particles) and break chemical bonds. Also ionizing radiation includes various sub-atomic particles, such as neutrons, electrons (β-particles) and α-particles. These make up cosmic rays coming from outer space, and are also emitted by radioactive metals (such as uranium that we saw earlier). Lower energy, non-ionizing radiation includes the ultraviolet radiation, the major source of which is exposure to the sunlight. UV radiation from the sun is intimately linked with the formation of melanomas and other skin cancers, which is why the use of high UV protection factor lotions is recommended when we are exposed to the sunlight.

Exposure to radiation is inevitable. The highest exposure to radiation is from natural sources, such as cosmic rays, radiation emitted by metals in rocks and soil, and for UV radiation from the sun. However, exposure to radiation can be from man-made sources, such as from weapons, medical X-rays and the use of radiopharmaceuticals for the imaging and treatment of various diseases (including cancer; see Chapter 8), and of

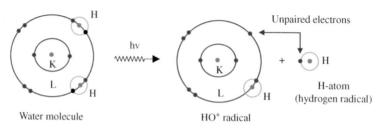

Figure 2.9 Schematic presentation of radiolysis of water molecules. The unpaired electrons are allocated at hydroxyl radicals and hydrogen atom

course nuclear accidents (such as the one in Chernobyl) or occupational exposure (for industrial workers and medical staff).

In a complex system such as the living cell, the molecules that are most likely to become ionized from the ionizing radiation are those that are more abundant. It follows that, when a cell is irradiated, the water molecules will take up most of the absorbed energy.

The primary products of radiolysis of water are hydroxyl free radicals and hydrogen atoms (radicals) as shown in Figure 2.9 and Box 2.3.

Box 2.3 The radiolysis of water

The final products of radiolysis of water are hydroxyl radicals, hydrogen atoms, hydrated electrons, and the molecular product, hydrogen molecule and hydrogen peroxide, according to the general equation (Equation 2.9) (the numbers in parentheses represent the radiation yield of the products):

$$H_2O \rightsquigarrow \cdot HO \cdot (2.8), H(0.45), e_{aq}^- (2.7), H_2, H_2O_2, H_3O^+ \tag{2.9}$$

The radical species produced this way may also react with biological molecules, thus resulting in new radical species:

$$RH + \cdot OH \rightarrow R \cdot + H_2O \tag{2.10}$$

$$RH + H \cdot \rightarrow R \cdot + H_2 \tag{2.11}$$

Radiobiologists have suggested that in a complex system such as the living cell, the action of radiation is both direct and indirect. Direct action is the interaction of radiation with the biomolecules, thereby inflicting direct damage to the biomolecule; the molecules become ionized or excited, leading to the formation of other stable products. Indirect action is the reaction between solute biomolecules and reactive species of solvent molecules formed by direct action of radiation. Since water is the main solvent in living cells, most of the indirect action in a cell involves reactive species derived from water molecules. Therefore, Equations 2.10 and 2.11 represent indirect damage to biomolecules. From the point of view of biological damage, it does not matter at all whether a biomolecule is damaged directly or indirectly. However, it does seem more likely that much of the damage is a consequence of indirect action since cells and tissues are composed of ~80 per cent water.

Among the various biomolecules, DNA is of unique importance because it is the repository of genetic information and several of the ROS-induced modifications have been shown to be mutagenic. Figure 2.10 shows the direct and indirect actions of radiation on the DNA molecule.

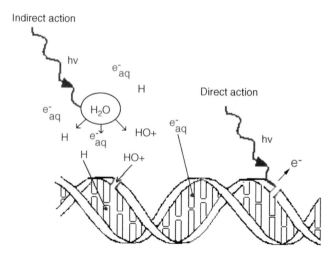

Figure 2.10 Effect of direct and indirect action of radiation, inducing damage to the DNA molecule

Oxidative stress in cells leads also to DNA damage and it occurs when reactive oxygen species are not removed or if antioxidants are depleted and the defenses cannot cope with this. DNA damage is often measured as a formation of single-strand breaks, double-strand breaks, or chromosomal aberrations. Exposure to elevated oxygen concentrations induces oxidative stress in cells. DNA damage in human cells may be produced by exposure to cigarette smoke (as we have seen before), asbestos, and ozone or to carcinogenic metals, such as some compounds of Ni or even essential life metals at above-normal concentrations. Many types of DNA modifications are produced by ROS, which include base damage, single strand breaks (ssb), double strand breaks (dsb), base and sugar damage on opposite strands, base damage and single strand break on the opposite strand, base damage in both strands (Figure 2.11).

The most common ROS-induced DNA alterations are base modifications (Figure 2.12), of which more than 20 have so far been determined. One such

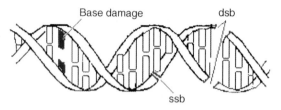

Figure 2.11 Possible patterns of DNA damage from free radical attack: base damage, in one or both strands, single strand breaks (ssb), double strand breaks (dsb) of the same or the opposite strands or any combination of them

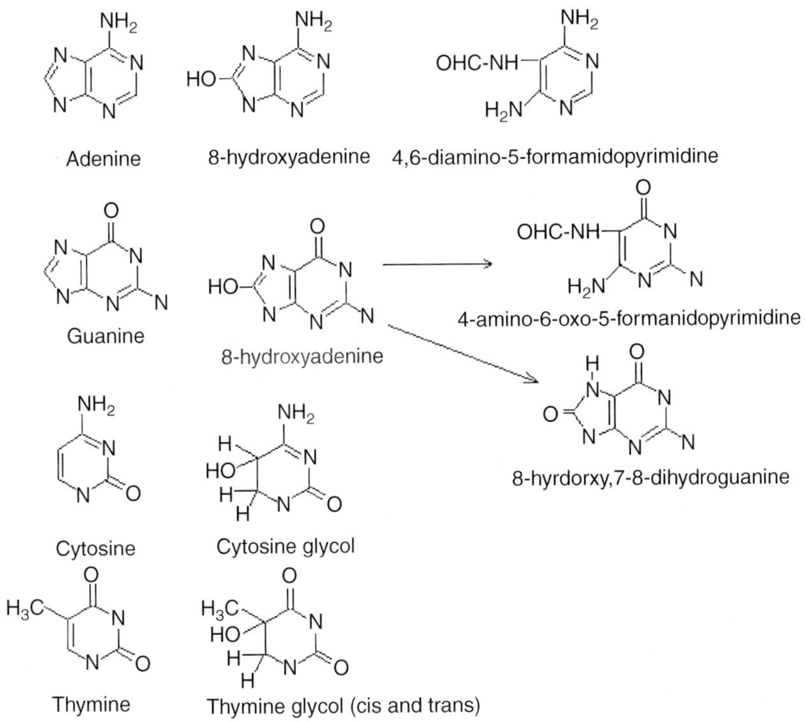

Figure 2.12 General patterns of nucleotide damage induced by the addition of hydroxyl radical on DNA bases and some of the products

modification (8-oxodG) is considered to be one of the DNA products generated by the reaction with active oxygen species and is a ubiquitous biomarker of DNA oxidation damage. However, the hydroxyl radicals can react with the DNA sugar-phosphate groups, also causing ssb or dsb. It is well established that breaks of the DNA phosphodiester backbone, with one or more lesions, may also be induced by several therapeutic drugs, such as bleomycin and neocarzinostatin, in the presence of copper ions.

The presence of metal ions during irradiation could affect the sensitization or resistance of the biological system. Thus, irradiation of 5′-guanosine monophosphate in the presence of cis-platinum (an anticancer drug) showed an increase of the nucleotide damage. On the contrary, the presence of magnesium ions showed a protection of the nucleotide upon irradiation (decrease of 8-oxodG).

The damaging effects of ionizing radiation are amplified by the presence of oxygen molecules. This increased effectiveness is known as the 'oxygen effect' and may involve the increased yield of damaging free radicals formed in the presence of oxygen (see Box 2.4).

Box 2.4 Free radical formation in the presence of oxygen

Oxygen can interact with H atoms and hydrated electrons to produce hydroperoxyl radicals (HO_2) and their superoxide anions ($O_2^-\cdot$).

$$O_2 + H\cdot \rightarrow HO_2\cdot \tag{2.12}$$

$$O_2 + e_{aq}^- \rightarrow O_2^- \tag{2.13}$$

$$O_2^-\cdot + H^+ \rightarrow HO_2^- \tag{2.14}$$

$$2HO_2^- \rightarrow H_2O_2 + O_2 \tag{2.15}$$

Moreover, if a biological molecule becomes a free radical it may interact with oxygen to give peroxides, as follows:

$$R\cdot + O_2 \rightarrow ROO\cdot \tag{2.16}$$

It is proposed that these reactions are tantamount to the fixation of biological damage and thus repair of the affected molecule (e.g. by GSH or ascorbic acid) is prevented. The reaction (Equation 2.16) is also observed in lipid peroxidation and it plays a critical role for the fluidity of cell membranes and their permeability of calcium ions.

2.7 Biomolecular targets of free radicals

As discussed above, ROS are the most frequent molecular entities likely to be formed during free radical chain reactions. In a biological system they are able to react with many small organic molecules (e.g. vitamins, sugars, amino acids, lipids), as well as with macromolecules (proteins, nucleic acids) and organized molecular and macromolecular systems (e.g. biological membranes). Such reactions may participate in the propagation stage of the radical chain reaction or in its termination process. In the context of metal ions, however, only oxidation of lipids, DNA and proteins will be discussed as they are linked to several pathologic states in humans (including cancer, atherosclerosis, Parkinson's and Alzheimer's disease).

The presence inside the protein of a complexed iron or copper ion that catalyses the decomposition of hydrogen peroxide (H_2O_2) may facilitate the initiation of a chain radical reaction, according to reaction (Equation 2.17):

$$Fe^{2+}(\text{protein bound}) + H_2O_2 \rightarrow Fe^{3+} + HO\cdot + OH^- + \text{protein} \tag{2.17}$$

H_2O_2, which readily crosses biological membranes, enters the nucleus and reacts with copper or iron ions to form the free radical $HO\cdot$. Because of its high reactivity, $HO\cdot$ does not diffuse away but it rapidly reacts with the DNA molecule. Copper(II) was shown to bind to DNA with higher affinity than any other divalent cation studied, which also explains why H_2O_2-dependent DNA oxidation has been reported to be 50 times faster than that of iron. The presence of iron in the nucleus has been proven; however, its direct binding to DNA is still a matter of speculation. The requirement of a catalytic metal ion for the generation of HO· from H_2O_2 has been demonstrated experimentally. ·OH formation was detected in the presence of H_2O_2 and a metal ion (either iron or copper), while no HO· was detected when H_2O_2 alone or an iron or copper salt, alone, were added to the reaction mixture.

'Free' or 'catalytic' transition metal ions (TMIs), if present in biological systems are able to autoxidise, catalyse the Fenton and Haber–Weiss reactions (Boxes 2.1 and 2.2), and the autoxidation of endogenous substrates. Thus, aerobic biological systems have developed highly sophisticated systems to keep the 'free' concentrations of TMIs as low as possible.

More specifically, iron ions are strongly bound to proteins, which, in their native form, do not participate in any deleterious reactions. About 70 per cent of iron ions in humans are stored in iron-containing proteins, the majority being in haemoglobin, and the rest in myoglobin and other proteins. From the remaining 30 per cent, the majority is stored intracellularly in ferritin, while the rest is transported to cells via transferrin or is bound to other proteins such as lactoferrin or haemosiderin (insoluble form of ferritin, found in lysosomes). There has been reported that a very small, yet poorly characterised, low molecular mass pool of iron ('transit pool') also exists in the cells, and these may represent iron ions attached to phosphate esters (e.g. ATP, ADP, GDP, etc.), organic acids (e.g. citrate) and perhaps to the polar head groups of lipids, or even DNA. This low molecular mass iron pool, however, could be a potential catalyst of free radical (·OH) formation *in vivo*. It is this form of iron that is considered as 'free' since these ligands of iron do not prevent its deleterious redox cycling.

In most cells, ferritin represents the most abundant and concentrated form of iron. Stored in ferritin, this iron species is relatively inert as a promoter of ROS formation, yet ferritin has been shown to stimulate formation of ·OH radicals from H_2O_2 and O_2^- under reductive conditions. The physiological reductant O_2^- can release a minor proportion of ferritin iron, which is sufficient to promote lipid peroxidation. Hence, generation of O_2^- and H_2O_2 adjacent to ferritin can cause extensive tissue damage. Transferrin is an iron-binding protein involved in the extracellular transport of iron. Binding of iron to transferrin is very tight at physiological pH (7.4) and requires the presence of carbonate or bicarbonate. Moreover, transferrin shows only 30 per cent saturation in body fluids, which allows it to bind any 'free' iron in the plasma, thus minimizing the catalytically active forms of iron. Furthermore, bound to transferrin, iron is not easily released in the presence of H_2O_2 or O_2^- unless a strong chelating agent is present, especially if the proteins are incorrectly loaded with iron. However, iron ions can be released from transferrin at pH values of 5.6 and below, as occurs in the microenvironment of activated phagocytic cells or in ischaemic tissues. In a similar way, iron can be released from lactoferrin, even though the pH value required for release of its iron is lower (pH 4.0).

Ferritin and transferrin are examples of proteins whose function is to keep iron in a redox-inactive form prior to it being used for the synthesis of iron-containing proteins. The 'low molecular mass' or 'transit' pool of iron supplies iron from ferritin for the biosynthesis of essential proteins.

Haemoglobin and myoglobin are such iron-containing essential proteins. Iron, coordinated in the porphyrin rings of haemoglobin and myoglobin, is crucial, as it serves in the transport of oxygen. It is held there by interactions with the haem rings of haemoglobin or myoglobin. However, even the iron in these two essential proteins can be removed from the porphyrin ring by highly reactive oxygen species and hydroxyl radicals. Even hydrogen peroxide and other organic peroxides can release iron from haemoglobin, but actually degrading the protein. Iron released from haemoglobin and myoglobin passes in the pool of 'free' iron, which is potentially dangerous for further generation of free radicals, as discussed above (Box 2.5).

Box 2.5   The release of iron from haemoglobin and myoglobin

The iron in the haem rings of haemoglobin and myoglobin is in the ferrous state and remains so when oxygen binds to its sixth coordination site. However, due to delocalization of the electron, an intermediate structure may occur:

$$\text{Haem} - Fe^{2+} - O_2 \rightarrow \text{Haem} - Fe^{3+} - O_2^- \tag{2.19}$$

It has been estimated that every day, about 3% of the haemoglobin undergoes oxidation such that O_2^- is released and haem is left with ferric iron, which is biologically inactive:

$$\text{Haem} - Fe^{2+} - O_2 \rightarrow \text{Haem} - Fe^{3+} + O_2^- \tag{2.20}$$

It was demonstrated in *in vitro* studies that the release of iron from the porphyrin ring is increased with increasing concentrations of O_2^-, as shown below [10]:

$$\text{Haem} - Fe^{2+} - O_2 \rightarrow \text{Haem} - Fe^{3+} + O_2^- \tag{2.20}$$

$$\text{Haem} - Fe^{3+} \rightarrow Fe^{3+} + \text{iron-free -haem} \tag{2.21}$$

The above oxidation and subsequent ejection of Fe^{3+} from the porphyrin ring can also be done by $\cdot OH$ radicals, as follows:

$$\text{Haem} - Fe^{2+} + \cdot OH \rightarrow \text{Haem} - Fe^{3+} + OH^- \tag{2.22}$$

$$Haem - Fe^{3+} \rightarrow Fe^{3+} + iron\text{-}free\text{-}haem \qquad (2.23)$$

Among H_2O_2, O_2^- and $OH\cdot$, H_2O_2 causes deoxygenation of oxymyoglobin to ferrimyoglobin as well as the removal of haem from oxymyoglobin, while both H_2O_2 and O_2^- release free iron from the haem nucleus. Thus a proposed scheme for the overall effects of oxyradicals on oxymyoglobin could be the following:

$$My - Fe^{2+} - O_2 \overset{H_2O_2}{\longrightarrow} My - Fe^{3+} \qquad (2.24)$$

$$My - Fe^{2+} - O_2 \overset{H_2O_2}{\longrightarrow} My - Fe^{3+} + apomyoglobin \qquad (2.25)$$

$$My - Fe^{3+} (haem - Fe^{3+}) \overset{O_2^-}{\longrightarrow} Fe^{2+} + iron\text{-}free\text{-}haem\ or\ myoglobin \qquad (2.26)$$

2.8 Free radicals and metal ions in cancer

ROS and other free radicals have long been known to be mutagenic, as a result of changes they cause to DNA, as discussed earlier. Furthermore, they are mediators of other genotypic and phenotypic changes that ultimately lead to cancer. The intake of transition metals, which facilitate the production of ROS, is correlated with development of cancer in both humans and animals.

Epidemiological studies conducted in order to measure the iron status and cancer risk showed that the mean total iron-binding capacity was significantly lower and transferrin saturation was significantly higher in men who developed cancer, while they concluded that high body iron stores increase the risk of cancer in men and increase overall death rates. These findings can be explained by the following lines of evidence(iron catalyses the formation of ROS and lead to mutations that may increase the chances that cancer cells will survive and proliferate.

Thus, as discussed above, ROS can induce DNA damage, and mutations in cancer cells were shown to have the characteristics of ROS attack. For example, 8-hydroxy-guanine induces G:(C to T:(A transversion at the time of DNA replication and such transversions are seen in the p53 gene in liver cancers and in other tumour suppressor genes, which become inactive. Furthermore, iron reduces some of the antioxidant defensive mechanisms of the cell, while it specifically activates others such that tumour cells acquire self-protective mechanisms for oxidative stress.

Other mechanisms of iron-induced carcinogenesis involve suppression of the immune response against tumour cells, activation of transcription factors such as c-fos, and mechanisms of enhanced iron uptake, necessary for increased proliferation. A hypothetical scheme for iron-induced carcinogenesis is shown in Figure 2.14.

It is proposed that the carcinogenicity of other metals, such as nickel and copper is also due to their capacity to enhance oxidative stress, a route possibly being by induction

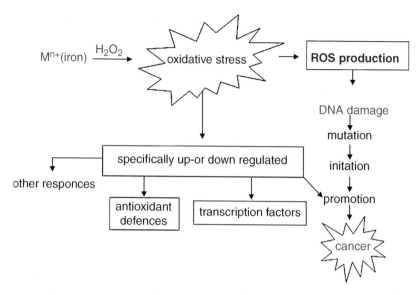

Figure 2.14   Hypothetical model of metal ions-induced carcinogenesis

of iron accumulation. The role of free radicals in tumour promotion through oxidative stress in the later stages of carcinogenesis has been well characterized. It is clear that tumour promotion *in vivo* takes place through a series of complex molecular events involving DNA damage.

Not only the excess but also the deficiency of metal ions induces cancer. There is evidence, both epidemiological and experimental, supporting the hypothesis that chronic magnesium deficiency causes leukemia and other cancers. The relationship to tumour formation is more complex and magnesium appears to be protective at early stages but promotes the growth of existing tumours. Cittadini *et al.* (1991) have found that in tumour cells extracellular magnesium concentration specifically affects and regulates cell energy metabolism. Durlach (1990) reported that magnesium deficiency may promote both anticancer and carcinogenic effects. The carcinogenic action of magnesium is suggested to link with amino acid metabolism and the immune system. It was shown that rats with a magnesium-deficient diet induce apoptosis as well as free radical production. Other investigators have shown that magnesium deficient diet induces an increase of tumour necrosis factor-α (TNF-α), an inflammatory cytokine known to increase inflammation and important in tumour metastases.

2.9   Conclusions

The use of TMIs is extensive in experimental systems, where production of free radicals is wanted. This does not exclude their relevance *in vivo*, in the augmentation of ROS production, even though evidence for their availability is, in many cases, lacking. The importance of iron and copper in the *in vivo* production of ROS appears to be more important compared to other metal ions, as observed by the wealth of publications on the potential toxicity of these trace elements. This may be attributed to their higher abundance and complex homeostasis in tissues. Studies performed with the rest of the trace metals involve their mechanisms in terms of excess concentrations in tissues, such as in cases of poisoning.

Iron and copper are endogenous factors that contribute to oxidative stress that accompanies various pathologic states. Thus, leakage of metalloproteins and 'free' TMIs from sites of sequestration stimulates the conversion of H_2O_2 to $\cdot OH$, lipid hydroperoxide breakdown and autooxidation reactions. Furthermore, release of haem proteins (haemoglobin, myoglobin, cytochromes) can lead to release of iron and haem, both of which are able to stimulate free radical damage, if excess H_2O_2 is present.

These factors, along with others also mentioned earlier (e.g. leakage from the mitochondrial electron transport chain and oxidoreductase active sites, ionizing radiation, UV light) may interact mutually and lead to the increased generation of radical species that will react with polyunsaturated fatty acid chains of lipids, with the amino acyl side chains of proteins and with the base and sugar residues of nucleotides and nucleic acids. Accumulation of 'free' TMIs and oxidative damage to biologically important biomolecules ultimately leads to extensive cell damage and tissue degeneration.

One point of debate between scientists is whether implication of TMIs and free radicals contributes significantly to the disease pathology or whether their appearance and formation is simply an epiphenomenon, i.e. a secondary and non-specific response to the already injured and malfunctioning tissue, organ or organism. In response to that, the following criteria have been established to determine the contribution of free radicals and/or metal ions in human disease:

- The suspected agent should be present at the site of injury with a time course of formation/appearance consistent with the time course of the tissue injury.

- Direct application of the agent to the tissue at concentrations relevant to those found during the disease should produce most, if not all, of the disease effects on the tissue.

- Removal or inhibition of the agent should diminish the injury to an extent related to the degree of removal or inhibition of that agent.

What is certain is that radiation, often emitted by metals, as well as the metals themselves, can lead to damage of DNA through formation of free radicals. This damage leads to mutations that are necessary for tumour initiation and progression, as we have already seen.

2.10   Self-assessment questions

Question: What is the percentage of metals in the Periodic Table?

Answer: The percentage of metals in the Periodic Table is 80 per cent. The rest is the metalloids and the non metals. The metals are also called the block s, d and f elements, whereas the non metals are called the block p elements and the metalloids are in between.(s, p, d, f are the outer valence orbitals).

Question: How are metals introduced in biological systems, i.e. humans, animals and plants?

Answer: The metals are introduced to the biological systems by oxidation. The metals are oxidized to give cations, which then react with the biological molecules (DNA, proteins), and membranes

Question: How are metals linked to biological molecules?

Answer: Metals are linked to biological molecules through ionic and covalent bonds.

Question: What is a free radical?

Answer: A free radical is any atom or ion or group of atoms that contains an unpaired electron.

Question: How can metal ions cause cancer?

Answer: The most common reason of metal ions causing or promoting cancer is their interaction with nucleic acids, causing DNA damage or various DNA adducts. Metal ions can do that either by direct or indirect interaction with the DNA, or through the formation of free radicals and reactive oxygen species that subsequently cause DNA damage. DNA damage subsequently leads to cancer promoting mutations the assist cancer initiation and progression.

Question: Name some forms of radiation and the sources by which we can get exposed to radiation.

Answer: We are constantly exposed to various forms of radiation. These include ionizing radiation such as X and γ radiation and sub-atomic particles, such as neutrons, electrons (β particles) and α-particles. Lower energy, non-ionizing radiation includes the ultraviolet (UV) radiation. Exposure to radiation can occur both from natural sources and from industrial, medical or other man-made sources. The highest exposure to radiation is from natural sources, such as cosmic rays, radiation emitted by metals in rocks and soil, and for UV radiation from the sun. However, exposure to radiation can be from man-made sources, such as the use in weapons, medical X-rays and the use of radiopharmaceuticals or nuclear accidents and occupational exposure.

2.11 Further reading and resources

Anastassopoulou J. In: *Spectroscopy of Inorganic Bioactivators*, ed. T Theophanides. D. Reidel Publishing Co, Dordrecht, Holland, 1989, p. 273.

Anastassopoulou J. Magnesium perchlorate and *cis*-platinum as radiosensitizers in in vitro radiolysis of nucleotides. *Magnesium Res* 1990, **3**, 19.

Anastassopoulou J. Radiolysis of aqueous solutions of guanosine-5′-monophosphate in presence of magnesium ions. *Magnesium Res* 1992, **5**, 97–101.

Anastassopoulou J. In: *Topics in Molecular Organozation and Engineering-Properties and Chemistry of Biological Systems*, eds N Russo, J Anastassopoulou and G Barone. Kluwer Academic Publishers, Dordrecht, 1994, p. 23.

Anastassopoulou J. Metal–DNA interactions. *J Mol Struct* 2003, **109**, 651–653.

Anastassopoulou J and Alexandrides J. *Metal Ions in Biology and Medicine*, Vol 8, MA Cser *et al.*, eds. John Libbey, Eurotext, 2004, pp. 250–253.

Anastassopoulou J. and Brekoulakis J. Radiation chemistry of *cis*-platinum-nucleotide complexes. *Anticancer Res* 1990, **10**, 983.

Anastassopoulou J. and Theophanides T. Magnesium–DNA interactions and the possible relation of magnesium to carcinogenesis. Irradiation and free radicals. *Crit Rev Oncol Heamatol* 2002, **42**, 79–91.

Anastassopoulou J, Chandrinos J and Rakintzis NTh. Radiolysis of triacetoneaminoxyl (TANO) and 2,2,6,6-tetramethylpiperidine-1-oxyl (TEMPO) in aqueous solutions. *Radiat Phys Chem* 1981, **17**, 55–61.

Anastassopoulou J, Chandrinos J and Rakintzis NTh. The behaviour of triacetoneaminoxyl (TANO) and 2,2,6,6-tetramethylpiperidine-1-oxyl (TEMPO) in irradiated aqueous solutions in the presence of oxygen. *Radiat Phys Chem* 1981, **17**, 119–121.

Anastassopoulou J, Rakintzis NTh and Theophanides T. The dose rate effects on the in vitro radiolysis products of magnesium-guanosine-5′-monophosphate complexes in aqueous solutions. *Magnesium Res* 1990, **3**, 15.

Anastassopoulou J, Brekoulakis J and Missailidis S. Role of magnesium as radiosensitizer in the in vitro radiolysis of aqueous solutions of guanosine-5′-monophosphate disodium. *Magnesium Res* 1993, **6/2**, 113.

Anastassopoulou J, Andreopoulos AG, Theophanides T. *Current Research in Magnesium*, eds MJ Halpern and J Durlach. John Libbey, London, 1996, Chap 33, pp. 137–140.

Anastassopoulou J, Barbarossou K, Korbaki V, Theophanides T, Legrand P, Huvenne J-P and Sombert B. In: *Spectroscopy of Biological Molecules*, Vol 7, eds. P Carmona, R Navarro and A Hernanz. Kluwer Academic Publishers, Dordrecht, 1997, p. 233–235.

Anastassopoulou J, Anifantakis B, Anifantakis Z-A, Dovas A and Theophanides T. The role of free radical reactions with haemoglobin and thalassaemia. *Bioinorg Chem* 2000, **79**, 327–330.

Anastassopoulou J, De Munno G and Theophanides T. In: *Metal–Ligand Interactions in Molecular-, Nano-, and Macro-Systems in Complex Environments*, eds. N Russo, DR Salahub and M Witko. Kluwer Academic Publishers, Dordrecht, 2003, pp. 285–300.

Armentano D, De Munno G, Regina M, Anastassopoulou J and Theophanides T. In: *Magnesium: Current Status and New Developments*, T Theophanides and J Anastassopoulou, eds. Kluwer Academic Publishers, Dordrecht, 1997, p. 47.

Anastassopoulou I, Banci L, Bestini I, Cantini F, Katsari E and Rosato A. Solution structure of the Apo and copper(I)-loaded human metallochaperone HAH1. *Biochemistry* 2004, **43**, 13046–13053.

Arnold LL, Eldan M, van Gemert M, Capen CC and Cohen SM. Chronic studies evaluating the carcinogenicity of monomethylarsonic acid in rats and mice. *Toxicology* 2003, **190**, 197–219.

Aruoma OI and Halliwell B. Superoxide-dependent and ascorbate-dependent formation of hydroxyl radicals from hydrogen peroxide in the presence of iron. Are lactoferrin and transferrin promoters of hydroxyl-radical formation? *Biochem J* 1987, **241**, 273.

Bagchi D, Stohs SJ, Downs BW, Bagch M and Preuss HG. Cytotoxicity and oxidative mechanisms of different forms of chromium. *Toxicology* 2002, **180**, 5–22.

Barbarossou K, Aliev A, Gerothanassis IP, Anastassopoulou J and Theophanides T. Natural abundance N-15 CP MAS NMR as a novel tool for investigating metal binding to nucleotides in the solid state. *Inorg Biochem* 2001, **40**, 3626.

Bois P. Tumour of thymus in magnesium deficient rats. *Nature* 1964, **204**, 1316–1320.

Bryant PE. In: *New Developments in Fundamental and Applied Radiobiology*, eds CB Seymour and C Mothersill. Taylor & Francis, London, New York, 1991, pp. 84–94.

Burdon RH. In: *Free Radical Damage and its Control*, eds CA Rice-Evans and RH Burdon. Elsevier, Edinburgh, 1994, p. 155–185.

Burkitt MJ. Copper-DNA adducts. *Methods Enzymol* 1994, **234**, 66.

Cerutti PAA. Oxyradicals and cancer. *Lancet* 1994, **344**, 862–866.

Chance B, Sies H and Boveriset A. Hydroperoxide metabolism in mammalian organs. *Physiol Rev* 1970, **59**, 527–606.

Cheeseman KH and Slater TF. *Free Radicals in Medicine.* Churchill Livingstone, Edinburgh, 1993.

Chiu TK and Dickerson RE. 1 angstrom crystal structures of B-DNA reveal sequence-specific binding and groove-specific bending of DNA by magnesium and calcium. *J Mol Biol* 2000, **301**, 915.

Cittadini A, Wolf FI, Bossi D and Calviello G. Magnesium in normal and neoplastic cell proliferation: state of the art on in vitro data. *Magnesium Res* 1991, **4**, 23–33.

Crichton RR and Charloteaux-Water M. Iron transport and storage. *Eur J Biochem* 1987, **164**, 485.

Davis CD and Newman S. Inadequate dietary copper increases tumorigeneis in the Min mouse. *Cancer Lett* 2000, **159**, 57–62, *Eur J Biochem* 1988, **173**, 345–347.

De Munno G, Medaglia M, Armentano D, Anastassopoulou J and Theophanides T. New supra-molecular complexes of manganese(II) and cobalt(II) with nucleic bases. Crystal structures of $[M(H_2O)(6)(1-MEcyt)(6)][ClO_4](2)\cdot H_2O$, $[Co(1-Mecyt)(4)][ClO_4](2)$ and $[M(H_2O)(4)(cyt)(2)[ClO_4](2)\cdot 2cyt\cdot 2H_2O$ [M = Co-II or Mn-II; cyt = cytosine; 1-Mecyt = 1-methylcytosine]. *Chem Soc, Dalton Trans* 2000; **10**, 1625–1629.

Denkhaus E and Salnikow K. Nickel essentiality, toxicity, and carcinogenicity. *Crit Rev Oncol Haematol* 2002, **42**, 35–56.

Duran HA and de Rey BM. Differential oxidative stress induced by two different types of skin tumor promoters, benzoyl peroxide and 12-O-tetradecanoylphorbol-13-acetate. *Carcinogenesis* 1991, **12**, 2047–2052.

Durlach J, Bara M, Guiet-Bara A. In: *Metal Ions in Biological Systems*, Vol 26, eds H Sigel and A Singel. Marcel Dekker Inc., New York, 1990, pp. 549–578.

Eagon PK, Teepe AG, Elm MS, *et al*. Hepatic hyperplasia and cancer in rats: alterations in copper metabolism. *Carcinogenesis* 1999, **20**, 1091–1096.

Egli M. DNA–cation interactions. Quo vadis? *Chem Biol* 2002, **9**, 277–286.

Eichhorn GL. *Inorganic Biochemistry*, Vols 1 & 2. Elsevier, Amsterdam, 1975, pp. 1191–1243.

Ei-Ichiro O. *Bioinorganic Chemistry: An Introduction*, Ally and Bacon, Inc. Toronto, 1966.

Farrell N. *Transition Metal Complexes as Drugs and Chemotherapeutic Agents*, Kluwer Academic Publishers, Dordrecht, Boston, 1989.

Fausto da Silva JJR and Williams RJ. *The Biological Chemistry of the Elements: The Inorganic Chemistry of Life*. Oxford University Press, Oxford, 1991.

Fenton HJH. Oxidation of tartaric acid in the presence of iron. *J Chem Soc* 1894, **65**, 899–910.

Fielden EM, Lillicrap SC and Robins AB. The effect of 5-bromouracil on energy transfer in DNA and related model systems: DNA with incorporated 5-BUdR. *Radiat Res* 1971, **48**, 421–431.

Flessel CP, Furst A and Radding SB. In: *Carcinogenicity and Metal Ions*, ed. H Singel. Marcel Dekker, Inc., New York, 1980, pp. 23–54.

Freedman SO and Krupey J. Respiratory allergy caused by platinum salts. *J Allergy* 1968, **42**, 233–237.

Gelagutashvili ES, Sigua KI and Sapojnikova NA. Binding and the nature of Cu(II) ion interaction with nucleosomes. *Biochemistry* 1998, **70**, 207–210.

Geday MA, De Munno G, Medaglia M, Anastasopoulou J and Theophanides TM. Supramolecular assemblies containing nucleic bases and magnesium(II) hexahydrate ions. *Angewante Chemie In. Ed Engl* 1997, **36**, 511.

Goldstein G, Meyerstein D and Czapski G. The Fenton reagents. *Free Rad Biol Med* 1993, **15**, 435–445.

Gutteridge JMC. Iron promotors of the Fenton reaction and lipid-peroxidation can be relaeased from hemoglobin by peroxides. *FEBS Lett* 1986, **201**, 291.

Gutteridge JMC and Wilkins SJ. Copper salt-dependent hydroxyl radical formation – damage to proteins acting as anti-oxidant. *Biochim Biophys Acta* 1983, **759**, 38.

Guy RH, Hostynek JJ, Hinz RS and Lorence CR. *Metals and the Skin: Topical Effects and Systemic Absorption*. Marcel Dekker, Inc. New York, 1999.

Guyton KZ and Kensler TW. Oxidative mechanisms in carcinogenesis. *Brit Med Bull* 1993, **49**, 523.

Haber F and Weiss J. The catalytic decomposition of hydrogen peroxide by iron salts. *Proc Roy Soc London* 1934, **A147**, 332–351.

Halliwell B and Gutteridge JMC. Role of free-radicals and catalytic metal-ions in human disease – an overview. *Methods Enzymol* 1990, **186**, 1–85.

Halliwell B and Gutteridge JMC. Biologically relevant metal ion-dependent hysroxyl radical generation – an update. *FEBS Lett* 1992, **307**, 108.

Halliwell B and Gutteridge JMC. *Free Radicals in Biology and Medicine*, third edition. Oxford University Press, Oxford, 1999.

Harrison PM and Arosio P. The ferritins: molecular properties, iron storage function and cellular regulation. *Biochim Biophys Acta* 1996, **1275**, 161.

Hippeli S and Elstner EF. Transition-metal ion-catalyzed oxygen activation during pathogenic processes. *FEBS Lett* 1999, **443**, 1–7.

Houee-Levin C, Gardes-Albert M, Rouscilles A, Ferradini C and Hickel B. Intramolcular semi-quinone disproportionation in DNA – pulse radiolysis of the one-electron reduction of Daunor-ubicin intercalated in DNA. *Biochemistry* 1991, **30**, 8216.

Housecroft C and Sharpe AG. *Inorganic Chemistry*, second edition, Pearson Education Ltd., England, 2005.

Hud NV and Polak M. DNA–cation interactions: the major and minor grooves are flexible ionophores. *Curr Struct Biol* 2001, **11**, 293–301.

Jahnova E. In: *Magnesium: Current Status and New Developments, Theoretical, Biological and Medical Aspects*, eds T Theophanides and J Anastassopoulou. Kluwer Academic Publishers, Dordrecht, 1997, pp. 321–323.

Kagawa TF, Geierstanger BH, Wang AH and Ho PS. Covalent modification of quinine bases in double-stranded DNA – the 1.2-A Z-DNA structure of D (CGCGCG) in the presence of $CuCl_2$. *J Biol Chem* 1991, **266**, 20175–20184.

Kawanishi S, Hiraku Y, Murata M and Oikawa S. The role of metals in site-specific DNA damage with reference to carcinogenesis. *Free Rad Biol Med* 2002, **32**, 822–832.

Kohli GS, Bhargava A, Goel H, *et al.* Serum magnesium levels in patients with head and neck cancer. *Magnesium* 1989, **8**, 77–86.

Kuwahara J, Suzuki T, Fukanoshi K and Sugiura Y. Photosensitive DNA cleavage and phage inactivation by copper(II) camptothecin. *Biochemistry* 1986, **25**, 1216–1221.

Liang Q and Dedon PC. $Cu(II)/H_2O_2$-induced DNA damage is enhanced by packaging of DNA as a nucleosome. *Chem Res Toxicol* 2001, **14**, 416–422.

Linder MC. Copper and genomic stability in mammals. *Mutat Res* 2001, **475**, 141–152.

Liochev SI. *Metal Ions in Biological Systems*, eds A Sigel and H Singel. 1996, 36, pp. 1–39.

Liochev SI and Fridovich I. The role of $O_2 \cdot$ in the production of $HO \cdot$ – in vitro and in vivo. *Free Rad Biol Med* 1994, **16**, 29–33.

Low LY, Hernandez H, Robinson CV, O'Brien R, Grossmann JG, Ladbury JE and Luisi L. Metal-dependent folding and stability of nuclear hormone receptor DNA-binding domains. *J Mol Biol* 2002, **100**, 87.

Lu X, Zhu K, Zhang M, Liu H and Kang J. Voltammetric studies of the interaction of transition-metal complexes with DNA. *J Biochem Biophys Methods* 2002, **52**, 189.

Macquet JP and Theophanides T. DAN–platinum interactions in vitro with *trans*-platinum and cis-$Pt(NH_3)Cl_2$. *Bioinorg Chem* 1975, **5**, 59–66.

Macquet JP and Theophanides T. Specificity of DNA–platinum interaction – level of platinum, pH measurement. *Biopolymers* 1975, **14**, 781–799.

Mainous AG, Gill JM and Everett Ch J. Trransferrin saturation, dietary iron intake, and risk of cancer. *Ann Fam Med* 2005, **3**, 131–137.

Marcus Y. A simple empirical model describing the thermodynamics of hydration of ions of widely varying charges, sizes and shapes. *Biophys Chem* 1994, **51**, 111.

Marrogi A, Khan MA, van Gjissel HE, *et al.* Oxidative stress and p53 mutations in the carcinogenesis of iron-overload-associated hepatocellular carcinoma. *J Natl Cancer Inst* 2001, **93**, 1652–1655.

Mello-Filho AC and Meneghini R. Iron is the intracellular metal involved in the production of DNA damage by oxygen radicals. *Mutat Res* 1991, **251**, 109.

Meneghini R. Temperature dependence of non-Debye disorder in doped manganites. *Free Rad Biol Med* 1997, **23**, 783.

Mercer JF. The molecular basis of copper-transport diseases. *Trends Mol Med* 2001, 7, 64–69.

Michaud DS, Spiegelman D and Clinton SK. Prospective study of dietary supplements, macro-nutrients, micronutrients, and risk of bladder cancer in US men. *Am J Epidemiol* 2000, **152**, 1145–1153.

Millard MM, Macquet JP and Theophanides T. X-ray photoelectron-spectroscopy of DNA. Pt complexes – evidence of O6(GUA).N7(GUA) chelation of DNA with *cis*-dichlorodiamine platinum(II). *Biochim Biophys Acta* 1975, **402**, 166–170.

Minotti G and Aust SD. Redox cycling of iron and lipid peroxidation. *Lipids* 1992, **27**, 219–226.

Mizuro S, Fujita K, Furuy R, Hishid A, Ito H, Tashim Y and Kumagai H. Association of HSP73 with the acquired resistance to uranyl acetate-induced acute renal failure. *Toxicology* 1997, **117**, 183–191.

Nordenskiold L, Chang D, Anderson C and Record TJ. Na-23 NMR relaxation study of the effects of conformation and base composition on the interactions of counterions with double-helical DNA. *Biochemistry* 1998, **37**, 16877.

Obata H, Sawada N, Isomura H and Mori M. Abnormal accumulation of copper in LEC rat liver induces expression of p53 and nuclear matrix-bound p21(waf1/cip1). *Carcinogenesis* 1996, **17**, 2157–2161.

Ogawa K, Hiraku Y, Oikawa S, Murata M, Sugimura Y, Kawamura J and Kawanishi S. Molecular mechanisms of DNA damage induced by procarbazine in the presence of Cu(II). *Mutat Res* 2003, **539**, 145–155.

Opie EL and Alford LB. The influence of diet upon necrosis caused by hepatic and renal poisons Part II. Diet and the nephritis caused by potassium chromate, uranium nitrate, or chloroform. *J Exp Med* 1915, **21**, 21–37.

Ozmen M and Yurekli M. Subacute toxicity of uranyl acetate in Swiss-Albino mice. *Env Toxicol Pharmacol* 1998, **6**, 111–115.

Prasad MR Jr, Engelman RM, Jones RM and Das DK. Effects of oxyradicals on oxymyoglobin. Deoxygenation, haem removal and iron release. *Biochem J* 1989, **263**, 731.

Pryor WA. *Free Radicals*. McGraw-Hill, New York, 1966.

Ravanat J-L, Di Mascio P, Martinez GM, Medeiros MHG and Cadet J. Singlet oxygen induces oxidation of cellular DNA. *J Biol Chem* 2000, **275**, 40601–40604.

Roberfroid M and Buc Calderon P. *Free Radicals and Oxidation Phenomena in Biological Systems*. Marcel-Dekker Inc., New York, 1995.

Rosenberg B, Renshaw E, VanCamp L, Hartwick J and Drobnik J. Platinum-induced filamentous growth in *Escherichia coli*. *J Bacteriol* 1967, **93**, 716–721.

Rueda M, Cubero E, Laughton ChA and Orozco M. Exploring the counterion atmosphere around DNA: what can be learned from molecular dynamics simulations? *Biophys J* 2004, **87**, 800–811 and references therein.

Scherer E, Tajmir-Riahi HA and Theophanides T. Synthesis, structure and a Fourier-transform infrared study of Pt(II), Cu(II), and Mg(II) complexes with xanthosine – 5′-monophosphate complexes. *Inorg Chim Acta* 1984, **92**, 285–292.

Shertzer HG, Bannenberg GL and Moldeous P. Evaluation of iron-binding and peroxide-mediated toxicity in rat hepatocytes. *Biochem Pharmacol* 1992, **44**, 1367–1373.

Shigenaga MK, Hagen TM and Ames BN. Oxidative damage and mitochondrial decay in aging. *Proc Natl Acad Sci U S A* 1994, **91**, 10771.

Singh KK. *Oxidative Stress, Disease and Cancer*. Imperial College Press, London, 2006.

Spins JW and Woods RJ. *An Introduction to Radiation Chemistry*, second edition. John Wiley & Sons, New York, London, 1976.

Stellwagen NC, Magnusdottir S, Gelfi C and Righeti PG. Preferential counterion binding to A-tract DNA oligomers. *J Mol Biol* 2001, **305**, 1025.

Stevens RG, Jone DY, Micozzi MS and Taylor PR. Body iron stores and the risk of cancer. *N Engl J Med* 1988, **319**, 1047.

Stohs SJ and Bagchi D. Oxidative mechanisms in the toxicity of metal-ions. *Free Rad Biol Med* 1995, **18**, 321–336.

Stryer L. *Biochemistry*. WH Freeman Co, New York, 1995, pp. 145–438.

Sun DF, Fujigaki Y, Fujimoto T, Yonemura K and Hishida A. Possible involvement of myofibroblasts in cellular recovery of uranyl acetate-induced acute renal failure in rats. *Am J Pathol* 2000, **157**, 1321-1335.

Szilágyi I, Nagy G, Hernadi K, Ladádi I and Pálinkó I. Modeling copper-containing enzyme mimics. *J Mol Struct (Theochem)* 2003, **666–667**, 451–445.

Tajmir-Riahi HA and Theophanides T. An FT-IR study of *cis*-dichlorodiammineplatinum(II) and *trans*-dichloroammineplatinum(II) bound to inosine-5′-monophosphate. *Can J Chem* 1984, **62**, 266, 1429–1440.

Tajmir-Riahi HA and Theophanides T. Magnesium–nucleotide interactions – synthesis, structure, H-1, C-13 nuclear magnetic resonance and Fourier-transform infrared studies of Mg-inosine-5′-monophosphate complexes. *Can J Chem* 1985, **63**, 2065–2072.

Tereshko V, Wilds CJ, Minasov G, *et al.* Detection of metal ions in DNA crystals using state-of-the-art A-ray diffraction experiments. *Nucleic Acids Res* 2001, **29**, 1208.

Theophanides T. Interactions des acides nucleiques avec les metaux. *Can J Spectrosc* 1981, **26**, 165–170.

Theophanides T. Fourier-transform infrared spectra of calf thymus DNA and its reactions with the anti-cancer drug cisplatin. *Appl Spectrosc* 1981, **35**, 461–465.

Theophanides T. FT-IR spectra of nucleic acids and the effect of metal ions. In: *Fourier Transform Infrared Spectroscopy, Industrial and Medical*, ed. T Theophanides. R Reidel Publishing Co Holland, 1984, pp. 105–124.

Theophanides T and Anastassopoulou J. In: *Spectroscopy of Biological Molecules – New Advances*, eds. ED Schmid, FW Schneider and F Siebert. Wiley, Chichester, 1987, pp. 433–436.

Theophanides T and Anastassopoulou J. In: *Equilibri in Soluzione, Aspetti Teorici, Sperimentali ed Applicaviti*, eds.C La Mesa, A Napoli, N Russo and M Toscano. Marra Editore, 1988, pp. 122–128.

Theophanides T and Anastassopoulou J. *Magnesium: Current status and New Developments*. Kluwer Academic Publishers, Dordrecht, 1997.

Theophanides T and Anastassopoulou J. Copper and carcinogenesis. *Crit Rev Oncol Haematol*, 2002, **42**, 57–64.

Theophanides T and Anastassopoulou J. In: *Oxidative Stress, Disease and Cancer*, ed. KK Singh. Imperial College Press, London, 2006, Chap. 28, pp. 807–823.

Theophanides T and Tajmir-Riahi HA. Flexibility of DNA and RNA upon binding to different metal-cations – an investigation of the B to A to Z conformational transformation by Fourier-transform infrared-spectroscopy. *J Biomolec Struct Dynam* 1985, **2**, 995–1004.

Theophanides T, Anastassopoulou J and Rakintzis NTh. In: *FEBS, Advanced Course on FT-IR of Biomolecules.* Berlin, 1993.

Theophanides M, Anastassopoulou J and Theophanides T. *Environmental science and pollution research*, 8th FECS Conference on Chemistry and the Environment, 2002, p. 131.

Toyokuni S. Iron-induced carcinogenesis: the role of redox regulation. *Free Rad Biol Med* 1996, **20**, 553–566.

von Sonntag C. *The Chemical Basis of Radiation Biology*. Taylor & Francis, London, 1987.

Vouk V. General chemistry of metals. In: *Handbook on the Toxicology of Metals*, second edition Vol I. eds. L Friberg, GF Nordberg and VB Vouk, Elsevier, Amsterdam, 1986, pp. 14–35.

Waggoner DJ, Bartnika TB and Gitlin JD. The role of copper in neurodegenerative disease. *Neurobiol Dis* 1999, **6**, 221–230.

Walker JM, Huster D, Ralle M, Morgan CT, Blackburn NJ and Lutsenko S. The N-terminal metal-binding site 2 of the Wilson's disease protein plays a key role in the transfer of copper from Atox1. *J Biol Chem* 2004, **279**, 15376–15384.

Wardman P and Candeias LP. Fenton chemistry: an introduction. *Radiat Res* 1996, **145**, 523–531.

Williams RJ. Bio-inorganic chemistry: its conceptual evolution. *Coord Chem Rev* 1990, **100**, 573–610.

Woods KK, McFail-Ison L, Sines CC, Stephens RK and Williams LD. Monovalent cations sequester within the A-tract minor groove of [d(CGCGAATTCGCG)](2). *J Am Chem Soc* 2000, **122**, 1546.

Yang C-Y and Chu H-F. Calcium and magnesium in drinking water and risk of death from rectal cancer. *Int J Cancer* 1998, **77**, 528–532.

Yang C-Y, Chiu H-F, Tsai S-S, Cheng M-F, Lin M-C and Sung F-C. Calcium and magnesium in drinking water and risk of death from prostate cancer. *J Tox Envir Health* 2000, **Part A**, 17–26.

Yang D and Wang AH-J. Structural studies of interactions between anticancer platinum drugs and DNA. *Prog Biophys Molec Biol* 1996, **66**, 81.

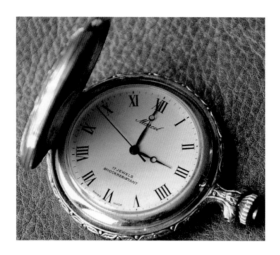

Cancer is often considered to be a genetic disease. The genetic origin of the disease can have a double meaning. We have seen in the two previous chapters, and we will see in the following two, that external factors such as diet, carcinogens, the environment, infection or inflammation can lead to cancer initiation and progression. However, most of these factors ultimately cause cancer through their effect on DNA, the genetic material inside the cell. One way or another, directly or indirectly, these factors can cause DNA damage that leads to mutations – the first stage in the initiation of cancer.

However, cancer is also a genetic disease in that there can be an inherited predisposition for the disease. Within families with cancer victims there is an increased risk of cancer that appears to be inherited from generation to generation. In this chapter we will have the opportunity to examine this phenomenon in some detail and link it with the external factors that we have encountered and will encounter later. Similarly, we will consider the relationship of genetics and genomics, a scientific discipline that has been of particular interest in the last few years. Even more specifically, we will consider the interaction of genetics and genomics with the environment through their relationship with diet and nutrition, as well as how genomics have given rise to a speciality area of oncogenomics and the design of modern therapeutic agents that take advantage of genetic differences in cancer cells and target them in a specific manner, resulting in drugs with improved specificity and reduced side effects than exist in traditionally used chemotherapy based on features such as the rapid division of the cancer cell as a means of effecting its selective cell kill action.

3

Genetics and cancer

Sotiris Missailidis

Chemistry Department, The Open University, UK

3.1 Introduction

We have seen in Chapters 1 and 2 how lifestyle and environmental factors, such as diet, smoking and alcohol, or exposure to chemicals and radiation can affect the onset of cancer. In fact, these factors account for a significant percentage of cancers, whilst another group of cancers is caused by infection and chronic inflammation, as it is discussed in the following two chapters (Chapters 4 and 5). However, most of these factors result in the initiation of disease through direct or indirect influence on DNA, which results in the increase of mutations, necessary for the various mechanisms of cancer to be set into motion. Such mutations can affect genes that control the DNA-repair mechanisms, or increase cell proliferation, or confer genetic instability that can lead to further mutations. Yet, such mutations are relatively rare, allowing only a small chance for a normal cell to give rise to a malignant tumour, and only because of the extreme amount of infections and the daily consumption of potentially harmful agents this becomes significant in terms of numbers of individuals affected by cancer. Most cancers arise from such somatically acquired mutations, which take place during the lifetime of the individual and appear only in the cancer cells.

On the other hand, if a genetic alteration in the form of a mutation on a particular gene is present in one of the parents and is inherited by the next generation, this mutation will appear in all the cells of the individual, giving the individual a greater propensity for the formation of cancer. A single critical mutation is not enough to convert a cell into a completely unregulated, proliferative state known as cancer. However, this critical mutation may increase the survival time or increase proliferation enough to give more opportunity for a second critical mutation to arise within the clone of cells (see Figure 3.1).

The Cancer Clock   Edited by Sotiris Missailidis

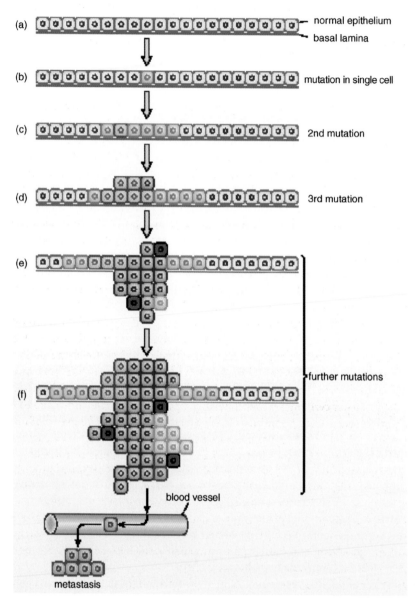

(a) — normal epithelium
— basal lamina

(b) mutation in single cell

(c) 2nd mutation

(d) 3rd mutation

(e)

further mutations

(f)

blood vessel

metastasis

Figure 3.1 The clonal evolution of a tumour. (a) A mutation in a single cell gives rise to increased cell proliferation. (b–d) Cells with further mutations may acquire other growth advantage characteristics and their progeny become the dominant cell clone in the tumour (purple in d). (e, f) Mutations may also lead to genetic instability, enhancing the probability of DNA mutations, which can either lead to growth advantage (red) or cell death (black). Successive rounds of cell division and gene mutation leads to the formation of different cell clones with multiple different mutations (yellow, brown and black cells), which may result in even more 'aggressive' growth properties such as metastatic capacity (brown) or in clonal extinction (black). Reproduced From OU course S377 Molecular and Cell Biology book 4. © 2004, The Open University

An individual containing such critical mutations is already more susceptible to further genetic changes caused by external factors and, in general, inherited forms of cancer occur at an earlier age than the sporadic or environmentally caused tumours.

3.2   Genes and cancer

The relationship between cancer and genetic predisposition was proposed as early as 1971 by Alfred Knudson, in the context of a childhood eye tumour, retinoblastoma. Later on, a relationship between inheritance and breast cancer was observed in a family with many cases of early onset breast cancer, liver cancer and other tumours. Today, a number of genes have been identified that can be inherited and confer high susceptibility of cancer to a family. These genes are shown in Table 3.1, and there have now been tests available for individuals to identify the presence of mutations on those genes and establish their potential risk for developing cancer. Inherited cancers contribute only about 5 per cent of the total cancers, with the remainder depended upon somatic mutations, mutations that happen during the lifetime of a person and are not passed on to the next generation, as they usually occur to a cell and are not part of the genetic makeup of the individual. These can be caused by a number of external factors, or may be spontaneous mutations that occur during cell division.

As we see in Table 3.1, the most common cancers that might arise due to inherited mutation are breast, ovarian, prostate, colorectal and endometrial cancers. However, inheriting a gene mutation that confers susceptibility is not the same as inheriting cancer, and in fact, not all people who inherit a known cancer gene will get cancer. Still, the lifetime risks of such patients can be very high, with women inheriting the *BRCA1* gene having a 70 per cent higher lifetime risk of developing cancer compared to women that they do not have such mutations. This often leads to the dilemma of the individual as to whether to progress into preventive surgery (radical mastectomy and removal of the ovaries) to eliminate this risk (see Chapter 8). The chances of inheriting such a mutation are relatively small and can range from 1/100 000 for individuals with rare syndromes to 1/1000 for genes such as *BRCA1* and *MLH1*.

Table 3.1 Cancer risk associated genes and their related tumours (World Cancer Report, 2003)

Gene	Associated tumours
BRCA1	Breast, ovary, colon, prostate
BRCA2	Breast, ovary, pancreas, prostate
P16 INK4A	Melanoma, pancreas
CDK4	Melanoma, other tumours
hMLH1	Colorectal, endometrial, ovarian cancer
hMSH2	Colorectal, endometrial, ovarian cancer
hMSH6	Colorectal, endometrial, ovarian cancer
PMS1	Colorectal cancer, other tumours
PMS2	Colorectal cancer, other tumours
HPC2	Prostate

In addition to the genes confering high risk susceptibility for development of cancer, there are also some rare genetic disorders that can increase the risk of cancer at a young age. These include conditions such as retinoblastoma, neurofibromatosis, Li–Fraumeni syndrome, multiple endocrine neoplasia type 1 (MEN1), von Lippel–Hindau disease, Bloom's syndrome, familial adenomatous polyposis and others.

For an individual to consider themselves at high risk for inheriting cancer genes, it is not enough to have a close relative with cancer. As we have indicated in earlier chapters, cancer is a common disease and almost one in three individuals develops cancer during their lifetime. Thus, for an individual to be considered at risk of having inherited a genetic mutation, there needs to be at least two close blood relatives with the same cancer on the same side of the family. In fact, a cancer is more likely to be inherited if there are two or more close blood relatives on the same side of the family affected by the same type of cancer, a close relative had more than one primary tumour, members of a family get cancer at a younger than normal age (under 60 years), or certain cancers occur within together in a family. If these conditions apply, then the individual is under risk of having inherited mutations in cancer related genes. Such an individual has then a 50 per cent chance of passing on these genes to their progeny, as well as risk in developing cancer themselves and this would warrant genetic testing to verify if indeed this is the case. If the gene responsible is for breast and ovarian cancer, then men are not likely to be affected, but they can still pass on the inherited mutation to their children.

The first step of addressing any worries with regards to the potential inheritance of tumour-related gene mutations is to discuss this with the medical general practitioner (GP) who can advise and refer the individual to a genetic testing clinic. After that, it is possible that the genetic consultant will not agree with the assessment of proceeding with the testing, but it also likely that they will seek family history information and then progress to screening or genetic test (this process is shown in the flow chart opposite).

Genetic testing involves the analysis of DNA contained in a blood sample. It is an expensive and time-consuming process and can only identify a few of the genes that may be involved in increasing cancer risk. Genetic testing is mostly concerned with the search for a mutation within genes. On the other hand, if a particular mutation within a family has already been found, then other members of the family can be offered a genetic screening, which is a lot easier and faster as it just checks if they also carry the same mutation in the same gene.

If the testing is positive and a mutation is identified, the individual has inherited a genetic mutation that increases their risk of getting a specific cancer, although it usually does not mean that the individual will definitely get cancer. The increase in the risk varies between mutations and different types of cancer, and for breast cancer in women who bear the *BRCA1* gene mutation it means that they have an 80 per cent chance of getting cancer compared to the normal 10 per cent. Similarly, the individual can also pass this mutation to their children, although again this is only a 50 per cent chance.

If the test is negative and no mutation is found, then the test is considered inconclusive. This is because there is indeed no mutation to be found, but it may also mean that there is a mutation in a gene that is not known to be involved in hereditary cancer risk, or even because the test may not have picked up the mutation or has not tested 100% of the gene sequence.

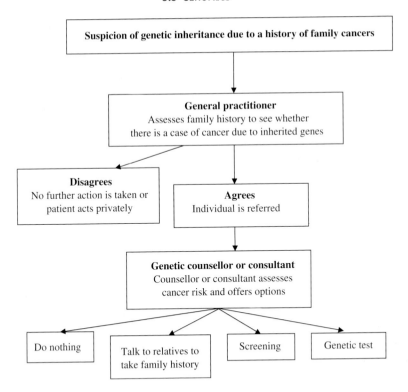

3.3 Genomics

The sequencing of whole genomes from various organisms, including the human genome, allows the unravelling of the biological capacity of the organism, their capability for protein synthesis and the identification and differentiation of genetic factors for the development of diseases, responses to treatments, or even the evolutionary progression of various species. Technological advances in sequencing instrumentation and bioinformatics, has offered the possibility of the sequencing of whole genomes from various organisms. These range from pathogenic microorganisms such as *Helicobacter pylori*, *Escherichia coli* and the malaria-causing parasite *Plasmodium falciparum*, to insects (such as the fruit fly *Drosophila melanogaster* and the malaria-carrying mosquito *Anopheles gambiae*), plants (such as the mustard weed *Arabidopsis thaliana* and rice *Oryza sativa*), animals such as the mouse (*Mus musculus*) and rat (*Rattus norvegicus*) and of course the human (*Homo sapiens*). By autumn 2003 the completed genome sequences were available for 18 Archaebacteria, 140 Eubacteria, 1364 viruses and 20 eukaryotes, including 4 plants. The identification of sequences from whole organisms gave rise to the field of genomics, which is a field of study that revolutionized biological and pharmaceutical research and was subsequently followed by various other research and scientific disciplines.

Genomics is the study of the whole set of genes, called the genome of an organism, including their sequence, structure, function and interactions.

Genomics created a revolution in our scientific thinking in general and in terms of drug discovery in particular. A range of other -omics were soon invented and, though still in their infancy, have been developing rapidly and are offering great promise in the prevention, diagnosis and treatment of diseases. These include proteomics, transcriptomics and metabolomics, dealing with the proteome, the total expressed proteins in a biological system, cell, tissue or organism, at a particular stage of its life cycle, the transcriptome, the complete set of RNA transcripts produced by the genome at any one time, and the metabolome, or the total number of metabolites and low molecular weight intermediates that is produced by the various cellular processes. In fact, even the general area of genomics itself has already been divided into subclasses, such as *functional, comparative* and *structural genomics.*

Functional genomics is concerned with the understanding of the function of genes and other parts of the genome. The Human Genome Project may have provided information on the sequence of the human genome, but has left many questions unanswered as to the function of most of the human genes, the role of gene polymorphism and single nucleotide polymorphisms and the role of the non-coding regions and repeats within the genome. Thus, functional genomics are not concerned solely with the sequence of the genome but with the genome's function, including the functional compatibility of genetic information, the expression profiles at the mRNA level, the resulting proteins expressed and the role these functions play in the organism's biochemical processes. Functional genetics utilized genetic technology and information provided by *structural genomics,* the area of genomics that is concerned with the three dimensional structural features of the resulting proteins, to elucidate the function and role of individual genes within an organism. Functional and structural genomics are particularly important in the identification of new targets for drug therapy.

The identification of the sequences from various organisms has allowed the development of another exciting area of study and biological research, *comparative genomics.*

3.3.1 Comparative genomics

Comparative genomics allows the comparison of genomes from different organisms as well as those from distinct individuals within a genome to identify regions of difference and similarity that can be used either in the development of strategies to combat disease or in the study of evolutionary changes among organisms. Comparative genomics offer a better understanding on how species have evolved and allows the determination of the function of genes and non-coding regions of the genome. This area of research has provided significant information about the function of genes by comparing them with their counterparts in simpler organisms and has helped elucidate various genetic traits: these include sequence similarity, gene location, the function, length and number of coding regions, exons, within the genes and the amount of non-coding DNA within the genome. Furthermore, it has provided information about highly conserved regions within genes that code for homologous proteins and have been maintained within millennia of evolution with great similarities between organisms ranging from bacteria to humans, or regions and genes that are significantly different and provide each organism with its unique characteristics and identity. Utilizing significant computational power, this field of genomics compares whole genome sequences from various species and can provide information on specific genes that are involved in the development and resistance to particular diseases. For example, although the human and chimpanzee genome sequences are differing in only 1.2 per cent, chimpanzees are resistant to various human diseases such as acquired immune deficiency syndrome and malaria. The identification of the genes responsible for this resistance and their comparison with the human gene may reveal the reasons for the species barrier to these diseases and suggest new genetic treatments to offer prevention of such diseases. Furthermore, comparison between individual genetic make ups and genetic profiling may eventually allow the development of the so sought after and long discussed personalized or patient-specific medicines, which will allow the treatment of individuals based on their genetic characteristics, specifically and efficiently and without the debilitating side effects that often accompany the treatment of some of the most serious diseases of our time, such as cancer. The seeking of such therapies has given rise to further subdivisions of genomics or their fusion with other disciplines, such as *pharmacogenomic* (pharmacology and genomics) or *nutrigenomics* (nutrition and genomics). These areas of research and their effect in the development of modern therapeutics and the treatment of the individual from a systemic perspective will be analysed in subsequent sections of this chapter.

3.3.2 Oncogenomics

The identification and description of the genetic aetiology or contribution to the onset and development of common complex diseases, such as cancer, mental illness and heart disease remains the main focus of modern genetic approaches to medicine and the pharmaceutical sciences. Cancer has been one of the first diseases where genomics have found wider applications in the molecular and genetic understanding of the disease and in the development of modern, gene-based drugs treatments such as Gleevec and Herceptin.

It is known that cancer is not a single disease, but hundreds of diseases with the common characteristic that they evolve as a result of the acquisition of genetic alterations that they confer to the cell, and its clones, growth advantages over normal cells. Ultimately, such alterations lead the cell to the ability to divide more rapidly, evade apoptosis and generate clones of cells, which, if not eliminated by the immune system, may accumulate further genetic changes and become malignant. Such changes further include the ability to produce inflammatory cytokines and chemo-kines that help the neoplastic cells evade recognition from the immune system and subsequently make alterations to their surrounding tissue that allows the generation of the tumour, its sustenance through angiogenesis and finally its spread through metastasis.

Several types of genetic alterations contribute to neoplastic transformation. Such alterations include loss of genes that control the fidelity of genome maintenance and checkpoint genes, responsible for quality control in cell division cycles, activa-tion of oncogenes and loss or mutation of tumour suppressor genes. Such altera-tions allow the tumour cell to bypass a number of controls available in the normal cells, which control the arrest of their division cycles when progression would lead to damaged progeny or to mitotic catastrophes, lead them to programmed cell death in response to developmental signals and irreparable damage and tightly define their migratory potential. Inherited or acquired mutations in DNA repair genes result in genetic diversity in the cell, from which subsequent genetic selections occur.

Particular genes in the tumour cells, termed oncogenes, become activated due to genetic alterations that are dominant and give rise to a gain of function at the gene level. Oncogenes can become activated by some type of mutation, such as a single point mutation, translocation to a highly active promoter, production of a consti-tutively active fusion protein, production of a truncated protein product that is hyperactive or genetic amplification. These mutation(s) are dominant with respect to the unaltered oncogene and can contribute to cell transformation. These muta-tions are almost never inherited, probably because if every cell in the body contained an activating mutation in an oncogene, the embryo would not develop normally. The fact that oncogenes are switched on in cancer, makes the oncoprotein products of oncogene mutations rational targets for genotype-specific drug design.

Another set of genes that are particularly important in the process of tumor-igenesis are the so-called tumour suppressor genes. These are genes that are generally responsible for the control mechanisms within the cell and keep in check abnormal growth, mutation, DNA damage and cell mobility. Tumour suppressor genes encode proteins that normally limit cell proliferation and would thus sup-press tumour formation. One well-studied example of tumour suppressor genes is the p53 tumour suppressor gene, whose central role is maintaining genetic stability by arresting proliferation and allowing repair of DNA damage or by inducing apoptosis, and which is the most frequently mutated gene in many human tumours. This is particularly significant, as almost any mutation in the p53 sequence will render it ineffectual as the 'guardian of the genome'. Such tumour suppressor genes, which become lost or inactivated in the development of cancer, are subject to cancer-associated mutations that are recessive at the gene level. These mutations occur both in sporadic cancers and in inherited cancer predisposition syndromes. Although typically two mutations are required to inactivate such genes in tumours that arise sporadically, if an individual is born heterozygous for such an inactivated gene, then there is an inherited susceptibility to cancer and a single alteration is adequate to produce a preneoplastic lesion. Such alteration may be either a second mutation or an epigenetic change, such as DNA methylation that reduces gene expression, or a gene conversion event that produces loss of heterozygosity at the locus. Such genetic and epigenetic changes are considered preneoplastic, because loss of the two copies of a single tumour suppressor gene is not fully transforming. Cancer is a multistage process that involves multiple genetic stages and the loss or inactivation of a single tumour suppressor gene may be necessary but it is not adequate for tumour development.

Some of the main characteristics of tumorigenesis are described below:

- *Genetic instability.* The cells acquire mutations in genes that normally check and enable repair of DNA before cell division.

- *Self-sufficiency in growth signals.* The cells acquire mutations in proto-oncogenes to produce their oncogenic versions. Oncogenes usually code for proteins involved in positively regulating signal transduction pathways in response to activation of growth factor receptors and for transcription factors and proteins involved in cell cycle control.

- *Insensitivity to tumour-inhibitory signals.* The cells acquire mutations that cause inactivation to tumour suppressor genes, which frequently help control cell division and sometimes operate in the same pathways as oncogenes. Often the pathways affected are also involved in gaining genetic instability, or in avoiding apoptosis and senescence.

- *Evasion of apoptosis.* The cells acquire mutations that result in the inactivation of death-related pathways, allowing them to escape apoptosis.

- *Limitless replicative potential.* The cells acquire mutations that allow them to escape from terminal differentiation states and from replicative senescence.

- *Sustained angiogenesis.* The cells in solid tumours can acquire mutations that enable them to establish a blood and lymphatic supply for themselves.

- *Tissue invasion and metastasis.* The cells acquire mutations that enable them to invade surrounding tissue and/or colonise other tissues at distant sites. Metastasis accounts for 90 per cent of cancer-related deaths in humans.

As the process of tumorigenesis, and ultimately cancer, is a genetic disease that is dependent on various genetic alterations, genetic analysis has been an important factor in the prediction, diagnosis and development or individual tailoring of its treatment. Though most treatments remain non-specific and were not developed against specific genotypes, molecular classifications of tumours in terms of, for example, oestrogen status in breast and cervical cancer, have long been used to tailor therapeutic regimes.

However, modern genomic approaches, with the use of developments in microarray technology and the progression in functional genomics, transcriptomics and proteomics, have revolutionized the areas of drug discovery and drug targeting through the continuous and rapid identification of new targets.

One of the important applications of such assays has been for the identification   of cancer-critical genes in tumorigenesis or cancer development. Additionally, tumours can be screened for somatic mutations, for protein or chromatin changes and for changes in genomic DNA methylation, or profiling of cancer stages.

A number of molecularly targeted drugs have been produced as a result of the expansion of oncogenomics and the identification of new targets for the treatment of tumours, either at the nucleic acid (DNA/RNA) level or at the protein level (this will be discussed in more detail in Chapter 9). Many previous systemic therapies, based on cytotoxic chemotherapeutic agents, acted on various points of DNA transcription and replication. Examples of such reagents include: doxorubicin, which stabilizes topoisomerase–DNA intermediate complexes; cisplatin and its derivatives that form intrastrand DNA crosslinks; topotecan, a topoisomerase I inhibitor; actinomycin D, an RNA synthesis inhibitor; alkylating agents such as nitrogen mustards; and anti-metabolites. Novel targets that have been identified using genomic and proteomic approaches in cancer include various protein kinases that have currently resulted in a number of drugs, including Herceptin, Gleevec (Box 3.1) and Iressa, with a great number of compounds either in the form of biological therapeutics or small molecules currently in clinical trials against various kinase targets such as EGFR, VEGFR, Chk-1 and CDKs. An example of such compounds, Gleevec, is presented in the case study below, whereas some of the other molecules are described in other parts of this book.

Box 3.1   Case study: Gleevec (imatinib)

Human chronic myelogenous leukaemia (CML) is generally considered a rare malignancy that is highly dependent on a single genetic mutation: a translocation between chromosomes 9 and 22, resulting in a distinct cytogenetic phenotype, known as the Philadelphia chromosome. This mutation leads to the synthesis of an oncogenic Bcr-Abl fusion protein, which is characteristic of the disease. Bcr-Abl is a tyrosine kinase with aberrant regulation of the kinase domain derived from the normal cellular Abl tyrosine kinase. A drug has been identified, named Gleevec, which specifically binds to the kinase domain of Abl in the Bcr-Abl fusion protein and blocks binding of ATP, thereby inhibiting its tyrosine kinase activity.

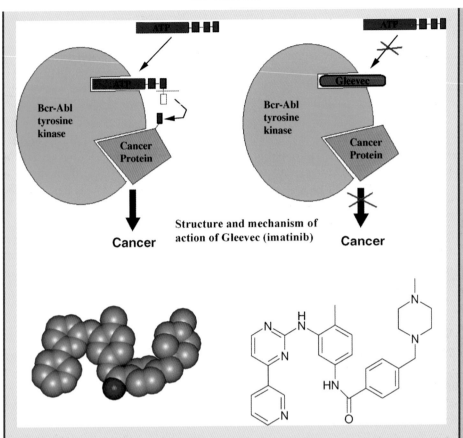

Structure and mechanism of action of Gleevec (imatinib)

Gleevec was approved by the FDA in 2001 after demonstration of marked efficacy in early and late stage CML. Like most kinase inhibitors, Gleevec binds the kinase in the ATP-binding pocket, the catalytic domain of the protein. Kinases need to bind ATP and act as a phosphotransferase when in their active shape, which makes them structurally very similar whilst in this conformation. Gleevec, however, binds to the catalytic domain on its inactive state, it stabilises it and thus prevents ATP binding and kinase function. This avoids great lack of specificity for Gleevec and limits its action mostly to the desired target. Inhibition of c-kit and PDGF receptor tyrosine kinases by Gleevec has actually demonstrated a beneficial effect and made Gleevec effective in the treatment of Gastrointestinal stromal tumours and chronic myeloproliferative malignancies. In addition, Gleevec was found to have only very mild side-effects, such as skin rashes and edemas, which only rarely necessitate the disruption of the therapeutic regime and has been one of the top three blockbuster drugs in 2005.

3.3.3   Nutrigenomics

Nutrigenomics is the study of how different foods and common dietary chemicals can affect health by altering gene expression and/or the structure of an individual's genetic makeup. Nutritional genomics or nutrigenomics is the second wave of personalized medicine to result from the bloom of genomics and the identification of the human genome. Just as oncogenomics and pharmacogenomics have led to the concept of 'personalized medicine' and 'designer drugs', so does the new field of nutrigenomics open the way for 'personalized nutrition'. By understanding our nutritional needs, our nutritional status, and our genotype, nutrigenomics aims to enable individuals to manage better their health and well-being by precisely matching their dietary needs with their unique genetic makeup.

Thus, nutrigenomics can have a profound effect on our understanding, preventing or even curing complex diseases, such as cancer, heart diseases, diabetes or obesity. Diet has been shown to be a big factor in many chronic diseases and perhaps responsible for even a third of all types of cancer (see also Chapter 1). Furthermore, dietary chemicals have the ability to change the expression of various genes and thus affect the transcriptome and proteome of the organism and perhaps even affect the genome itself.

The influence of diet on health has been shown to depend on an individual's genetic makeup. Thus, under certain circumstances, diet can be a serious risk factor for a number of diseases. Common dietary chemicals can act on the human genome, directly or indirectly through interactions mainly with the proteome, to affect and/or alter gene expression, with further implications on all downstream process and products: m-RNA expression, protein expression, metabolites. The degree to which diet influences such processes and can alter the balance between healthy and disease states largely depends on the individual's genetic make-up. However, the influence of diet and dietary chemicals on specific genes can play a role in the onset, incidence, progression and severity of complex and chronic diseases and thus, dietary intervention based on the individual nutritional requirements, nutritional status, genotype and phenotype (personalized nutrition) can be used to prevent, control or even cure such diseases.

Food was originally considered to be mainly our source of energy. It is metabolized by the body to provide energy for the cells and the necessary components we need, such as proteins (or amino acids for the synthesis of our proteins), vitamins, etc. However, a number of dietary chemicals can, either themselves or through their metabolic products, interact with proteins involved in the 'turning on' of particular genes to various degrees. This gene activation will then cause gene expression of products that can cause further changes in both genetic and metabolic pathways and thus lead towards chronic illness. Tailor-made or 'intelligent' diet, designed and based on the individual's genetic profile and determined by the specific demands of the genetic signature can reverse such effects and balance the micro- and macronutrient needs of the organism, thus preventing disease onset or restoring good health. One such example of the individual nature of nutritional needs based on genetic profiling is the case of genistein, a chemical in soy, which has the ability to attach to the oestrogen receptors, thus regulating particular genes. However, the interaction of genistein with oestrogen receptors is different between individuals, thus affecting the maintenance or gain of weight.

A particular issue that is related to nutritional genomics and has come to life with a great degree of controversy, is the fact that genetic variation between ethnic groups is part of the principle of nutrigenomics that focuses on such genetic variations and a 'systems biology' approach to identify foods and their effect on health and disease. One common example of such variations is the ability to digest milk. Most people of northern European ancestry have the ability to digest milk, whereas many individuals of south-east Asian origin can not, due to a genetic variation in the gene that encodes for the enzyme lactase, responsible for the breaking down of lactose in the milk. In most mammals, this gene for lactose tolerance switches off once an animal is weaned. Humans shared this genetic trait until a mutation in the DNA of an isolated population of northern Europeans around 10 000 years ago introduced an adaptive tolerance for nutrient-rich milk. Thus, the likelihood of milk tolerance depends largely on the genetic ancestry.

A number of similar examples have become apparent. As humans lived and interacted with their environment and consumed different foods within their particular habitat in each of the continents, selected variants that were better suited for their environment evolved naturally. In modern times, when travel has become so much easier and migration has brought people to live in places which were perhaps unthought-of by their ancestors, such variants have led certain populations, when exposed to western-type food, fatty, overprocessed and high in calories, towards obesity and disease (the effects of migration on cancer have also been discussed in Chapter 1). Many examples have demonstrated these genetic variations, suggesting a relationship between genes and nutrition. Such examples include the Japanese population that has relocated to the US and are now presented with high cholesterol problems, the Alaskan Inuit, who upon living in heated homes and travelling with snowmobiles are now showing high levels of obesity, diabetes and cardiovascular disease, and the Masai of east Africa, who are now suffering ill health, after abandoning their traditional diet of meat, blood and milk for corn and beans. These types of genetic variation are central to the field of nutrigenomics, where individual dietary needs are sought out and addressed.

Genetic researchers found in 2001 that the human genome appears to consist of and be organized in blocks, known as haplotype blocks, with limited number of common variations, which suggests that the genetic variants that put people at risk for common diseases might also be widely shared. Haplotype blocks vary from 10 000 to 50 000 bases in length, neatly organizing the three billion bases in the human genome. This suggests a far simpler structure for the human genome than previously thought. Based on this model, it would not be necessary to identify millions of base variants, which would be both time consuming and extremely expensive with current technologies, but would suffice to identify only the particular bases on each block and any variants around it. This would make both pharmacogenomic and nutrigenomic development much simpler and has spurred an international project, called HapMap, with participating laboratories from the US, UK, China and Japan to identify these haplotype blocks in various human populations. Analysis of samples includes hundred of blood samples from Nigeria, Japan, China and the US and uses highly automated genomic tools for the identification of haplotype patterns among a number of the world's population groups. This has been a very controversial project that has met with lots of criticism from geneticists, since it is viewed by some as a very simplistic and highly speculative approach to be used in drug discovery and target identification. Further, it is criticized as a means of racial discrimination between ethnic groups, and even the way the groups are selected for testing has been a point of debate. However, advocates of the HapMap project claim that the HapMap will be at least a particularly useful genetic tool for the study of genetic variation and perhaps reveal subtle differences in genetic patterns that will allow medical researchers and practitioners to treat common diseases like diabetes, schizophrenia, obesity and hypertension more effectively. Such genetic information, although it should be used with caution and avoid generalization based on statistical differences, can make significant changes in the future development of pharmaco- and nutrigenomics. As it is already recognized that members of different subpopulations tend to respond to different diets and environmental conditions and members of various ethnic backgrounds present different degrees of diet-related health issues, physicians already consider this in their treatment of diseases and prescriptions. For example, BiDil, a controversial heart disease treatment specifically meant for African Americans has already appeared in the market. In fact, a number of early start-up biotechnology and genomics companies have already been formed and provide either genomic profiling services with personalized diet and nutritional supplements, or tools based on fibre-optics, microarrays and mass spectrometry to scan and rapidly identify genetic variations for use in the pharmaceutical industry and the clinic.

The area of oncogenomics and nutrigenomics research is still on its very first steps, but it has the potential for great development in the future, ultimately leading to the prevention of many common illnesses and the patient-specific, personalized treatment of the occurring ones. It will allow the development of new drugs within the next decade or so, that will provide the ultimate advantages of treating specifically and with minimum side effects.

3.4 Summary

Genetic testing has been a reality for the last few years, and it has been well documented that there are genetic factors that can increase the risk for cancer onset. A number of genes have been identified that, when mutated, can increase the risk of cancer. These genes can be inherited from generation to generation and can increase the risk of cancer within family members, as well as cause cancer in younger age. Cancers caused from inherited genes account for only 5 per cent of the total number of cancers. However, genetic testing causes a significant amount of anxiety, as it results in a number of tests that often can lead to preventive surgery to reduce risk, but not without significant psychological cost, but they can also lead to uncertainty when results are inconclusive. Genetic and genomic developments, however, apart from prophylactic and diagnostic uses, they have given rise to areas such as oncogenomics, which have had a profound effect on the novel anticancer drug development that has improved therapeutic potential and reduced side effects. Similarly, genomics and nutrition can also lead to a better knowledge of the appropriate dietary factors that can prevent a number of diseases, including cancer.

3.5 Self-assessment questions

Question: Why is cancer considered a genetic disease?

Answer: Cancer can be considered a genetic disease for two reasons. The first is that for cancer to occur, genetic mutations need to accumulate within the cell. Such mutations may be caused by a number of external factors, or rise spontaneously. The second is that damage or mutation to some genes can be inherited between generations within a family, carrying a significant increase in the risk for the onset of the disease.

Question: Name some genes that are mutated and, when inherited can increase the risk of cancer.

Answer: Some of the genes that can be inherited and cause an increased risk of cancer onset are mentioned in Table 3.1. Briefly, these include *BRCA1* and *2*, *P16 INK4A*, *CDK4*, *hMLH1*, *hMSH2*, *hMSH6*, *PMS1* and *2*, and *HPC2*. They are involved in breast, ovarian, endometrial, colorectal, colon and pancreatic cancers as well as melanoma.

Question: What is genomics?

Answer: Genomics is the study of the whole set of genes, called the genome of an organism, including their sequence, structure, function and interactions.

Question: What are the main characteristics of tumorigenesis?

Answer: Genetic instability, self-sufficiency in growth signals, insensitivity to tumour-inhibitory signals, evasion of apoptosis, limitless replicative potential, sustained angiogenesis, tissue invasion and metastasis.

Question: Tamoxifen is a known anti-oestrogen drug, known as selective oestrogen receptor modulator (SERM), that binds to the oestrogen receptor and, although it allows its dimerization and DNA-binding function, it blocks the transcription of the oestrogen-responsive genes. Can you define how genetic analysis may assist on the decision of whether tamoxifen is an appropriate agent as part of a therapeutic regime for the treatment of breast cancer?

Answer: Genetic profiling and molecular classification of the tumour can identify its oestrogen status. Thus, it can determine whether the tumour is oestrogen positive and therefore will respond to tamoxifen treatment or not, in which case tamoxifen would not be an appropriate agent and alternative regimes should be sought.

Question: What is nutrigenomics?

Answer: Nutrigenomics is the study of how different foods and common dietary chemicals can affect health by altering gene expression and/ or the structure of an individual's genetic makeup.

3.6   Further reading and resources

Brenner C and Duggan D (eds) *Oncogenomics: Molecular Approaches to Cancer,* Wiley, Chichester, 2004.

Debouck C and Metcalf B. The impact of genomics on drug discovery. *Annu Rev Pharmacol Toxicol* 2000, **40**, 193–208.

Kaput J and Rodriguez RL. Nutritional genomics: the next frontier in the postgenomic era. *Physiol Genomics* 2004, **16**, 166–177.

Murcko M and Caron P. Transforming the genome to drug discovery. *DDT* 2002, **7**, 583–584.

Ohlstein EH, Ruffolo RR Jr and Elliott JD. Drug discovery in the next millennium. *Annu Rev Pharmacol Toxicol* 2000, **40**, 177–191.

Romero I (ed.) *Molecular and Cell Biology, The Interactive Cell.* The Open University, Milton Keynes, 2004.

Steward BW and Kleihues P (eds) *World cancer report,* WHO, IARC press, Lyon, 2003.

Tribut O, Lessard Y, Reymann JM, Allain H and Bentue-Ferrer D. *Pharmacogenom Med Sci Monit* 2002, **8**, 152–163.

http://www.cancerbackup.org.uk/, (accessed February 2007).

http://www.hapmap.org/ (accessed February 2007)

www.nugo.org/, (accessed February 2007)

http://nutrigenomics.ucdavis.edu/, (accessed February 2007)

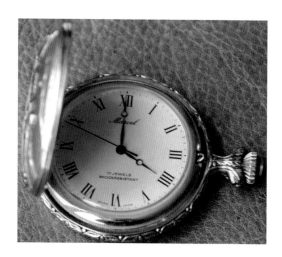

In the previous chapters we have seen how cancer can be caused by diet, smoke and alcohol, environmental factors, or how specific genes are inherited to give higher vulnerability to the changes necessary for cancer initiation. We have thus encountered the genetic factors responsible for cancer initiation, the various oncogene and tumour suppressor genes, with their activation or silencing respectively. However, in this chapter we will see another very important reason for cancer initiation, also linked with inflammation that will be discussed in Chapter 6. This is infection. We are all subjected to various infections and we live most our lives hosting friendly and unfriendly bacteria in our system. Similarly, all too often we are subjected to viral infections, mostly thinking nothing of them as a reason to develop cancer. However, this is not always the case. There are a number of infections, both viral and bacterial, that have now been associated with cancer development, either through their direct action or through the causing of inflammation, as will be discussed in the next chapter. Preventing or treating these early on, to avoid chronic infection, can lead to the prevention of various forms of cancer. Also, identifying these infections can often provide diagnostic assays for cancer risk, as some of these infectious agents are so closely associated with cancer development (as we shall discuss in Chapter 6). Thus, infection is a very important part in cancer development and the fight against the disease.

4
Infection and cancer

Toni Aebischer[1] and Thomas Rudel[2]

1. *Institute of Immunology and Infection Research, University of Edinburgh, UK*
2. *Max-Planck-Institute for Infection Biology, Department of Molecular Biology, Germany*

4.1 Viral infection as a cause of cancer

4.1.1 Introduction

At the end of the nineteenth century, Luis Pasteur and Robert Koch discovered infectious agents as the cause of diseases such as rabies, dysentery and cholera. At that time, where important human diseases were discovered to be caused by infections, cancer was also considered a candidate infectious disease. Initial experiments performed in the 1870s with tumour tissue transferred from one animal to another demonstrated the general principle of limitless growth intrinsic to tumours. However, those findings were not rated as proof for an infectious agent causing cancer, because transplantations of normal, non-cancerous tissue, has been demonstrated before. It was Peyton Rous from the Rockefeller Institute in New York who is credited as being the first person to show that cancer could have an infectious origin. In 1910, Rous prepared cell-free filtrates of sarcomas from chickens and injected them into another chicken, which too developed sarcomas. He could even transfer the induced sarcomas by injecting homogenates of them into other chickens. These findings revolutionized the field. First, cancer could be induced at wish within a predictable timeframe and so, from then on, could easily be made available for research. More importantly, the cancer-inducing agent was shown to be small enough to pass through a filter. In those days, infectious material was categorized by behaviour upon filtration. If the infectious

The Cancer Clock Edited by Sotiris Missailidis
© 2007 John Wiley & Sons Ltd

agent could be passed through a filter, it was presumed to contain viruses. If the material was trapped in the filter it was graded as bacteria. Based on this simple test, the agents causing rabies and smallpox were classified as viruses. Rous' findings, therefore, strongly suggested a virus-like agent as the cause of cancer. And indeed, Rous' discovered soon thereafter oncogenic viruses. However, the field of infection and cancer research experienced a drawback, which prevented the acknowledgement of Rous' work at that time. Johannes Grib Fibiger reported in 1913 that the parasite *Spiroptera carcinoma* caused stomach cancer in rats and, finally, received in 1926 the first Nobel Prize in the field. However, it later turned out that the reason why the rats developed cancer was malnutrition and not a parasite. This scandalous finding paralysed the field for decades.

Then, in the 1950s, the tide began to turn again to favour infectious agents as the cause of cancer. RSV (Rous sarcoma virus) was introduced into isolated chicken fibroblasts and a series of experiments unveiled the principles of tumour genesis, previously only observed in animals, now at the cellular level. The most important principles of tumorigenesis, such as extended lifespan, change in cell morphology, or loss of contact inhibition, to name only a few, were recognized as features of transformed cells by studying oncovirus infection. Moreover, electron microscopy was developed that finally allowed visualization of the first virus in 1957. As a result, intensive research started again leading to the discovery of more than two dozen oncoviruses by 1970. As one consequence of this race for new oncoviruses, Rous' work was rediscovered and found the attention it deserved. He received the Nobel Prize in 1966 for his discovery of the first tumour-inducing RNA virus, RSV. These successful findings paved the way for an era during which an infectious origin for cancer became a dominant hypothesis. Huge research programmes were started to investigate the basis of infectious agents and carcinogenesis. Most of the molecular principles for cell transformation were elucidated as a consequence of research in the tumour virus field. For example, it was observed that certain viral genes had transforming potential, whereas others were required for the replication of the virus. The first described viral oncogene identified in RSV was *src*. Soon thereafter, a cellular homologue for the viral *src*, *c-src*, was discovered. This finding shifted the focus of research dramatically. Apparently, oncogenes already present in the host cell were picked up by an ancestor of the virus during infection.

The difference between the gene involved in normal cell function and the viral oncogene could be explained if the viral gene was altered. As a consequence of this hypothesis, the cellular homologues, called proto-oncogenes, could have the intrinsic potential to induce cancer. A similar alteration in the proto-oncogene as in the viral oncogene could induce the formation of cancer even in the absence of infection.

Research into viral oncogenes has led to the discovery of a large group of proto-oncogenes. Indeed, numerous mutations have been discovered in the oncogenic versions of these proto-oncogenes. It is therefore fair to say that the research on tumour viruses has also substantially influenced the current view on infection-independent cancer as the consequence of the accumulation of genetic alterations in genes controlling proliferation and survival of cells.

4.1.2 Principles of oncogenic transformation by virus infection

Integrating viruses

Intensive research into infectious agents as a cause of cancer has lead to the discovery of oncogenes as the cause for cell transformation. Oncogenes emerge from mutations, which very often lead to the permanent activation of factors driving proliferation or cell survival. Another possible reason for cancer development is the inactivation of tumour suppressor genes by mutations. Tumour suppressors are part of highly sophisticated cellular machinery involved in the deletion of damaged, potentially pro-cancerous cells. However, oncogenes as well as inactivated tumour suppressor genes can only support cancer formation if the damaged genes are passed to the progeny of the transformed cell. A very important principle of cancer formation by infection is therefore the requirement of the permanent action of a viral oncogene to keep the transformed state of a cell. Moreover, the virus and thereby also the oncogene have to be passed from the transformed mother cell to the daughter cells and further to their descendants. The loss of viral oncogenes would inevitably lead to the reversion of a transformed cell to normality. One way that tumour viruses achieve their transmission is by integration into the host cells' chromosomes. They thereby become part of the host's genome and are passed to progeny through the process of chromosomal DNA replication. The process of genomic integration was first discovered for a DNA tumour virus called simian virus 40 (SV40). In the case of SV40, the integration was easy to envisage since, both the virus and the host genomes consisted of DNA. A similar process could not however be responsible for the transmission of RSV genomes because they consist of single stranded RNA. It turned out that RSV uses a complex backward reaction of the normal flow of genetic information and produces double stranded DNA from the RNA molecule. The double stranded DNA incorporates into the genome and is used to transcribe viral mRNAs as well as the viral genomes. The finding that tumour viruses integrate into the host's genome was a very important observation, because it not only explained the passage of the virus and the continuous activity of viral oncogenes in transformed cells. It also offered an explanation on how tumour viruses acquired host proto-oncogenes. If a virus integrates close to a cellular proto-oncogene it may acquire the gene during the virus maturation process and transfer it as part of a newly formed virus to other host cells (Figure 4.1). To date numerous viral oncogenes have been identified which were acquired by viruses in a similar way (Table 4.1).

However, viruses do not need to transfer oncogenes to transform host cells. Often the integration of the virus or parts thereof close to a cellular proto-oncogene is sufficient to drive its uncontrolled expression (Figure 4.2). The behaviour of some integrating oncoviruses to activate cellular proto-oncogenes, for example by strongly inducing their transcription, was even used by investigators to systematically screen for cellular proto-oncogenes. Meanwhile large cohorts of proto-oncogenes were identified to drive cellular transformation if activated by oncoviruses (Table 4.2).

But introducing viral or activating cellular oncogenes to transform cells is not the only mechanism by which viral infection may transform cells. In the broader sense, any integrating virus could act as a tumour virus, for example if the integration destroys

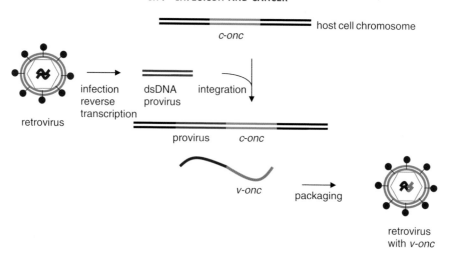

Figure 4.1 Capture of a cellular proto-oncogene by a retrovirus. The figure schematically illustrates how retroviruses may acquire cellular proto-oncogenes. The viral provirus (red) randomly integrates into the host chromosomes. In rare cases, the provirus may integrate close to a cellular proto-oncogene (green) from where both are co-transcribed into a single hybrid RNA transcript (blue and orange). The hybrid transcript is then packaged into a virion which may carry the proto-oncogene eventually as part of the viral genome

cellular tumour suppressor genes (Figure 4.2). As a consequence of the inactivation of tumour suppressor genes, or anti-oncogenes, as they are sometimes called, cells with damaged DNA and mutated genes survive and may eventually become cancer cells.

Non-integrating viruses

At this stage, all explained principles of tumorigenesis induced by viruses depended on their behaviour to integrate into the genome of the host cells. However, there are at least two other general principles of how viral and bacterial infections may cause cancer. First, infections may induce chronic inflammation accompanied by the formation of reactive oxygen (ROS) and nitrogen species (RNOS) by phagocytes at the site of inflammation, which, as we have seen in Chapter 2 can also lead to DNA damage and carcinogenesis.

Table 4.1 Examples of acutely transforming retroviruses and the oncogenes they have acquired

Virus	Oncogene	Type of oncoprotein
Rous sarcoma virus	v-src	Non-receptor tyrosine kinase
Simian sarcoma virus	v-sis	Growth factor
Avian erythroblastosis virus	v-erbA or v-erbB	Hormone receptor
Kirsten murine sarcoma virus	v-kras	Small G protein
Moloney murine sarcoma virus	v-mos	ser/thr kinase
MC29 avian myelocytoma virus	v-myc	Transcription factor

Abbreviations: G, GTP-binding; ser/thr, serine/threonine.

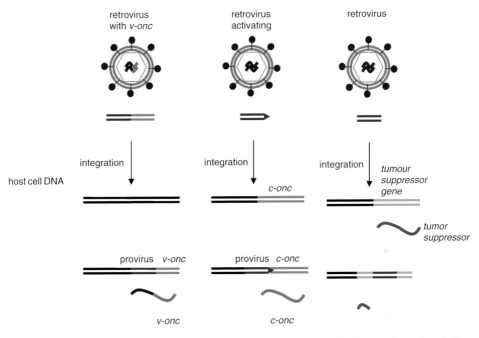

Figure 4.2 General principles of how integrating viruses may lead to cellular transformation. A virus may carry viral oncogenes which lead to cellular transformation upon integration of the virus (left scenario). Some integrating viruses have the potential to activate cellular proto-oncogenes (middle scenario). Integration close to a cellular proto-oncogene may lead to transcriptional activation of an otherwise stringently regulated gene controlling e.g. proliferation. Also the integrative inactivation of anti-oncogenes and tumour suppressors may ultimately prone a cell to transformation (right scenario)

Table 4.2 Examples of acutely transforming retroviruses and the oncogenes they have acquired

Gene	Virus	Tumour type	Type of oncoprotein
Myc	Avian leukosis virus	B-cell lymphoma	Transcription factor
erbB	Avian leukosis virus	Erythroblastosis	Receptor tyrosine kinase
Wnt-1	Mouse mammary tumour virus	Mammary carcinoma	Growth factor
Bmi-1	Moloney murine leukaemia virus	T-cell lymphoma	Transcription factor
K-Ras	Friend murine leukaemia virus	T-cell lymphoma	Small G protein
CycD1	Friend murine leukaemia virus	T-cell lymphoma	G1 cyclin

Abbreviations: G, GTP-binding.

Chronic inflammation may cause an environment of increased mutagenesis which supports oncogenic transformation (see Chapter 5). Chronic inflammation may also support the proliferation of pre-cancerous, not fully transformed cells, which gradually acquire more mutations on their way to become cancer cells. Recent research has unveiled a very important role for immune cells secreting factors which support the proliferation of these cells.

The other mechanism depends on severe and long term immunosuppression by viruses such as human immunodeficiency virus (HIV). The immune surveillance hypothesis – first raised by Paul Ehrlich in 1909 – proposed that one role of the immune system was to destroy tumours that arise spontaneously on a continued and frequent basis. The discovery of tumour-specific antigens and the ability to prevent tumour development in mice by inducing immunity against such antigens supported this theory. At first glance, the increased risk of cancer in immunosuppressed patients is in line with the immune surveillance hypothesis. However, immunosuppressed individuals are not at an increased risk of developing some of the most common malignancies like breast, prostate and colon cancer. Most of the cancers that do develop during stages of immune suppression are rare cancers associated with viral infection.

4.1.3 Human pathogenic viruses causing cancer

Most principles of virus-induced tumorigenesis have been discovered by the study of animal viruses. The question of whether human pathogenic viruses are cancer inducing agents can, for ethical reasons, not be addressed in a causative manner as it was done for most of the animal viruses. Causation can be examined by addressing Koch's postulates as modified by Rivers for viral diseases. According to them, a virus has to be isolated from the diseased host, has to have the capacity to grow in host cells, retain their activity after filtering away bacteria, and has to produce disease in the host or related species. The virus has to be re-isolated and should elicit a specific immune response. Several of these postulates can not be tested in humans. That is why we heavily depend on epidemiological data and laboratory studies to provide the mechanistic basis for cellular transformation by human viruses. In the following section, we will review the most important human viruses and their association to cancer formation (Table 4.3). Where possible, the most likely mechanism of cancer induction by a given virus will be discussed.

Hepatitis B virus (HBV)
HBV is the smallest known virus with a clear association to cancer development. The 3.4 kilobase circular DNA genome codes for only four proteins, the envelope protein (HBsAg), the nucleocapsid (core), a polymerase/reverse transcriptase and the 'X' protein. Infection with HBV is extremely prevalent with an estimated 200 million people infected worldwide. About 350 million people – mainly from Asia and Africa – are chronically infected carriers of the virus. Chronic infection with HBV is a definite cause of hepatocellular carcinoma in humans, one of the most common cancers worldwide with 560 thousand new cases each year, 83 per cent in developing countries. The risk

Table 4.3 Human viruses implicated in cancer development

Virus	Non-tumour diseases	Tumour associated with infection
Hepatitis B virus	Hepatitis, liver cirrhosis, liver failure	Liver cancer
Hepatitis C virus	Hepatitis, liver cirrhosis, liver failure	Liver cancer
Epstein–Barr virus	Infectious mononucleosis ('kissing disease')	Burkitt's lymphoma Non-Hodgkin's lymphoma, Hodgkin's disease Nasopharyngeal carcinoma
Human papillomavirus	Warts	Cervical carcinoma Head and neck cancer
Human herpes virus 8	Castleman's disease	Kaposi's sarcoma Body cavity lymphoma
HTLV-1	Tropical spastic paraparesis	Adult T cell leukemia
HIV	Acquired immune deficiency syndrome (AIDS)	Kaposi's sarcoma Non-Hodgkin's lymphoma Cervical cancer

to develop liver cancer is nearly 14 times higher for carriers than for non-carriers and 50 per cent of all liver cancers are therefore caused by chronic HBV infection.

HBV may integrate into the chromosomes of infected cells and thereby cause a variety of alterations, such as gene inactivation. In addition, genomes containing HBV DNA tend to frequently rearrange, a phenomenon called genetic instability which is often found in cancer cells. Moreover, the HBV X protein directly affects the activity of cellular genes. For example, the cellular proto-oncogene *c-myc* is activated by HBV protein X. It may also bind and inactivate the important cellular tumour suppressor p53.

All these direct effects of HBV on human cells may support the initiation of hepatic cancer. However, not all hepatocellular carcinoma tumours contain integrated HBV DNA. Therefore, the tumour promoting effect of HBV may rather depend on the virus-induced liver damage, chronic inflammation and regeneration leading to the accumulation of damaged cells with multiple genetic alterations. In this sense, HBV is a classic carcinogen with tumour-initiating and promoting capabilities.

Hepatitis C virus (HCV)

HCV has a single, positive sense RNA genome of about 9.6 kilobases. The viral genome has only one long open reading frame coding for one large polyprotein, which is processed to ten individual proteins. HCV infects approximately 170 million people worldwide and causes chronic liver damage. Primary infection with HCV is predominantly asymptomatic and, in the majority of cases, leads to persistent infection. These patients have an increased risk to develop cirrhosis, liver failure and hepatocellular carcinoma after prolonged chronic infection, sometimes decades after the initial infection. HCV is often found in association with so-called 'cryptic' HBV infection, a situation where no viral protein is produced although HBV DNA is detectable. Cryptic HBV infection is an important risk factor for the development of hepatocellular carcinoma in patients with HCV infections.

HCV does not integrate into the host cells' chromosomes. Hepatocellular carcinoma evolves after many years of chronic infection and is generally preceded by the development of cirrhosis. Chronic liver injury is followed by regeneration, cirrhosis and the development of hepatocellular carcinoma. Increased cell turnover in the context of inflammation and DNA damage facilitating the accumulation of genetic alterations is very likely the main mechanism of carcinogenesis. However, recent evidence has also suggested a more direct role for viral proteins in promoting malignant transformation and hepatocellular carcinoma, mainly based on two observations: HCV replication occurs within hepatocellular carcinoma tumours; and HCV can induce hepatocellular carcinoma even in the absence of cirrhosis. Experimental evidence suggests the activation of cellular proto-oncogenes and the inhibition of apoptosis by the HCV core protein as possible mechanisms.

Epstein–Barr virus (EBV)

EBV is a member of the herpes family of viruses. The virus harbours a 172 kilobase genome made up of double stranded, linear DNA encoding for more than 100 genes. After entry into the cell, the virus becomes circular to form so-called EBV episomes – non-integrating replicating viral genomes. EBV infects more than 90 per cent of the world's population. In developing countries most children are already infected by the age of 2, whereas infections occur later in life in developed countries. EBV is an established carcinogen for three types of cancer: non-Hodgkin's lymphoma, Hodgkin's disease and nasopharyngeal carcinoma. EBV was first isolated from tissue of Burkitt's lymphoma, a rapidly growing B-cell lymphoma highly prevalent in Africa. Although nearly 100 per cent of the Burkitt's lymphoma patients in Africa contain EBV episomes, the fraction is much smaller in other countries, suggesting that the same tumour may be caused by EBV infections as well as independent of infections with EBV.

B lymphocytes become infected with the virus, resulting in latent infection and the strong stimulation of B-lymphocyte proliferation. In some cases, EBV-infected B lymphocytes escape their destruction by the immune system. In these cases, persistent infection is maintained through the EBV episome, giving raise to a permanently proliferating subpopulation of B lymphocytes. This form of lymphoproliferative disease may be linked to the onset of B-cell lymphomas many years after the initial infection.

Human papillomavirus (HPV)

More than 100 different HPV genotypes have been defined, of which about 40 infect the genital mucosa. They are small DNA viruses with a circular, double-stranded genome of about 8 kilobases. HPV is sexually transmitted with a prevalence of about 7 per cent in developed and 15 per cent in developing countries. Genital HPV types have been clearly associated with cervical cancer. It has been estimated in 2002 that 493 000 new cervical cancers develop each year, which lead to 274 thousand deaths, 80 per cent of which occur in developing countries. Individual HPV genotypes are classified into low or high risk by their propensity to cause cervical cancer. Low-risk HPV, like HPV6 and HPV11, produce benign genital warts whereas the high risk types, HPV16 and HPV18, are the etiological agents of cervical cancer. HPV16 accounts for about half of all cervical cancers and HPV18 an additional 20 per cent, but there are at least 15 known oncogenic HPV types. HPV are highly tissue-specific and infect only the basal cells of the squamous epithelium in the genital tract, skin and upper respiratory tract.

The carcinogenic potential of HPV is related to its ability to integrate into host genomes, since cancer is rare in the absence of integration. There are two viral proteins with outstanding importance for the development of cervical cancer: The E6 and E7 proteins. Both genes retain their functionality in nearly all cases of cervical cancer. Their enormous potential as viral oncogenes is further underlined by the observation that they alone are necessary and sufficient to immortalize primary human genital keratinocytes in cell culture plates. E6 and E7 have a different function in the development of cervical cancer. E6 is a strong repressor of the tumour suppressor p53 which is the 'genome guardian protein' and has an important role to play in the destruction of cells with damaged DNA. As a consequence of the E6 action, the genomic instability and the accumulation of mutations are enhanced. The E7 protein interacts with the retinoblastoma protein (RB), which controls the cell cycle and DNA replication. Inactivation of RB by E7 forces the cell to enter the cell cycle and to proliferate. Both E6 and E7 may act via additional mechanisms to immortalize cells since interactions with numerous other proteins have been observed.

Screening programs have strongly reduced the number of cervical cancer cases in developed countries. Cells from a woman's cervix are collected by Pap smears and screened for abnormal cells. Women with abnormal cells are then further diagnosed by, for example biopsies, and therapeutic approaches can be initiated at early stages of cancer development. Despite the success of this approach, many women do not have access to the screening process and consequently the impact of cervical caner is highest in this group. Supported by the success of the screening program, a vaccine for the prevention of HPV infection has been developed and approved. There is now the hope that HPV vaccination may provide an opportunity to profoundly affect cervical cancer incidence worldwide.

Human herpes virus 8 (HHV8)

HHV8, also known as Kaposi's sarcoma-associated herpes virus (KSHV) is a gamma-herpes virus only found in humans. The HHV8 genome consists of double-stranded DNA and contains at least 80 open reading frames, including genes with transforming potential.

Overwhelming evidence documents HHV8 as the cause of Kaposi's sarcoma (KS), a multiple pigmented sarcoma of the skin. There are four types of KS: classic, endemic, post-transplant and AIDS-associated KS. Classic and endemic KS occur in patients of southern European, Arabic or Jewish ancestry and some equatorial countries of Africa, respectively. Both classical and endemic KS were known of long before the emergence of HIV, but even today the reason for these types of KS is not really understood. In contrast, the onset of post-transplant and AIDS-associated KS is clearly the consequence of

immunosuppression. Post-transplant KS is mainly found in people receiving immu-
nosuppressive therapy (e.g. transplant patients) where the incidence to develop KS
increases about 150 times over average. Also, HHV8 is the most frequent cause of
malignancy in patients with AIDS. In certain parts of Africa, due to the AIDS epidemic,
KS is the most common cancer. HHV8 was identified in 100 per cent of AIDS patients
with KS and in 15 per cent of non-KS tissue samples from AIDS patients. In addition to
KS, HHV8 may also cause other tumours such as primary effusion lymphoma (PEL) and
multicentric Castleman's disease (MCD), two rare lymphoproliferative disorders.

KSHV has pirated cellular cDNAs from the host genome. Many of the viral regulatory
homologues encode proteins that directly inhibit host adaptive and innate immunity.
For example, v-Bcl-2 is a viral homologue of an important class of human regulators of
apoptotic cell death, the Bcl-2 family of proteins. Other viral proteins may target RB and
p53 control of tumour suppressor pathways, which play key effector roles in intracellular immune responses. The immune evasion strategies used by KSHV in targeting
tumour suppressor pathways, activated during immune system signalling, may lead to
inadvertent cell proliferation and tumorigenesis in susceptible hosts.

Human thymus-derived-cell leukaemia/lymphoma virus-1 (HTLV-1)

HTLV-1 is a retrovirus with a single-stranded RNA of about 9 kilobases. The virus
preferentially infects CD4-positive T cells and integrates randomly into the genome.
HTLV-1 is associated with two fatal human diseases, adult T-cell leukaemia (ATL), a
clonal malignancy of infected mature $CD4^+$ T cells and tropical spastic paraparesis, a
neurodegenerative disease. The number of infected people is estimated to be 10–20
million worldwide but the prevalence is highest in parts of Japan, South America, Africa,
and the Caribbean. Children are probably infected by their mothers through breast
feeding, adults by sexual contact or blood transfusions. The infection remains asymptomatic in the majority of individuals, but approximately 2–5 per cent of HTLV-I carriers
develop disease 20–40 years post infection.

As it can also immortalize CD4 T cells *in vitro*, and is clearly associated with ATL,
HTLV-1 is rated as a definite carcinogen. The long clinical latency and low percentage of
individuals who develop leukemia suggest that T-cell transformation occurs after a series
of cellular alterations and mutations. The viral *tax* gene thereby appears to play an
outstanding role. Tax expression itself promotes transformation of normal cells *in vitro*
and transgenic mice which produce Tax develop tumours. Multiple interactions for Tax
have been described, leading to an inactivation of tumour suppressors, DNA repair and
apoptotic responses and an increased expression of proto-oncogenes and enhanced
proliferation.

Human immunodeficiency virus (HIV)

HIV belongs to the group of retroviruses with a single-stranded RNA genome. After
entry into host cells, a DNA intermediate is made by reverse transcription, which
integrates into the host's genome. HIV causes AIDS, characterized by severe depletion
of functional T cells. The virus is transmitted sexually, from mother to child, and
parenterally. More than 40 million people have been infected worldwide with HIV.

Several different types of cancers are observed at an increased frequency in AIDS patients, most of which are virus-associated cancers. The most common cancer found in AIDS patients is Kaposi's sarcoma caused by HHV8. Non-Hodgkin's lymphoma, mainly caused by EBV and/or HHV8 infection, is another significant source of morbidity and mortality in AIDS patients. HPV-induced cervical cancer and EBV-caused Hodgkin's disease are also significantly increased in AIDS patients.

The enormous potential of HIV to cause cancer is clearly a consequence of the dramatically compromised immune system of infected individuals. This is also in line with the observation of an overall drop in the incidence for AIDS-related cancer in AIDS patients treated with highly active antiretroviral therapy (HAART). This therapy includes both HIV reverse transcriptase and protease inhibitors. Established KS lesions usually resolve when patients begin HAART and survival of patients with lymphomas has dramatically improved through HAART-induced immune restoration. There may also be a direct effect of HIV infection such as insertional mutagenesis and upregulation of oncogenes and growth factors.

4.2 Bacterial infection as a cause of cancer

4.2.1 Introduction

Virchow, the eminent german pathologist of the nineteenth century, had postulated that infections and inflammation are at the source of cancer development. Epidemiologists have gathered evidence over the last two decades that viral and bacterial infections probably cause one of every five tumours! In 1984 Barry Marshall, an Australian physician, drank a suspension of *Helicobacter pylori* that he had isolated from patients and over the next few days developed gastritis. This 'gutsy' self experiment rightly earned him the Nobel Prize in Medicine in 2005 because *H. pylori* was subsequently found in epidemiological studies to be linked to gastric cancer development. Infection with *H. pylori*, a spiral shaped, flagellated Gram-negative bacterium triggers gastritis, which over a sequence of pathological changes in the mucosa – pan-gastritis, atrophy of the mucosa, build up of intestinal type mucosa tissue (intestinal metaplasia) – leads to gastric cancer in about one of every 100 infected humans. Because more than 50 per cent of humans are infected, this means that since you started reading this paragraph somebody died of gastric cancer and, for example, in China alone this will be tragically repeated every 2 minutes.

H. pylori is a compelling example linking bacterial infection to cancer development in humans. This connection is firmly based on epidemiological evidence but the exact molecular mechanisms leading to malignancy still remain to be deciphered. In fact, this is true for most of the examples that will be presented below, although we possess strong hypotheses on how bacteria could cause cancer. Bacteria affect several properties of host cells that are conceptually linked to carcinogenesis and instructive examples will be discussed in the next sections. These properties refer to three to seven traits that are needed for malignant cell growth and are often captured as *hallmarks of cancer*: independence of growth signals; non-responsiveness to growth limiting signals;

limitless replication potential; evasion of apoptosis; ability to sustain angiogenesis; and capacity to metastasize.

Our knowledge of the molecular basis for how bacteria may affect these traits has been boosted tremendously in the past 10 years with the revolution in genomics. Today, the complete information on the genes making up pathogenic bacteria is available for many species (for the extent of this resource see http://www.ncbi.nlm.nih.gov/genomes/lproks.cgi) and comparative analyses of benign and pathogenic bacterial relatives has accelerated the discovery of virulence and pathogenic factors. Bacteria seem to have integrated these factors as islands in their chromosomes (called PAI for pathogenicity island(s)), or retain them lined up on self-contained units such as plasmids. Individual genes or gene arrays in these horizontally acquired genetic elements can vary from pathogenic isolate to isolate creating diversity and in the interaction with genetically non-identical hosts this increases complexity. The quest for deciphering cause and effect relationships therefore becomes formidable. Although integrating this knowledge and linking virulence/pathogenicity gene sets in bacteria to disease manifestations in patients will require much more research, the fact that we begin to understand the toolkits that bacteria use creates fascinating opportunities.

4.2.2 Bacterial infection causing malignancies: examples and evidence

To date we link a handful of bacterial infections to tumours in humans or model animals (Table 4.4). The evidence for this link differs for the individual bacterial species and

Table 4.4 Bacterial infections implicated in cancer development

Bacterium	Primary disease	Tumour associated with	Host infection
Bartonella spp. (henselae, quintana, bacilliformis)	Cat scratch disease, trench fever, Carrion's disease	Angioma	Immunosuppressed Humans
Citrobacter rodentium	Colitis	Colon carcinoma	Inbred mice
Chlamydophyla pneumoniae	Pneumonia	Lung cancer	Humans
Helicobacter pylori	Gastritis, duodenal ulcer, gastric ulcer	Gastric adenocarcinoma (diffuse and intestinal type) MALT lymphoma	Humans
Helicobacter hepaticus	Hepatitis, typhlitis, colitis	Hepatocarcinoma	Inbred mice
Salmonella enterica Serovar typhi	Typhoid fever	Gall bladder cancer (hepatocellular carcinoma)	Humans
Streptococcus bovis	Colitis	Colorectal cancer	Humans

MALT, mucosa-associated lymphoid tissue.

ranges from weak or questionable in the case of *Chlamydophyla pneumoniae* and lung cancer, to strong and partly understood at the molecular level in the case of *Bartonella* and angioma (see below). A common feature of these bacterial infections, however, is that they can become chronic and it is chronic infection that is linked to cancer development. Another shared aspect is that tumours do not invariably develop and, in fact, in most patients luckily will not develop. Therefore, other factors must contribute to push cells to pass the hurdles towards malignancy. These factors may be linked to the host's immune response to infection (see later chapters in this book for a discussion of host factors) but may also invoke environmental stress such as exposure to noxious substances in the diet or when smoking.

Bartonella spp. and angioma

Bartonella spp. are Gram-negative facultative intracellular bacteria, transmitted by blood-sucking arthropods such as cat fleas, body lice or certain sandflies. They establish themselves basically in two niches by infecting (i) endothelial cells and (ii) erythrocytes. While the latter is important for their mode of transmission and closing the infectious cycle, it is the intra-epithelial cell infection that is associated with tumour formation in the chronic stages of infection with one of the three species *Bartonella henselae*, *B. quintana* or *B. bacilliformes*. The tumours are vascular tumours, angiomas that require the presence of bacteria and often only form under conditions of immunosuppression such as in AIDS patients, who develop bacillary angiomatosis. The tumours are benign and antibiotic treatment will lead to their regression.

Citrobacter rodentium and colon cancer

Epidemics of colonic hyperplastic disease and diarrhoea with high mortality in mouse colonies in Japan and the USA in the 1960s lead to the identification of *Citrobacter rodentium*, a Gram-negative bacterium of murine intestines, as the culprit. Experimental infection with this bacterium is often self limiting and resolves over the course of 4 weeks. Colonic hyperplasia builds up after 1 to 2 weeks but does not lead to full malignant transformation by itself. However, if animals have existing precancerous lesions these are promoted by the infection. *C. rodentium* infection is therefore used as a model for human disease. Furthermore, since acute disease symptoms are shared with human gastrointestinal infections with enteropathogenic or enterohaemorrhagic *E. coli*, it is also used as a model for this family of pathogens.

Chlamidophyla pneumoniae and lung cancer

Infection with the Gram-negative *Ch. pneumoniae* occurs via aerosols and can cause lower respiratory tract disease. Infection is widespread with more than 50 per cent of adults presenting evidence of persistent or past infection. The bacteria replicate only within a vacuole inside host cells. These bacteria can be driven to severely reduce their metabolic activity by antibiotic treatment, whereby they resist elimination and establish persistent infections. Several epidemiological studies link chronic infection with lung cancer since lung cancer patients showed higher antibody titres in their serum. However, the evidence is currently purely epidemiological, and some studies in fact contradict such an association.

Helicobacter pylori and gastric cancer or mucosa-associated lymphoid tissue (MALT) lymphoma

In the case of the Gram-negative *H. pylori* infections are acquired in infancy by oral/oral or faecal/oral transmission within families and infections persist for life. Acute infection leads invariably to gastritis but the outcome of chronic infection is much more variable. Patients may develop symptomatic diseases such as gastric and duodenal ulcers or, worse, gastric cancer or MALT lymphoma. The latter two may take 50 to 60 years to develop and affect 1–3 per cent of patients, indicating again that additional factors contribute to malignant transformation. Infection is said to increase the risk to develop gastric cancer at a younger age by greater than 20-fold and, in 1994, *H. pylori* was therefore classified as a carcinogen. The very protracted onset of cancer development highlights, however, an important general aspect in this field: Not enough time has passed yet since the discovery of *H. pylori*'s role in gastric malignancies to give a final assessment of the efficacy of disease prevention by antibiotic eradication. Clinicians struggle to justify broad application of antibiotic therapy since there is little information on the point in time after infection when the carcinogenic process cannot be reversed and antibiotic treatment would not be effective as a cancer preventing measure. The answer will come from prospective epidemiological studies that have been initiated but will not be finished before the next decade. Fortunately, animal models were developed in the early 1990s to study this infection and its link to cancer in more detail. These models indeed experimentally link infection and gastric malignancy. In addition, they support the hypothesis that infection acts in concert with host genetic factors responsible for a high inflammatory response and factors in the diet to cause and promote gastric cancer. Importantly, the models now provide the tools to dissect the molecular mechanism whereby the bacteria may promote or initiate cancer.

Helicobacter hepaticus and liver cancer

H. hepaticus is a Gram-negative natural pathogen of mice and present in many colonies of experimental mice. Depending on the genetic background of the mice, but found in particular in A/JCr mice, predominantly in males, the infection causes chronic active hepatitis and hepatocellular carcinoma. In humans, extra-intestinal *Helicobacter* species were also found in liver and gall bladder of liver cancer patients. It is thus possible that these bacteria are responsible for part of the non-viral infection-caused hepatic cancers. Thus, *H. hepaticus* infection in mice is believed to model the emerging liver infections with human hepatic *Helicobacter*.

Salmonella enterica serovar typhi and cancer of the gall bladder

Salmonella enterica serovar *typhi* is better known as the cause of typhoid fever in humans. However, after acute oral infection these Gram-negative bacteria can establish a persistent infection in gall bladder and patients therefore become carriers. These carriers can initiate epidemics by the faecal/oral route under conditions of low hygiene as they shed bacteria. Retrospective epidemiologic studies on two epidemics of typhoid fever, one in 1922 in New York and one in 1964 in Aberdeen, traced an increased risk of developing gall bladder cancer back to such *S. typhi* carriers. The studies showed that the risk of developing gall bladder cancer was roughly six-fold higher in carriers but not in patients that cleared the *Salmonella* infection and did not become carriers.

Streptococcus bovis and colorectal cancer
S. bovis, is a Gram-positive bacterium that, unlike the name suggests, is also a frequent inhabitant of the human gastrointestinal tract. However, it can leave this niche and cause bacteraemia and infectious endocarditis. Epidemiological studies that analysed cases of *S. bovis* bacteraemia found a correlation with colonic neoplasia. About 25–80 per cent of patients that had suffered from *S. bovis* bacteraemia develop a colonic tumour. Moreover there is experimental credit to link the infection with this bacterium with promotion of tumorigenesis since rats treated with azomethane, a carcinogen, and then given cell wall extracts of *S. bovis* or the bacteria showed increased progression of precancerous lesions.

4.2.3 Common molecular machines linked to pathogenesis: Type 3 and 4 secretion systems

In 1907 Smith and Townsend published on a plant tumour that was linked to bacterial infection, Crown Gall tumours caused by *Agrobacterium tumefaciens*. Since then, the pathogenesis of this process has been elucidated and, on a molecular level, this became by far the best understood and, therefore, exemplary case of bacterial infection-triggered tumorigenesis.

Virulent *A. tumefaciens* harbour a tumour-inducing, so-called Ti plasmid. This plasmid encodes for structural genes that form a molecular syringe, a critical device to deliver transforming protein–DNA complexes into host cells (Figure 4.3). Both the genes encoding the proteins that bind the transferred DNA and this DNA are also part of the plasmid. The syringe is a so-called type 4 secretion system (T4SS). These systems are thought to have evolved from bacterial conjugation systems mediating DNA exchange between bacteria. In the case of the Ti type 4 secretion machinery, DNA is translocated from the bacterium to a eukaryotic cell and becomes integrated into this host cell's chromosomal DNA. The transferred DNA encodes enzymes needed to synthesize plant growth hormones, such as auxin, which support tumorigenic growth of the transformed cells. In addition, transferred DNA holds the genetic information for proteins catalyzing the induced synthesis of amino acid sugar conjugates – opines – which provide an extra source of carbon and nitrogen for the bacteria and allow them to gain a selective growth advantage. Transformation is thus a means whereby the bacteria induce a self-renewing, expanding source of nutrients.

The strategy used by *A. tumefaciens* relies on its capacity to directly deliver genetic information into the host cell, as bacteria deficient in structural components of this syringe are no longer tumour inducing. The genomes of other bacteria were searched for similar devices and the presence of genes encoding orthologues for molecular syringes to deliver factors directly into host cells were found to be a theme that recurs again and again in these pathogens. Furthermore, the delivery of effector molecules changes

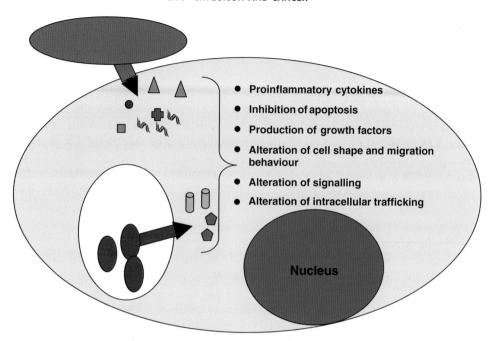

Figure 4.3 Bacterial Type 3 and 4 secretion systems transfer effector proteins that disturb cellular processes implicated in cancer development. Bacteria assemble molecular syringes to deliver factors directly to a host cell cytoplasm or integrate them into the host cell membrane. They may do so being either extracellular (e.g. *Helicobacter*) or in a vesicular compartment inside an infected cell (e.g. *Chlamydia, Salmonella*)

cellular functions that are implicated in tumour development (Figure 4.3). The syringes can be classified according to their homologies. Type 4 secretion systems (T4SS), like in the case of *A. tumefaciens*, share properties with the conjugation apparatus of bacteria, and so called type 3 secretion systems (T3SS) share homologies to another common structure in bacteria, the flagellum. Most of the time, the genes encoding these injection machines are found integrated into the bacterial chromosome and are not encoded on a plasmid like the Ti plasmid in *A. tumefaciens*. However, a closer analysis of the DNA base composition in these chromosomal regions, the pathogenicity islands or PAI, shows that the $G + C$ content is different from the rest of the genetic information. Thus, it is thought that these devices were acquired during evolution by horizontal gene transfer as functional units. Type 3 or 4 secretion systems are present in many bacteria and in all gram negatives with a link to tumour development. As these injection machines become more and more understood, it transpires that their function appears to be directly linked to virulence and to contribute to tumour formation, as in the reference case of *A. tumefaciens*. In the next section we will see how the bacteria we examined above use such mechanisms and secretion systems and their potential link to cancer development.

Bartonella spp.

Bartonella spp. harbour genes for two types of T4SS, one called VirB4/D4 and one called Trw. Both systems are related to genuine bacterial conjugation systems. The VirB4/D4 system forms a PAI on the chromosome, consisting of 10 structural genes encoding proteins used to build the syringe and seven genes encoding proteins that the needle injects into a host cell. Therefore, here the T4SS translocates not protein/DNA complexes but proteins. Bartonellae that lack a functional syringe and do not inject the bacterial proteins fail to induce changes in endothelial cells that contribute to angiomatosis, the inhibition of apoptotic cell death or synthesis of proinflammatory cytokines. The T4SS is critical for virulence and establishment of the chronic infection, but additional factors further contribute to angiomatosis by inducing endothelial cells to proliferate due to expression of VEGF, a key vascular growth factor.

Citrobacter rodentium

Virulence of C. rodentium, in particular the ability to cause lesions in bowel mucosa, is linked to the presence of a PAI that stretches over some 41 genes on the chromosome. This PAI is called locus for enterocyte effacement and is present not only in C. rodentium but also in human pathogens such as enterohaemorrhagic E. coli that cause similar enterocyte effacement during acute infections. Genes that belong to this PAI encode a T3SS, a critical machine that again translocates effector proteins into host cells. The action of these proteins leads to lesions in the mucosa. Besides this, Citrobacter also transfer their own receptor, Tir, to host cells and binding to Tir triggers actin condensation, whereby cells change their shape. Colonic hyperplasia caused by C. rodentium only happens if they possess the T3SS.

Chlamydophyla pneumoniae

The genome of C. pneumoniae also contains a T3SS and more than 20 proteins may be translocated from the intracellular hideout of these bacteria to the host cell cytoplasm. A consequence of chlamydial infection is the inhibition of programmed cell death, which is thought to be relevant for cancer development. Research to find out if proteins injected into the host cell are needed for this effect, is hampered because it is not yet possible to genetically manipulate Chlamydophyla. Therefore, the cause and effect of the relationship between these proteins and cellular functions are not yet established.

Helicobacter pylori

In the early 1990s a protein called CagA was identified from H. pylori because gastric cancer patients had antibodies against this protein present in their serum. The cagA gene was then cloned and later found to be part of a PAI in the chromosome. This PAI was called cag PAI and is a 40 kB long stretch of DNA that is either functionally present in H. pylori isolates or not. The presence of this PAI in the bacteria is correlated with patients developing gastric cancer. Similar to the examples described above, genes in this PAI encode a T4SS syringe that injects the protein CagA into host cells. By interaction of CagA with host cell proteins, cell growth, death and migration is disturbed. In addition, the synthesis of proinflammatory cytokines is increased in cells when the T4SS is present. Thus, several characteristics belonging to the hallmarks of cancer (that we saw earlier) are critically influenced by the T4SS and its translocated proteins. It is, however, currently unclear whether the cag PAI has to be active at all or only at a particular stage of cancer development.

Helicobacter hepaticus

When the genome for this mouse pathogen was sequenced in 2003 it was found to contain a 71 kB long PAI encoding a T4SS. Since then, the relevance of this PAI was tested by constructing mutants that lack this genetic element and testing them in mice. Indeed, in comparison to the wild type bacteria, these mutants induced markedly less severe hepatitis, indicating that the PAI is important for cancer development.

Salmonella typhi

Salmonellae harbour the information for two T3SS on separate PAIs on their chromosome. These syringes are critical for individual stages of the infectious cycle. One, called SPI-1, is relevant during the transfer from the gut lumen into epithelial cells and the other, SPI-2, is relevant for survival inside macrophages and bacterial persistence. Numerous effector proteins are translocated by these two T3SS and they also affect cell shape, intracellular signalling, proinflammatory cytokine synthesis, and vesicular trafficking. It is likely, but difficult to prove, that the syringes and translocation of the effector proteins are relevant for the induction of hepatocellular carcinoma, because there is no animal model available for testing mutants of this strictly human pathogen.

In summary, the direct delivery of effector proteins into host cells to manipulate cellular functions such as growth, cell death, signalling cascades, synthesis of cytokines and cell migration is a common aspect of the bacterial infections implicated in cancer development discussed here.

4.2.4   Other bacterial effects potentially contributing to cancer

Besides the elaborate nature of their secretion systems, bacteria synthesize other molecules, such as toxins, that could contribute to cancer development. For example, H. hepaticus and H. pylori produce toxins that are important to maintain chronic infections. It is thought that the chronic inflammatory response, sustained by bacterial infections, can induce mutations via reactive oxygen and nitrogen metabolites (such as ROS, discussed extensively in Chapter 2) produced by activated inflammatory cells. Such mutations, though, are critical for malignant transformation. Although direct induction of mutations has only been observed in the case of A. tumefaciens, where translocated bacterial DNA is inserted into the host cell genome, bacterial infections may reduce the ability of host cells to repair genetic damage. For example, H. pylori-infected cells show a reduced ability to repair DNA mismatches. Indeed, genes that are prone to accumulate mutations when the DNA mismatch repair system is not working properly have been found mutated in gastric cancers. Therefore, although not inducing mutations directly, infection may favour conditions where mutations become stabilized and inherited by daughter cells.

4.2.5 Anti-infection strategies to prevent infection related cancer

The realization that 20 per cent of cancers are probably caused by an infection has direct relevance for cancer prevention. Antibiotic treatment may be used to prevent or treat the respective cancers. Gastric cancer, which is the third most common cause of cancer in males, may in practice become preventable by treating *H. pylori* infections with antibiotics. This will cut stomach cancer incidence significantly, as a direct result of Marshall's discovery. It may also be feasible to eradicate the *Helicobacter* species that colonize the liver and prevent hepatic tumours. Antibiotics are already known to cure angiomatosis bacilliformes due to infection with *Bartonella*. In contrast, antibiotics may not be a promising strategy to interfere with chlamydial infections, as these organisms evade treatment and persist.

Thus, developing vaccines is an alternative strategy and this is currently being attempted to prevent or treat *H. pylori* infection. Vaccines against typhoid fever are in use but their efficacy may have to be improved. In contrast, vaccines against human hepatitis virus A and B are established and, recently, vaccines against HPV infection became available. Overall, these are promising strategies to curb the future cancer burden.

4.3 Summary

More than 15 per cent of all malignancies worldwide – a total of 1.2 million cases per year – can be attributed to infectious agents. The types of cancers induced by infections are diverse as are the inducing organisms. In general, the mechanisms by which infectious agents induce cancer include insertion or activation of oncogenes, inhibition of tumour suppressors, chronic inflammation and the induction of immunosuppression. Infectious agents connected to tumour formation are generally highly prevalent in the population and have the potential to persist over a long period of time inside their host. We have highlighted the principles of cancer formation induced by viral and bacterial infection and present examples for infectious agents and their association to cancer formation.

4.4 Self-assessment questions

Question: What is the evidence for the notion that cancer is an infectious disease?

Answer: The clearest support for the notion that infection is a cause of cancer can be provided if Koch's postulates are fulfilled, as for example sarcomas induced by Rous sarcoma virus. If this is not possible, a clear epidemiological link between an infectious agent and a certain type of cancer is a strong support for an infection – cancer connection. The infectious agents suspected to be oncogenic are often highly prevalent in the host population. This is additional evidence for a cause of cancer by this infectious agent. Another support of an infection link with cancer is the strong increase in the incidence of a cancer and a special type of infection in immune-suppressed patients as for example KS and HHV-8, or the strong reduction of the incidence for a special type of cancer and infection by anti-infective therapies.

Question: What type of studies provides most of the current evidence for a link between cancer and infections?

Answer: Epidemiological studies should clearly link an infectious agent to a particular form of cancer. The relationship should be plausible and if possible supported by animal experiments. When a virus is the infectious agent, the presence of viral nucleic acids in tumour probes further supports the link. *In vitro* studies demonstrating the ability of the infectious agent to stimulate the proliferation or transformation of cells strengthen the connection of infection and cancer formation.

Question: Which viruses are currently implicated with cancer development?

Answer: Hepatitis B virus (HBV), hpatitis C virus (HCV), Epstein–Barr virus (EBV), human papillomavirus (HPV), human herpes virus 8 (HHV8), human thymus-derived-cell leukaemia/lymphoma virus-1 (HTLV-1)

Question: Which bacteria are currently implicated with cancer developments?

Answer: *Helicobacter pylori*, *Bartonella* spp., *Chlamydophyla pneumoniae*, *Salmonella enterica* serovar *typhi*, *Streptococcus bovis*

Question: Given the high prevalence of cancer-associated infectious viruses and bacteria, why is infection-associated cancer so rare?

Answer: The immune system is very effective in fighting the infectious agent and the infected cell. Moreover, it recognizes precancerous and cancer cells and effectively clears them from the body. Therefore, one of the main reasons for the relatively low incidence of cancer (compared to infections) is an efficient immune response against all stages of infection and carcinogenesis.

Question: What are the mechanisms of cellular transformation by virus infection?

Answer: Integrating viruses introduce viral oncogenes into the host cell, activate host proto-oncogenes or inactivate tumour suppressors. Non-integrating viruses may cause a chronic inflammation, which generates an environment of increased mutagenesis and oncogenic transformation. Severe immune suppression by viral infection (HIV) is another mechanism strongly supporting the formation of cancer.

Question: What evidence suggests that HHV-8 is the cause of Kaposi's sarcoma?

Answer: HHV-8 is associated with 100 per cent of the Kaposi sarcomas (KS) of AIDS patients and with many KS of non-AIDS patients. In addition there is a strong geographical correlation between HHV-8 prevalence and risk for KS.

Question: Given that 1–3 of 100 patients infected with *Helicobacter pylori* will develop gastric cancer during their life time, can you give an estimate for the number of cases worldwide? Not all patients develop cancer, what could this mean?

Answer: If we assume that half of the current world population of 6600 million people is infected and that we could observe these people over their life time, 33–99 million people may develop gastric cancer. This is of course too simple a calculation but the order of magnitude is right as it is estimated that up to 1.2 million people develop gastric cancer each year and with an average life expectancy of 67 years young infected people are likely to live the 50–60 years after which the infection may lead to cancer. The fact that not all infected persons will suffer in that way illustrates the fact that other factors contribute to cancer development such as host genes (e.g. regulating inflammation) or cultural and behavioural factors (smoking, diet).

Question: Infection with a handful of bacterial species is linked to cancer, is there any common aspect to these infections?

Answer: Common aspects to bacterial species associated with cancer are that they can produce chronic infections and the majority possess genes organized in pathogenicity islands – genetic elements linked to virulence and likely acquired by horizontal DNA transfer – that encode molecular syringes whereby the bacterial can alter host cell biology.

Question: What is a type 3 or type 4 secretion system?

Answer: Both secretion systems are molecular syringes whereby the bacteria can translocate molecules such as proteins or DNA directly into host cells. Type 4 systems are evolutionarily related to bacterial conjugation systems, type 3 secretion systems to flagella.

Question: What cellular functions can be affected by bacterial infections and how are they related to steps in tumour formation?

Answer: Bacterial infections affect, e.g. control of DNA damage, cell proliferation, cell death programmes, cell morphology and migratory behaviour and can induce vascularization. According to Hanahan and Weinberg (in *Cell* 2000, **100**, 57) tumours progress from cells that become independent for growth, insensitive to death signals, invasive, and can induce vascularization to support further growth. Therefore, bacterial infection directly or indirectly can contribute to each of these tumour features.

Question: Antibiotics cure bacterial infections, but are they necessarily a remedy against bacterial infection-related cancers? Are there alternative preventive strategies?

Answer: No, antibiotics are not necessarily a remedy against cancers caused by bacterial infections, since they are used as a therapy, i.e. after an infection has been diagnosed and the cancer inducing or promoting step may have already occurred. In contrast, vaccines ideally do not only prevent infections but will prevent infection induced cancers as well.

4.5 Further reading and resources

Boshoff C and Weiss R. AIDS-related malignancies. *Nat Rev Cancer* 2002, **2**, 373–382.

Boshoff C. Kaposi virus scores cancer coup. *Nat Med* 2003, **9**, 261–262.

Bruix J, Boix L, Sala M and Llovet JM. Focus on hepatocellular carcinoma. *Cancer Cell* 2004, **5**, 215–219.

Christie PJ, Atmakuri K, Krishnamoorthy V, Jakubowski S and Cascales E. Biogenesis, architecture, and function of bacterial type IV secretion systems. *Annu Rev Microbiol* 2005, **59**, 451–485.

Cornelis GR. The type III secretion injectisome. *Nat Rev Microbiol* 2006, **4**, 811–825.

Coussens LM and Werb Z. Inflammation and cancer. *Nature* 2002, **420**, 860–867.

Dehio C. *Bartonella*–host-cell interactions and vascular tumour formation. *Nat Rev Microbiol* 2005, **3**, 621–631.

Hatakeyama M. *Helicobacter pylori* CagA – a bacterial intruder conspiring gastric carcinogenesis. *Int J Cancer* 2006, **119**, 1217–1223.

Karin M, Lawrence T and Nizet V. Innate immunity gone awry: linking microbial infections to chronic inflammation and cancer. *Cell* 2006, **124**, 823–835.

Kuper H, Adami HO and Trichopoulos D. Infections as a major preventable cause of human cancer. *J Intern Med* 2000, **248**, 171–183.

Lax AJ and Thomas W. How bacteria could cause cancer: one step at a time. *Trends Microbiol* 2002, **10**, 293–299.

Levrero M. Viral hepatitis and liver cancer: the case of hepatitis C. *Oncogene* 2006, **25**, 3834–3847.

Lloyd AR, Jagger E, Post JJ, Crooks LA, Rawlinson WD, Hahn YS and Ffrench RA. Host and viral factors in the immunopathogenesis of primary hepatitis C virus infection. *Immunol Cell Biol* 2007, **85**, 24–32.

McCullen CA and Binns AN. *Agrobacterium tumefaciens* and plant cell interactions and activities required for interkingdom macromolecular transfer. *Annu Rev Cell Dev Biol* 2006, **22**, 101–127.

Roden R and Wu TC. How will HPV vaccines affect cervical cancer? *Nat Rev Cancer* 2006, **6**, 753–763.

Rogers AB and Fox JG. Inflammation and Cancer. I. Rodent models of infectious gastrointestinal and liver cancer. *Am J Physiol Gastrointest Liver Physiol* 2004, **286**, G361–G366.

Stehelin D, Varmus HE, Bishop JM and Vogt PK. DNA related to the transforming gene(s) of avian sarcoma viruses is present in normal avian DNA. *Nature* 1976, **260**, 170–173.

Zur HH. Viruses in human cancers. *Science* 1991, **254**, 1167–1173.

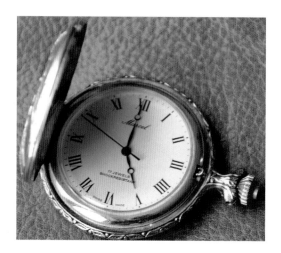

Inflammation has strong links with infection, which we discussed in the previous chapter. Furthermore, it is linked to trauma as well as exposure to many carcinogenic substances that we have analysed in Chapters one and two. These include tobacco smoke, asbestos, iron-induced irritants and others. Inflammation has been a protective mechanism of the body against infection or exposure to such substances. However, it has been clearly shown that when inflammation becomes chronic, it generates an environment that supports tumour development and can help in the initiation of the disease. This chapter will mostly focus on the relationship between inflammation and cancer initiation and describe the links between the two. But the relationship of inflammation with cancer goes much deeper. Not only inflammation can cause cancer, as we'll see in this chapter, but cancer also causes inflammation around the tumour site. This offers many advantages to the progression of the disease, as cancer can use the inflammation mechanisms of increased blood flow and emission of pro-inflammatory molecules described in this chapter, to protect itself from the immune system and spread through metastasis to other sites in the body.

It has even been demonstrated that the inflammatory response in cancer can greatly affect the efficacy of chemotherapy on cancer treatment. There is thus a strong clinical link between inflammation and cancer treatment, which will also be discussed in this chapter to some degree, as well as the use of drugs in inflammation and cancer.

5

Inflammation and cancer

Nigel Courtenay-Luck

Antisoma Research Ltd., London, UK

5.1   Introduction

The immune system can be thought of as a surveillance system, which ensures that tissues of the body are free of invading organisms and pathogens. Another function is to remove cells that have been damaged through injury to a tissue, or by infection.

In many cases, the inflammation that is mediated through a number of cytokines (low molecular weight proteins that stimulate or inhibit the differentiation, proliferation or function of immune cells) and chemokines (cytokines which selectively induce chemotaxis and activation of leukocytes and play a vital role in wound healing), produced by many of the cells which together form a large part of the immune system, can lead to further destruction of tissues and cells. In this chapter, an introduction into how an inflammatory response, which is aimed at protecting the body, in fact, can, and often does lead to the development of tumours, and the ultimate demise of many of those developing such tumours.

Inflammation can be divided into two parts, acute and chronic.

5.1.1   Acute inflammation

In acute, or short lived, inflammation, a number of inflammatory cytokines are produced, which include interleukin-1 (IL-1), IL-6, IL-8, IL-11 and tumour necrosis factor-α (TNF-α), as well as other chemokines such as granulocyte colony-stimulating

The Cancer Clock   Edited by Sotiris Missailidis

© 2007 John Wiley & Sons Ltd

factor (G-CSF) and granulocyte–macrophage colony-stimulating factor (GM-CSF). In chronic or long-term inflammation, there are a larger number of cytokines produced, which can mediate both humoral (antibody producing) and cellular (for example: T-cells and antigen-presenting cells, such as macrophages) immune responses. These include IL-1, IL-2, IL-3, IL-4, IL-5, IL-6, IL-7, IL-9, IL-10 and IL-12, together with many other soluble factors which mediate different immune responses, such as interferon (IFN), transforming growth factor-β (TGF-β) and TNF-α and -β).

5.1.2   Chronic inflammation

It is well known that the longer inflammation, and hence injury to tissues, persists, the higher the risk of cancer developing is. As long ago as 1863, Rudolph Virchow showed that leukocytes where present in neoplastic tissue, and many groups have demonstrated the emergence of cancers following long-term inflammation. The causes of inflammation are numerous and include infections (see Chapter 4) by bacteria, viruses and parasites, as well as chemical irritants such as asbestos and those chemicals found in cigarette smoke (see Chapter 1). In inflammation there is an infiltration into the tissue by mononuclear cells, such as macrophages and lymphocytes. Macrophages play a key role in chronic inflammation by the release of many of the cytokines mentioned above. It is this persistent activation of these macrophages that results in further and continued damage to the tissues.

These macrophages not only release cytokines, they also produce chemokines, matrix remodeling proteases and reactive oxygen species (see Chapter 2), which have a profound effect on the nature of the environment that the damaged tissue is in. Other significant effects are protein and DNA damage, caused largely by the production of nitric oxide (see Chapter 1). Nitric oxide and its products can induce a number of oncogenic effects, which include DNA damage, inhibition of apoptosis and DNA mutations. In addition to this, nitric oxide may also effect cellular repair functions such as p53 and promote angiogenesis (the formation of new blood vessels), all factors critical for the development of tumours.

5.2   Acute inflammation

The onset of acute inflammation may occur within minutes or hours following injury to tissues of the body. Acute inflammation normally persists from hours to days, depending on the rate at which the tissue damage caused by trauma or infection is repaired. When tissue damage occurs there are a number of events which follow. First, there is dilation of the arterioles, which allows an increase in blood flow to the damaged tissue. Gaps between the capillary endothelial cells, which line the blood vessels, then occur, allowing protein rich plasma to get to the tissue. Red blood cells flood into the vessels and form a plug, which in turn stems the blood flow into the damaged tissue. This is rapidly followed by neutrophils making contact with the endothelial cells, a process which is vital for the resolution of the inflammatory response. The neutrophils bind to the endothelial cells by means of adhesion proteins found on the neutrophil membrane. These adhesion proteins then bind to complementary receptors on the endothelial cells.

5.2.1 Mediators of acute inflammation

Numerous mediators are involved in the acute inflammatory response, some acting directly on the smooth muscle wall surrounding the arterioles, to alter blood flow, as discussed above. One of the first events to occur is the up-regulation of molecules on the endothelial cells that line the venules. Two molecules, P-selectin and platelet-activating factor (PAF) are up regulated in response to the production of histamine and thrombin, which are released in response to an inflammatory stimulus. Migrating neutrophils bind firmly to the endothelial cells by engagement of the lectin-like domain of P-selectin binding to the sialyl Lewis carbohydrate determinates on the mucin like P-selectin glycoprotein ligand-1 (PSGL-1) on the neutrophil surface. This allows the neutrophils to slow and roll along the endothelial wall, helping PAF to bind to its corresponding receptor. This, in turn, leads to an increase in the expression of another molecule, known as the integrin lymphocyte function-associated molecule-1 (LFA-1), which allows the neutrophils to bind even more tightly to the endothelial cell surface.

Once activated, the neutrophils increase their response to chemotactic agents, and due to the complement component C5a and leukotriene-B4, these neutrophils can exit the circulation, and pass through the gaps between the endothelial cells, across the basement membrane. This is a fundamental process involved in the resolution of acute inflammation, and is referred to as *diapedesis*, which serves to increase the chemotactic gradient at the site of inflammation. Endothelial cell produced PAF leads to the aggregation of platelets and the formation of a thrombus, through adherence of platelet glycoproteins 1b with von Willebrand factor on the vascular surface. This thrombus formation serves to control blood loss from the damaged vessel at the site of inflammation. In the venous system, fibrin clots occur, to achieve the same thing, due to the activation of the intrinsic clotting system via contact with factor XII. Activated factor XII then triggers the kinin and plasma systems and several of the resulting products affect the inflammatory process by events such as, increasing vascular permeability, activating endothelium, increasing further the production of factor XII and the cleaving of the complement protein C3.

IL-1 and TNF produced by macrophages act later to maintain the inflammatory process by up-regulating E-selectin and sustaining the expression of P-selectin. E-selectin binds to the E-selectin ligand-1 (ESL-1) on neutrophils. Chemokines or chemotactic cytokines such as IL-8 and epithelial derived neutrophil attractant-78 (ENA-78) also enhance neutrophil attraction. Both IL-1 and TNF act on endothelial cells, fibroblasts and epithelial cells to stimulate the production of monocyte chemoattractant protein (MCP-1), another chemokine, which in turn attracts mononuclear phagocytes to the inflammatory site, in order to deal with any infectious organisms, such as bacteria.

The production of chemokines induced by pro-inflammatory cytokines, such as IL-1, TNF and IFN-γ are chemotactic for a wide range of cells of the immune system, such as T cells, monocytes, dendritic cells, natural killer (NK) cells, basophils and eosinophils, all recruited to the site of acute inflammation. Recruitment of lymphocytes to the site of infection is in response to up regulation of vascular cell adhesion molecule-1 (VCAM-1) on the endothelial cells, which acts as a homing receptor for very late antigen-4 (VLA-4)-positive activated regulatory T-cells.

Control of the inflammatory response is essential, to prevent the development of chronic inflammation and, as discussed later, the possible development of tumours. Control of this inflammatory process is regulated by a number of compliment regulatory proteins, such as C1 inhibitor, C4b-binding protein, C3 control factors H an I, complement receptor CR1, decay accelerating factor (DAF), MCP, and immuncon-glutinin, in addition to other proteins which block the membrane attack complex, such as CD59, are all produced to regulate the inflammatory response. Lymphocyte proliferation is controlled by prostaglandin E2 (PGE2), which blocks the production of cytokines from both T-cells and macrophages.

TGF-β inhibits the production of potentially dangerous reactive oxygen intermediates, described earlier, from macrophages and down-regulate major histocompatability complex (MHC) class II expression on immune cells, as well as controlling IFN-γ-activated NK cells. In addition, endogenous glucocorticoids are produced via the hypothalamic–pituitary–adrenal axis, which controls inflammation by repression of a number of genes, such as for the pro-inflammatory cytokines, and adhesion molecules. They also induce inflammation inhibitors such as lipocortin-1, secretory leukocyte proteinase inhibitors and IL-1 receptor antagonists. IL-10 inhibits antigen presentation, cytokine production and nitric oxide killing by macrophages, and has been used in a number of clinical trials, in an attempt to control inflammatory conditions.

5.3   Chronic inflammation

It is often said that acute and chronic inflammation are distinguished only by the time course of the inflammatory response; this could not be further from the truth. Failure of the immune system to deal with the cause of acute inflammation results in progression to the chronic stage, due to the persistence of the original stimulus, repeated episodes of acute inflammation or defective acute inflammatory responses. If the chronic inflammatory response is not dealt with by the body, or by appropriate treatment, tumorigenesis could occur (See Figure 5.1). An example of an ongoing infection, which leads to chronic inflammatory disease, is infection by *Helicobacter pylori*. In patients with this bacterium, inflammation of the gut (gastritis) is common, and the immune system appears unable to clear the infection. For these patients, there is a doubling in the risk of developing cancer.

As previously stated, there are wide arrays of pro-cytokines and chemokines produced in the inflammatory environment, and if these responses are not down regulated,

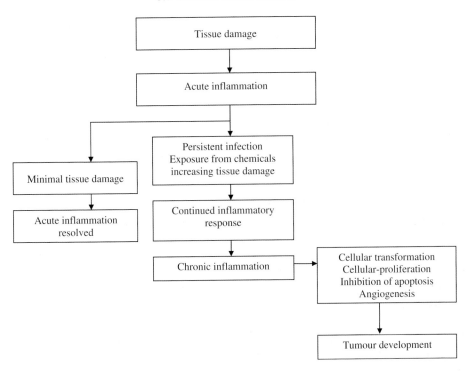

Figure 5.1 The progression from chronic inflammation to tumour development

the risk of tumour genesis increases. Persistent production of nitrogen and oxygen intermediates by phagocytes (neutrophils and macrophages) has a detrimental effect, causing tissue damage and damages the DNA of cells. Damage to the DNA can lead to mutations, as well as altering cellular repair mechanisms and may also lead to the inhibition of cell death by apoptosis, allowing the continued growth of mutated cells, a key hallmark in tumour development. IL-10, which is produced by macrophages, has been shown to be pro-angiogenic allowing for the formation of new blood vessels, essential for both the development and growth of tumours. IL-10 also inhibits T cells, which are one of the immune system's main cell types thought to be involved in tumour killing. Hence this immune suppression by IL-10 actually facilitates the development of tumours in this context.

Prostaglandins, as mentioned in the section on acute inflammation, are continuously produced in chronic inflammation, and have also been shown to favour the development of tumours. Inhibition of COX-2, a cyclooxygenase enzyme involved in the synthesis of prostaglandins, has been shown to have an inhibitory role in the development of tumours. This has been illustrated by the use of COX-2 inhibitors in the prevention of cancer. Patients taking COX-2 inhibitors have shown a reduction in the risk of developing Barrett's cancer, as well as other cancers, and will be discussed later in this chapter.

Activation of nuclear factor (NF)-κB, discussed later, is another hallmark of cancer development and growth. TNF-α, in a recent study, was shown to increase gene mutations, gene amplification, micronuclei formation and chromosomal instability in cultured cells, again all hallmarks of cancer cells. This study also showed that TNF-α treatment of mouse embryo fibroblasts also led to an increase in malignant transformation. Another recent study looking at fibroblast-like synovicytes from patients with rheumatoid arthritis (RA) showed that stimulation with TNF-α led to an increase in production of vascular endothelial growth factor-c (VEGF-C). In oncology, the inhibition of members of this vascular endothelial growth factor family, has led to improved responses of patients with cancer, and are now an important target in the development of new therapies for human neoplasia.

In summary, the progression from acute to chronic inflammation is associated with continued production of pro-inflammatory cytokines that instead of resolving the inflammatory condition may, in many circumstances, assist with the development of tumours. Inhibition of many of these cytokines, and other proteins, is a major goal in the development of new anti-cancer drugs.

5.4 Drugs used in inflammation and cancer

5.4.1 COX-2 inhibitors

Both osteoarthritis and rheumatoid arthritis, common inflammatory diseases, have been treated with non-steroidal anti inflammatory drugs (NSAIDs) for decades. These drugs, such as aspirin and ibuprofen, work by inhibiting COX-2, a cyclooxygenase enzyme involved in the production of prostaglandins, which as described, can modulate inflammation. A major draw back to their long-term use is the development of stomach irritation and gastrointestinal bleeding. These side effects are due to the NSAIDs inhibiting another cyclooxygenase enzyme, COX-1. The protective role of COX-1 is illustrated by the fact that the prostaglandins it produces have been shown to reduce ulcer formation.

It has been known for some time that inhibiting the formation of prostaglandins may be beneficial in the treatment of cancer. In 1988 two new drugs that specifically inhibited COX-2 became available. These drugs were Vioxx and Celebrex. Huge interest was raised in these among cancer researchers, as these drugs could be used without the detrimental effects of inhibiting COX-1 as seen with earlier NSAIDs. Numerous clinical trials were initiated to investigate the use of these drugs in the prevention of cancer.

Both Vioxx and Celebrex entered clinical trials for the prevention of colon cancer. Additional studies were also undertaken to look at the prevention of other cancers. These included bladder, breast, cervical, colorectal, oesophageal, head and neck, skin, lung oral and prostate cancer. In September 2004 the makers of Vioxx withdrew the drug from the market, due to fact that the colon cancer trial had shown that patients on this drug had twice the risk of developing heart attacks and strokes. Within 3 months the makers of Celebrex announced that they, too, were stopping its colon cancer trial, as a study had also shown that Celebrex was linked with increased risk of heart attack and stroke. Many cancer trials using Celebrex alone or in combination with other cancer therapeutic drugs also had to be suspended.

In oncology, cardiovascular risks are not foreign, and are seen with other drugs used to treat cancer, such as doxorubicin (Adriamycin), used widely in the treatment of breast cancer. In cancer treatment the risk benefit is different from that in relatively healthy people. Side effect profiles of drugs used to treat cancer are often more severe than seen for drugs used to treat other non-life threatening conditions. It will be interesting to see the long-term follow-up results, from trials where COX-2 inhibitors were used, to see if there is a case for the continued use of such drugs in cancer prevention and treatment.

5.4.2 Antihypertensive drugs

Box 5.1 illustrates the use of antihypertensive drugs in the treatment of cancer.

Box 5.1 Cancer and hypertension drug therapy

Angiotensin is a powerful chemical, formed in the blood by the action of the angiotensin-converting enzyme (ACE), which attaches to the angiotensin receptors found in many tissues, but primarily on smooth muscle cells of blood vessels. Angiotensin's attachment to the receptors causes the blood vessels to narrow, leading to an increase in blood pressure (hypertension). Various hypertensive drugs have been developed, usually either blocking the ACE inhibitors, thus preventing the formation of angiotensin, or blocking the angiotensin receptors (angiotensin receptor blockers; ARB), thus inhibiting the action of angiotensin. A study undertaken in 1998 suggested that hypertensive patients taking ACE inhibitors were significantly less at risk of developing cancer than those taking other hypertensive treatments. Similarly, use of ARB, has been hypothesized as the mechanism to overcome cancer associated complications in organ graft recipients, and tumour progression has been significantly slowed with their use. It is interesting to note that the rennin–angiotensin system is not only involved in vasoconstriction, but it is a key mediator of inflammation, with the receptors governing the transcription of pro-inflammatory mediators and production of inflammatory cytokines and chemokines both in resident tissue and in infiltrating cells such as macrophages. These include the inflammatory cytokine TGF-β and the mediators reviewed by Suzuki *et al.* (2003), as well as IL-1β in activated monocytes, TNF-α, MCP-1, plasminogen activator inhibitor type 1 (PAI-1), adrenomedullin, and various surface adhesion molecules involved in inflammation, all of which have been shown to have active participation in various aspects of cancer development.

So far, cancer immunotherapy (see Chapter 10) has had limited success. It has long been established that the body does have the capability to recognize cancer cells and develop antibodies. Based on this knowledge, dendritic cell vaccines have been developed and have demonstrated limited effect in treating established tumours. This effectiveness was, however, greatly enhanced leading to complete regression of tumours in 40 per cent of cases when the dendritic cell vaccine was used in combination with monoclonal antibodies that neutralised the actions of the multi-functional inflammatory cytokine TGF-β.

It has been clearly demonstrated that tumour cells over-express angiotensin receptors and preferentially one of the two, the AT1 receptor, and evidence has shown implication of AT1 in cancer progression. It has thus been proposed by Smith and Missailidis (2004) that effective blockade of AT1 with a tight binding receptor antagonist, such as candesartan, losartan, ibersartan, or other ARB, in combination with NSAIDs and standard immunotherapy or chemotherapy could significantly improve current therapeutic outlook.

5.5   Evidence for a molecular link between inflammation and cancer

Recent studies have highlighted that the molecular link between inflammation and cancer involves a gene much studied in the development of neoplasia; this gene is I-κ-B kinase, or Iκk beta. Iκk beta is essential for the activation of NF-κB. NF-κB is known to turn on inflammation in response to either bacterial or viral infection. NF-κB plays a major role in the development of tumours derived from epithelial cells, by inhibiting the natural cell killing process known as apoptosis. Cell death due to apoptosis prevents the development of unwanted cells in the body. This normal process is responsible for the body killing any mutated or transformed cells, or cells which have outlived their usefulness or purpose. Evading apoptosis by activation of NF-κB is one of the key hallmarks of cancer.

de Visser and co-workers demonstrated the link between inflammation and cancer, using colitis-associated cancer (CAC) as their animal model, by administering two compounds to mice. The first was azoxymethane (AOM), a known pro-carcinogen widely used to induce colon cancers in animal models. The second compound was dextran sulfate sodium salt (DSS), a pro-inflammatory irritant that erodes the epithelial cells of the intestinal tract, which then allows enteric bacteria to infiltrate into the intestinal tract. This infiltration of bacteria induces inflammation as a means of the body attempting to fight the resultant infection.

Three groups of mice where given the two compounds, the first being normal mice, the second being mice that had been bred without the Iκk beta gene in the intestinal epithelial cells, and the third a group of mice which lacked the Iκk beta gene in their myeloid cells, which generate macrophages, which, as stated above, are key in the development of inflammation.

In those mice lacking the Iκk beta gene in their epithelial cells of the intestine, DSS induced inflammation without activation of the NF-κB, but the incidence of tumours was 80 per cent lower than found in the control group. Further studies on this group of mice showed that the decrease in tumour development was due to the activation of apoptosis. This increase in apoptosis was demonstrated by the observed increase in pro-apoptotic proteins Bak and Bax, and a corresponding decrease of a protein known to inhibit apoptosis, known as Bcl-xl.

In the third group of mice whose myeloid cells were deficient in Iκk beta, a 50 per cent reduction in tumours developing was seen compared to the control group. Those tumours that did develop were noted to be smaller than tumours developing in the normal control group mice. Further studies of this group demonstrated that the inactivation of Iκk beta in the myeloid cells had reduced the expression of a number of genes that play a significant role in the development of inflammation. There was clear evidence of a decrease in the expression of a number of pro-inflammatory molecules such as COX-2 and IL-1 and -6, which are key in the inflammatory process. In this group of mice there appeared to be no link between Iκk beta deletion and apoptosis, which nicely demonstrates the role of myeloid cells in inflammation associated tumour promotion, progression and invasiveness. The authors of this study quite rightly concluded that 'in addition to identifying a key molecular mechanism connecting inflammation and cancer, our results suggest that specific pharmacological inhibition of Iκk beta may be very effective in prevention of colitis associated cancer'.

5.6 Clinical relationship between inflammatory disease and cancer

In the clinical setting, a large number of inflammatory diseases are monitored carefully in order to detect emerging cancers (Table 5.1).

5.6.1 Inflammatory bowel disease

Inflammatory bowel disease is one of the most widely studied and best established links between inflammation and cancer, such as chronic ulcerative colitis and Crohn's disease, which can lead to colon carcinoma. In inflammatory bowel disease there is disruption of the gastrointestinal barrier, which leads to infiltration of microbial pathogens from the lumen together with leukocytes in the lamina propria, producing an inflammatory response. Production of pro-inflammatory cytokines and chemokines in the area recruit further leukocytes, regulate the integrity of the epithelial barrier and stimulate the production of chemokines from epithelial cells. Together, these events lead to chronic inflammation of the bowel.

Table 5.1 Chronic inflammatory conditions and their associated cancers

Inflammatory condition	Associated cancer
Marjolin's ulcer.	Skin cancer
Asbestosis	Mesothelioma
Cigarette smoking induced bronchitis.	Lung cancer
Chronic asthma	Bronchial cancer
Human papillomavirus infection	Penile cancer
Schistomiasis	Bladder cancer
Pelvic inflammatory disease	Ovarian cancer
Ovarian epithelial inflammation	Ovarian cancer
Epstein–Barr virus infection	Nasopharyngeal carcinoma
Barrett's metaplasia	Oesophageal cancer
H. pylori gastritis	Gastric cancer
Chronic pancreatitis	Pancreatic cancer
Chronic cholecystitis	Gallbladder cancer
Hepatitis	Liver cancer
Inflammatory bowel disease	Colorectal cancer
Proliferative inflammatory atrophy of the prostate	Prostate cancer

5.6.2 Prostate cancer

In a recent study by Sanjay Gupta, chronic inflammation may also be tied to prostate cancer. In this study, initial biopsies showed that 144 patients had chronic inflammation out of a total of a 177 patients. In a 5-year follow up of these patients, 20 per cent of those with chronic inflammation of the prostate went on to develop adenocarcinomas while only 6 per cent (2 patients) from the remaining 33 patients, who did not have inflammation, developed adenocarcinomas, and of these 2 patients, one had high grade prostatic intraepithelial neoplasia at initial diagnosis, and the other had atypical small acinar proliferation at initial diagnosis. These findings are highly indicative of a strong association between chronic prostatic inflammation and premalignant and malignant changes in prostatic epithelium.

In a separate study, Sarma *et al.* have shown that men with a history of the sexually transmitted disease gonorrhoea may face an increased risk of prostate cancer, as the infection leads to chronic inflammation of the prostate gland. The link between these two studies is chronic inflammation. In this study of over 800 African-American men, 78 per cent of those between 40 and 79 were more likely to develop prostate cancer than men who had never had sexually transmitted disease.

Work carried out at the Hopkins Kimmel Cancer Center indicated that a hyper methylation of a gene called glutathione S-transferase P (GSTP1) may be a key event in the transition from chronic inflammation of the prostate, to prostate cancer. GSTP1 is normally involved in the detoxification of environmental carcinogens, and therefore protects against cancer. This study looked at GSTP1 hypermethylation in normal and prostate cancer tissue samples as well as inflammatory prostate lesions known as PIA (proliferative inflammatory atrophy) and PIN (prostate intraepithelial neoplasia). Results showed GSTP1 methylation in 17.6 per cent of PIA lesions, in 60 per cent of high-grade PIN lesions and 100% of prostate cancers. No GSTP1 methylation was seen in the normal prostate tissues. Although this was quite a small study, its findings suggested that increased levels of GSTP1 methylation in PIA lesions, which are associated with inflammation, might be the starting point for the development of prostate cancer. As a result of this study, it was suggested that the effects of anti-inflammatory agents, and anti-oxidants on PIA lesions, be investigated in animal models.

5.7 Discussion

The aim of this chapter is to give the reader an introduction to inflammation and the consequences of not resolving such inflammation. It is not intended to go into the complex pathways that lead to acute inflammation, chronic inflammation and tumour development. There are many inflammatory conditions which are resolved by the simple use of NSAIDs and never give rise to any complications, there are others which, if not corrected either by removal of the agent causing the inflammation, or by treatment, can develop into life threatening conditions, such as cancer. Cigarette smoking, continued exposure to asbestos or other carcinogenic agents can all lead to the development of cancer affecting various tissues of the body, for example the lungs and skin.

Infections by one of many infectious organisms, if not treated, or inadequately treated, can give rise to continued or chronic inflammation. As has been highlighted in this chapter, many types of tumours are now associated with prior inflammatory conditions, which were either inadequately treated or, worse still, not treated at all. The immune system has evolved to defend the body against invading organisms, and has sophisticated mechanisms for dealing with cells of the body that are altered in any way, or have died. For the majority of people, both components of the immune system, the humoral (antibody producing) and cellular (various cell types which deal with foreign antigens) work well and result in a strong defence mechanism against illness. However, if the immune system is continuously turned on, as in chronic inflammation, and produces many of the cytokines and chemokines mentioned in this chapter, the results can be devastating.

In medicine, inflammation is often seen as a non-life threatening condition, and insufficient emphasis is put on its treatment. Infection with the bacterium *H. pylori*, which is thought to infect about 50 per cent of the population, has been shown to increase the risk of colon cancer and other cancers (see previous chapter). Screening for continued inflammation is a must, and new non-invasive tests, such as blood tests are needed. It is expensive to follow people up by the use of methods such as endoscopy on a continued basis, but the development of new reliable blood assays, which look for markers of inflammation, would result in significant savings in both time and money to the health services, as well as reduce the stress and inconvenience caused to patients.

Preventive medicine is a natural way forward for the health care of the population, and as such should include long-term follow-up of patients treated for inflammatory conditions. If we are to reduce, or hopefully eradicate certain cancers from the population, we need to be far more aware of the causes of such cancers, and implement ways of detecting early signs of potential tumour development. Put simply, the screening for indicators of chronic inflammation could prevent a non-life threatening condition becoming an all too often, life threatening one.

5.8 Self-assessment questions

Question: What is inflammation caused by?

Answer: Inflammation can be caused by injury to tissue, by viral or bacterial infection, or due to exposure to various inflammatory agents, chemicals, metals, etc.

Question: By what mechanisms could chronic inflammation lead to cancer?

Answer: There is a wide array of pro-cytokines and chemokines produced in the inflammatory environment that can increase the risk for tumorigenesis. Persistent production of nitrogen and oxygen intermediates by phagocytes causes tissue damage and damages the DNA of cells. Damage to the DNA can lead to mutations, as well as altering cellular repair mechanisms and may also lead to the inhibition of cell death by apoptosis, allowing the continued growth of mutated cells, a key hallmark in tumour development. IL-10, which is produced by macrophages, has been shown to be pro-angiogenic allowing for the formation of new blood vessels, essential for both the development and growth of tumours. IL-10 also inhibits T cells, which are one of the immune systems main cell types thought to be involved in tumour killing. Finally, chronic inflammation can contribute to the onset and progression of cancer through angiogenesis and increased blood supply to the tumour site, through increased production of members of the vascular endothelial growth factor family.

Question: How could anti-inflammatory drugs help in the treatment of cancer?

Answer: The use of anti-inflammatory drugs, such as COX inhibitors, or anti-hypertensive drugs with anti-inflammatory action, can alleviate the symptoms of inflammation that have been described above, thus blocking this mechanism of assisting tumour progression through the use of inflammatory cytokines and chemokines, angiogenesis and reduced apoptosis. This would also allow other treatments to act better against the tumours and improve cancer treatment.

Question: Give examples of chronic inflammatory conditions that are associated with tumour development.

Answer: All the examples presented in Table 5.1 are clear examples of chronic inflammatory conditions and cancer. It is worth noting that some of the examples shown are clearly infectious diseases as much as inflammatory conditions and you have seen those in the previous chapter of infection and cancer.

5.9 Further reading and resources

Aust AE and Eveleigh JF. Mechanisms of DNA oxidation. *Proc Soc Exp Biol Med* 1999, **222**, 246–252.

Babbar N and Casero RA Jr. Tumor necrosis factor-alpha increases reactive oxygen species by inducing spermine oxidase in human lung epithelial cells: a potential mechanism for inflammation-induced carcinogenesis. *Cancer Res* 2006, **66**(23), 11125–111230.

Babior BM. Phagocytes and oxidative stress. *Am J Med* 2000, **109**, 33–44.

Balkwill F, Charles KA and Mantovani A. Smouldering and polarised inflammation in the initiation and promotion of malignant disease. *Cancer Cell* 2006, **7**, 211–217.

Basran GS, Morley J, Paul W and Turner-Warwick M. Evidence in man of synergistic interaction between putative mediators of acute inflammation and asthma. *Lancet* 1982, **1**, 935–937.

Beebe-Dimmer JL, Lange LA, Cain JE, Lewis RC, Ray AM, Sarma AV, Lange EM and Cooney KA, Polymorphisms in the prostate-specific antigen gene promoter do not predict serum prostate-specific antigen levels in African-American men. *Prostate Cancer Prostatic Dis* 2006, **9**(1), 50–55.

Blakwill F and Coussens LM. An inflammatory link? *Nature* 2004, **431**, 405–406.

Botting RM. Inhibitors of cyclooxygenases: mechanisms, selectivity and uses. *J Physiol Pharmacol* 2006, **57**(Suppl 5), 113–124.

Cha HS, Bae EK *et al.* Tumour necrosis factor-a induces vascular endothelial growth factor-C expression in rheumatoid synoviocytes. *J Rheumatol* 2007, **34**(1), 16–19.

Chen R, Alvero AB, Silasi DA and Mor G, Inflammation, cancer and chemoresistance: taking advantage of the toll-like receptor signaling pathway. *Am J Reprod Immunol* 2007, **57**(2), 93–107.

Coussens LM and Werb Z. Inflammatory cells and cancer: think different. *J Exp Med* 2001, **193**, F23–F26.

de Visser KE, Eichten A and Coussens LM. Paradoxical roles of the immune system during cancer development. *Nat Rev* 2006, **6**, 124–135.

Faghali CA and Write TM. Cytokines in acute and chronic inflammation. *Front Biosci* 1977, **1**, d12–26.

Fitzgerald GA. Prostaglandins: modulators of inflammation and cardiovascular risk. *Clin Rheumatol* 2004, **10**(3 Supp), S12–7.

Greten FR, Eckmann L *et al.* IKKb links between inflammation and tumourgenesis in a mouse model of colitis associated cancer. *Cell* 2004, **118**(3), 285–296.

Grosch S, Maier TJ, *et al.* Cyclooxygenase-2 (COX-2)-independent anticarcinogenic effects of selective COX-2 inhibitors. *J Natl Cancer Inst* 2006, **8**(11), 763–747.

Half E and Arber N. Chemoprevention of colorectal cancer: two steps forward, one step back? *Future Oncol* 2006, **2**(6), 697–704.

Huang EH, Park JC, Appelman H, Weinberg AD, Banerjee M, Logsdon CD and Schmidt AM. Induction of inflammatory bowel disease accelerates adenoma formation in Min +/– mice. *Surgery* 2006, **139**(6), 782–788.

Kontoyiannis D, Pasparakis M, *et al.* TNF biosynthesis in gut associated immunopathologies. *Immunity* 1999, **10**, 387–398.

Kulbe H, Levinson NR, Blakwill F and Wilson JL. The chemokine network in cancer – much more than directing cell movement. *Int J Dev Biol* 2004, **48**, 489–496.

Ling FC, Baldus SE, *et al.* Association of COX-2 expression with corresponding active and chronic inflammatory reactions in Barretts metaplasia and progression to cancer. *Histopathology* 2007, **50**(2), 203–209.

Macarthur M, Hold GL and El-Omar EM. Inflammation and cancer II. Role of chronic inflammation and cytokine gene polymorphisms in the pathogenesis of gastrointestinal malignancy. *Am J Physiol Gastrointest Liver Physiol* 2004, **286**, G515–G520.

Mohseni H, Zaslau S, McFadden D, Riggs DR, Jackson BJ and Kandzari S. COX-2 inhibition demonstrates potent anti-proliferative effects on bladder cancer in vitro. *J Surg Res* 2004, **119**(2), 138–142.

Mon NN, Ito S, Senga T and Hamaguchi M, FAK signaling in neoplastic disorders: a linkage between inflammation and cancer. *Ann N Y Acad Sci* 2006, **1086**, 199–212.

Nelson WG, De Marzo AM, DeWeese TL, Lin X, Brooks JD, Putzi MJ, Nelson CP, Groopman JD and Kensler TW. Preneoplastic prostate lesions: an opportunity for prostate cancer prevention. *Ann N Y Acad Sci* 2001, **952**, 135–144.

Roitt IM and Delves PJ. *Roitts Essential Immunology*, tenth edition. Blackwell Science, Oxford, 2001.

Romano M, Ricci V and Zarrilli R. Mechanisms of disease: *Helicobacter pylori*-related gastric carcinogenesis – implications for chemoprevention. *Nat Clin Pract Gastroenterol Hepatol* 2006, **3**(11), 622–632.

Sarma AV, McLaughlin JC, Wallner LP, *et al.* Sexual behavior, sexually transmitted diseases and prostatitis: the risk of prostate cancer in black men. *J Urol* 2006, **176**, 1108–1113.

Shacter E and Weitzman SA. Chronic inflammation and cancer. *Oncology* 2002, **16**, 217–226.

Smith GR and Missailidis S. Cancer, inflammation and the AT1 and AT2 receptors. *BMC J Inflamm* 2004. http://www.journal-inflammation.com/content/1/1/3 [accessed 3 May 2007]

Sunjay Gupta. Chronic inflammation tied to prostate cancer. *J Urol* 2006, **176**, 1012–1016.

Suzuki Y, Ruiz-Ortega M, Lorenzo O, Ruperez M, Esteban V and Egido J. Inflammation and angiotensin II. *IJBCB* 2003, **35**, 881–900.

Virchow R. Standpoints in scientific medicine, 1877. *Bull Hist Med* 1956, **30**, 537–543,.

Warren JS, Ward PA and Johnson KJ. Tumor necrosis factor: a plurifunctional mediator of acute inflammation. *Mod Pathol* 1988, **1**(3), 242–247.

Yan B, Wang H *et al.* Tumour necrosis factor-alpha is a potent endogenous mutagen that promotes cellular transformation. *Cancer Res* 2006, **66**(24), 11565–11570.

Acute inflammation, healing and repair. Clinical features and nomenclature of acute inflammatory processes. www.fleshandbones.com/readingroom/pdf/221.pdf [accessed May 2007]

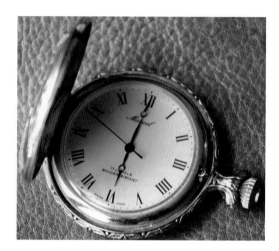

We have so far seen how cancer is developed, the aetiology behind the disease, as well as the biological mechanisms by which the disease is initiated, progresses and metastasizes. The first few 'hours' of this book were devoted to the initiation of the disease and subsequently its biology, so as to provide an understanding on the 'why' we get cancer and the 'how' the disease progresses.

However, cancer is not necessarily an incurable disease and the success or failure in eradicating the disease from the system and achieving complete clearance, or the control of the disease chronically is very much dependent on the time of the diagnosis. An early diagnosis of the disease offers significantly higher chances of success. One of the main problems in treating solid tumours is that we usually do not diagnose the cancer until the tumour is 3 mm in diameter, by which time the tumour has often entered the metastatic stage. A number of attempts have been made to develop methods that will help us achieve prognosis or early diagnosis of cancer, based on differences between the tumour cell or tumour environment and that of normal tissue. Some of the tests developed help in identifying agents that are known to cause cancer, such as particular strains of the human papillomavirus, whilst others are aimed at diagnosing cancer cells and tissue, or molecular and chemical entities secreted by the cancer cell and possibly picked up in biological fluids, such as blood and urine. Great progress has been made in the diagnosis of the disease in the recent years and current methodologies in genetics, genomics and proteomics lead constantly in the discovery of new such markers that may facilitate better prognosis, diagnosis and ultimately therapy for cancer.

6

Cancer diagnosis

Anna Batistatou[1] and Konstantinos Charalabopoulos[2]

1. *Department of Pathology, Ioannina University Medical School, Greece*
2. *Department of Physiology Clinical Unit, Ioannina University Medical School, Greece*

6.1 Blood tests for tumour markers

Tumour markers represent substances that may be found in blood, urine or body tissues, associated with cancer. Their identification and quantification in serum/urine/tissue aids greatly in patients' diagnosis, management, and prognosis. The ideal marker for cancer would be a blood test in which a positive result would be found only in patients with certain types of cancer, would be correlated with the stage and the response to treatment, and furthermore, it would be easily reproducibly measured. Until now, such a tumour marker is not available, since none of the available markers has adequate sensitivity and specificity. Tumour markers can be proteins, enzymes, biochemicals, or antigens. These substances are produced either by the neoplastic tissue or by the human body in response to the presence of cancer. It is a general phenomenon that tumour marker levels are lower at the early stages of the disease and higher in advanced disease. In addition, the levels decrease in response to treatment and increase when the cancer recurs.

Tumour markers are used to screen individuals at risk, to identify specific cancer subtypes, to monitor tumour progression and development of metastases, to detect response to treatment, to detect recurrence and, finally, to predict prognosis. The prostate-specific antigen (PSA), is an example of a tumour marker that is specific enough for one situation, the prostate cancer, and functions as a screening test for asymptomatic, men at risk, which in general refers to men over 50 years of age with at

The Cancer Clock Edited by Sotiris Missailidis
© 2007 John Wiley & Sons Ltd

least a 10-year life expectancy. Some types of cancer are divided into subtypes that may be more or less aggressive; thus, some tumour markers may be useful in distinguishing between various types of cancer and levels of the same tumour marker can be altered in more than one type of cancer. Finally, some tumour marker tests indicate the possibility of a negative or positive outcome, based on outcomes of other patients with similar results.

Tumour markers are not specific enough to be used alone for cancer diagnosis. This is due to several reasons, including the following: tumour marker levels can be elevated in people with benign lesions, they are not elevated in every person with malignancy, in particular those with an early stage disease, and they are not totally specific for a single condition. Indeed, many different types of neoplastic and non-neoplastic diseases can lead to increased levels of a certain tumour marker. In daily clinical practice, tumour markers must not be used in isolation to diagnose cancer, but their levels must always be evaluated in the context of the patient's history, symptoms, and other diagnostic procedures, such as a biopsy. Furthermore, serial measurements are more meaningful than a single measurement. Determination of the tumour marker levels must be done at the time of diagnosis, before, during, and after therapy, and finally periodically for monitoring the chance of a recurrence.

Nowadays, a great interest and search for potential new tumour markers is observed. Most tumour markers are proteins, but today the interest is also focused to desoxyribonucleic acid (DNA), with new methods to detect DNA being developed. Even in early-stage cancer, neoplastic cells may break away from the primary site and can be detected in blood, urine and body tissues. Abnormal DNA has been detected in the blood of individuals suffering from breast, liver, lung, and ovarian cancer as well as in patients with melanoma. Similar results have been achieved with urine tests in individuals with bladder cancer. In patients with cancer of the oral cavity, abnormal DNA has also been detected in their saliva. Accurate and useful information regarding screening, early detection, monitoring and planning management may be achieved using these techniques.

6.1.1 Established and novel tumour markers in serum

Tumour antigens

Carcinoembryonic antigen (CEA)   CEA, identified in 1965, represents one of the first oncofetal antigens, which was exploited in the clinical praxis. It is a glycoprotein associated with the plasma membrane of tumour cells, from which it may be released into the blood stream. It may also be released from the lung epithelial cells, so that it may be detected in the bronchoalveolar lavage of patients undergoing fiberoptic bronchoscopy. Although CEA was first identified and described from patients with colorectal cancer, an elevated serum CEA level is specific neither for colon cancer nor for any other malignancy specifically. Apart from colon cancer, a variety of other neoplasms, including pancreatic, gastric, lung, ovarian, cervical and breast carcinoma may lead to elevated serum CEA levels. In these cases, CEA can be used to monitor the progress of the disease and the response to treatment. Usually, CEA levels return to normal within 1–2 months after surgery. It must be mentioned, herein, that benign lesions such as chronic lung disease, inflammatory bowel disease, cirrhosis and pancreatitis may also represent conditions with increased serum CEA levels. In addition, CEA was found to be increased in up to 19 per cent of smokers and in approximately 3 per cent of the healthy control population. The measurement of serum CEA levels as a screening test is not satisfactory, since elevated CEA levels have unacceptably low positive predictive value with excess false positives. Furthermore, it has been shown that elevated CEA levels are found in advanced stages of incurable cancer but are low in the early curable disease; thus, the likelihood of a positive result affecting the patient's survival is diminished. In patients with colon cancer, serum CEA levels have a prognostic value. Preoperative CEA levels have been correlated positively with the disease stage and negatively with disease-free survival. CEA levels can be used in monitoring disease recurrence, since their increase precedes clinical relapse by several months. Thus, the opportunity for a 'second look' surgery is given early, with the hope that, relapse will be detected at the time when surgical resection for cure is still possible. Today we know that CEA belongs to the immunoglobulin gene superfamily of adhesion molecules (see below), but it is reported here for historical reasons.

Alpha-fetoprotein   Alpha-fetoprotein (AFP) is a protein synthesized by the liver, yolk sac and gastrointestinal tract of the developing fetus. A decrease in AFP levels is observed soon after birth, being undetectable in serum of healthy individuals, with only the exception of pregnancy. The AFP half-life is 3.5 days. A peak concentration of AFP is observed at 12 weeks of gestation. Elevated levels of AFP suggest a primary liver cancer or a germ cell tumour of the ovary or the testis. It is a useful screening marker in areas with populations at high risk of hepatocellular carcinoma and HbsAg positive individuals. In patients with germ cell tumours, AFP is a marker with high sensitivity, being a good indicator for relapse and response to the treatment. AFP is a marker of high sensitivity, but not of high specificity, since other neoplasms, such as gastro-intestinal and primary lung carcinomas and conditions associated with liver regeneration (hepatitis, cirrhosis) may also lead to increased serum levels of AFP. The presence and persistence of high levels of serum AFP in an adult with liver disease and without an obvious gastrointestinal tumour strongly suggests hepatocellular carcinoma. A rising level suggests progression of the tumour or recurrence after hepatic resection, chemotherapy or chemoembolization.

CA19-9   CA19-9 is produced in pancreas, bile ducts, stomach, colon, endometrium, and salivary glands. It is a glycoprotein with high molecular weight and represents a modified antigen of the Lewis A blood group. Five per cent of the population with Lewis A-B genotype do not produce CA19-9. Elevated levels of CA19-9 are found in cases of gastrointestinal tract malignancy. Among them, gastric, colon and pancreatic cancer are most commonly observed. In particular, elevated levels of CA19-9 are found in 80, 67, 30–50 and 30 per cent of patients suffering from pancreatic adenocarcinoma, cholangiocarcinoma, hepatocellular carcinoma, and colorectal cancer, respectively. Serum levels of CA19-9 are correlated with disease stage in pancreatic cancer. High levels suggest recurrence 1–7 months prior to the clinical/radiological disease detection; unfortunately until now effective treatment is not available. In gastric cancer, measurement of CA19-9 levels, in combination with CEA, consists of a useful diagnostic tool. The sensitivity for each marker is 18–30 per cent exceeding 50–60 per cent in a combined use. Excessively high levels of CA19-9 are suggestive of metastatic disease. Non-cancerous conditions with elevated CA19-9 levels are pancreatitis, ulcerative colitis, primary sclerosing cholangitis, and inflammatory bowel disease.

CA 125   CA 125 is an antigen found on 80 per cent of the non-mucinous ovarian carcinomas. In 80 per cent of women with ovarian cancer CA 125 is elevated. It is a good serum marker reflecting the clinical course of the disease and the response to surgical/chemotherapeutic treatment. CA 125 is elevated in 50 per cent of women with Stage I ovarian cancer, 90 per cent in Stage II and >90 per cent in Stages III and IV. Furthermore, there is a direct association between CA 125 serum levels and tumour mass. Sustained high levels are correlated with poor prognosis. Besides serum, CA 125 may be detected in ascetic fluid, in the liquid content of cysts, as well as in uterine and cervical excretions. Endometrial, breast, pancreatic, lung and colon cancer, as well as pregnancy, endometriosis and other conditions may lead to elevated CA 125 serum levels.

CA15-3   CA15-3 represents a tumour biomarker useful in monitoring the response to treatment and the detection of metastases in cases of breast, mainly, cervical and liver cancer. In the general population, 5–6 per cent of healthy women present slightly elevated levels of CA15-3. On the other hand a little as 23 per cent (range 23–70 per cent in different studies) of women with breast cancer has elevated levels of CA15-3. Thus, CA15-3 is not a useful marker for breast cancer diagnosis. Furthermore, low levels of CA15-3 in individuals with high suspicion for breast cancer, do not exclude malignancy. Serial measurements of CA15-3 are useful in early diagnosis of recurrence following radical therapy. Bone and liver metastases are detectable in 65–75 per cent and 85–90 per cent, respectively.

CA72-4   This cancer antigen is useful not only in the diagnosis of gastric cancer, but also mainly in monitoring the course of the disease and the response to treatment. High levels of CA72-4 are found in 3 per cent of healthy individuals and in 6.7 per cent of individuals with benign diseases of the gastrointestinal tract. High CA72-4 serum levels are detected in 40, 36 and 24 per cent of patients suffering from gastric, lung and ovarian cancer, respectively. The sensitivity in diagnosing gastric cancer rises up to 64 per cent when combined with CEA and CA19-9. This tumour marker has also been used in monitoring patients suffering from mucinous carcinomas of the ovaries, since the usefulness of the CA 125 antigen is somewhat limited.

CA27-29 CA27-29 is a recently identified tumour marker, for monitoring response to treatment and detecting metastases in breast cancer cases, as well as, in cervical cancer.

Prostate-specific antigen (PSA) PSA is a glycoprotein synthesized and secreted by the prostate tissue only. Therefore, it is a highly specific marker for prostate pathologies. Benign prostate hyperplasia (BPH) and prostate carcinoma lead to elevated serum levels of PSA. Serum PSA is mostly bound to α1-antichymotrypsin and/or α2-macroglobulin and only a small fraction circulates as free PSA. The ratio free PSA/bound PSA differs in BPH and prostatic adenocarcinoma, i.e. increased ratio favours BPH. The value of PSA in screening for prostate cancer is beyond doubt, particularly when combined with rectal digital examination. In men over 50 years of age, annual determination of serum PSA levels is strongly recommended. Of particular value are the estimation of PSA density (defined as the ratio of PSA levels/ prostate size, determined by transrectal ultrasound) and PSA velocity (the change in serum PSA levels over time).

Hormones

Human chorionic gonadotropin (HCG) HCG is a hormonal glycoprotein normally synthesized during pregnancy by the syncytiotrophoblastic cells of the placenta. It is a reliable marker in cases of trophoblastic tumours and its sustained high levels indicate poor response to treatment. HCG serum levels are correlated with tumour mass, having thus a prognostic value. Only occasionally, HCG serum levels are increased in tumours from other sites, such as lung, breast and gastrointestinal tract. In combination with AFP it is a useful tool in monitoring testicular cancer.

Other hormones Certain tumours produce hormones, which are released by the tumour cells in the blood circulation and may, thus, be used as specific markers in serum. Examples are the production of insulin, thyroglobulin, calcitonin, catecholamines, adrenocorticotropin hormone (ACTH) and antidiuretic hormone (ADH), by islet cell tumours, follicular thyroid carcinoma, medullary thyroid carcinoma, pheochromocytoma and primary lung cancer, respectively. Other markers are gastrin for gastrinoma and glucagon for glucagonoma.

Enzymes

Acid phosphatase (ACP) ACP is found in the lysosomes of the cells in all human tissues, especially in liver, spleen, bone marrow, erythrocytes, platelets and prostate. The majority of the non-inhibited by the tartaric serum ACP is of osteoclastic origin. In contrast, the inhibited by tartaric fraction of ACP is of platelet and prostate origin. High levels of the non-inhibited by tartaric ACP are found normally in adolescence, as well as in women suffering from metastatic breast cancer. ACP is of great interest in cases of primary and metastatic prostate cancer, being a useful screening marker for early detection of the disease and in the follow-up of patients with advanced disease. In particular, ACP levels are increased in the majority of cases with skeletal metastases. However, the enzyme may also be found elevated in cases of BPH.

Alkaline phosphatase (ALP)   ALP is produced by liver, bones and leukocytes and their malignant conditions. Nowadays, four genes encoding ALP isoenzymes are known to exist:

1. The non-specific tissue gene, found in kidneys, liver and bones. This gene encodes three ALP isoenzymes, which differ in the number of carbohydrates present in the side chains.

2. The placental gene, which encodes the placental ALP isoenzyme.

3. The gut gene, which encodes for the intestinal ALP isoenzyme.

4. The blastic gene, which encodes for the testis, thymus and lung ALP isoenzymes.

In healthy individuals, plasma total ALP is of liver and bone origin. Increased levels of total ALP are found normally during the second trimester of pregnancy and in growing children.

Neuron specific enolase (NSE)   NSE is an enzyme found in the brain and neuroendocrine tissues. It is used as a biomarker in cases of neuroblastoma, small cell lung carcinoma and melanoma, as well as other neuroendocrine tumours. Its value is limited, due to its poor sensitivity.

Lactic dehydrogenase (LDH)   LDH may also be elevated in many different neoplasms, therefore it lacks any specificity. It must be co-evaluated as part of a panel with other tumour markers. Particularly high concentrations of LDH are found in liver, myocardium, kidneys, skeletal muscles and erythrocytes. Tissue LDH concentrations are 500-fold those of serum. Thus, tissue destruction of any aetiology releases LDH in the plasma.

Galactosyl transferrase II   This is useful in the follow-up of gastrointestinal and pancreatic tumours.

Cathepsin D   Elevated levels of cathepsin D indicate a poor prognosis, particularly in breast cancer patients under chemotherapy.

Immunoglobulins
A paraprotein in the band of gamma-globulin in serum electrophoresis, of monoclonal type, characterizes multiple myeloma. Paraproteins may be isolated as light, kappa or lambda, or heavy chains of any immunoglobulin subtype.

Adhesion molecules

Substances belonging to integrins, cadherins, immunoglobulin gene superfamily, selectins and the CD44 molecule comprise the group of adhesion molecules. Until now, more than a hundred members of this group have been identified and fully characterized. Among them, epithelial E-cadherin, intercellular cell adhesion molecule-1 (ICAM-1), neural cell adhesion molecule (NCAM), VCAM and platelet endothelial cell adhesion molecule (PECAM), represent some putative serum biomarkers. NCAM in particular is considered today a better marker than NSE in cases of neuroendocrine tumours. PECAM is considered as a putative biomarker of neoangiogenesis. The adhesion molecules are the field with the most active research for putative new tumour markers in serum.

6.1.2 Various types of tumour markers in use

- *Beta-2 microgobulin* is elevated in malignancies, including lymphoproliferative diseases and carcinomas (e.g. lung cancer).

- Low levels of *ferritin*, an indicator of iron storage protein in sialic acid, are correlated with better prognosis in patients with head and neck malignancies.

- *Pancreatic polypeptide* (PP) diagnoses pancreatic gamma-cell islet tumours, being elevated in APUDomas, VIPomas and MEN.

- *Pro-insulin cell peptide* differentiates the cell types of endocrine secreting tumours, being elevated in insulinomas and islet cell tumours.

- *Tissue polypeptide antigen* (TPA) is an antigen marker for gynaecological, bladder and lung cancer, but lacks specificity. In men it is used to monitor bladder and lung cancer.

- *Chromogranin* A (CGA), B (CGB), and C (CGC) are found in neuroendocrine cells of the human body. Central nervous system and autonomic sympathetic system also contain chromogranins. Various types of endocrine neoplasms are associated with high levels of chromogranin concentrations. In contrast, normal values of chromogranins are found in neoplasias of non-endocrine origin, as well as in benign endocrine disorders. CGA, in general, represents a better tumour marker than CGB, showing high sensitivity in neuroblastomas, however their combined determination is necessary.

- Elevated *vanillylmandelic acid* (VMA) levels suggest a catecholamine-secreting tumour. VMA is the final product of catecholamine metabolism reflecting secretion from the adrenal chromaffin cells. Phaeochromocytoma are rare tumours found in adrenals, with the diagnosis based on the determination of high urine metanephrine levels, urine VMA, as well as catecholamine levels in plasma or urine. Determination of the homovanillic acid (HVA) levels is of low diagnostic value in patients suffering from phaeochromocytoma, but is of great interest in differential diagnosis between phaeochromocytoma and neuroblastoma. In gangliomas, which are well-differentiated tumours found in young adults, high levels of catecholamines and their metabolites are found in plasma and urine.

6.2   Urine tests for tumour markers

Urine testing is preferable to serum, since it is a non-invasive method. However, the presence of the kidney barrier prohibits most of the tumour markers found in serum from passing into the urine, due to their high molecular weight. Therefore, researchers are focusing their efforts in identifying new tumour markers in urine, mainly for diagnosing neoplasms of the urinary tract. Bladder cancer is the fifth most common malignancy. Quick, cheap, easy and pain-free screening tests are not available yet. Recently, researchers have reported the use of *Mcm5 protein* in the bloody urine of patients with bladder cancer. Mcm5 protein is involved in the normal replication of DNA in all cells. In cases of bladder cancer, Mcm5 protein is shed in large amounts into the urine. This protein is detectable microscopically after a special stain. *Bladder tumour antigen* (BTA) and *nuclear matrix protein 22* (NMP 22), also represent antigens found in bloody urine of patients with bladder cancer. *Fibrin/fibrinogen degradation products* (FDP), urine *telomerase activity* and urine ultra-sensitive assay for haemoglobin constitute other approaches used in bladder cancer detection. *BLCA-4* is another protein appearing to be expressed by the bladder only in patients suffering from bladder cancer; not in healthy population. All scientific efforts are focused in screening, initial diagnosis and monitoring recurrence.

In the future, biomarkers found in serum, urine and other biological fluids will change substantially clinical decisions, aiding in early cancer diagnosis, management and prognosis, in hope of eventually saving lives.

6.3   Smear tests and their association with tumour development

The interpretation of cells that spontaneously exfoliate from tissues or are removed from them by abrasion or fine needle aspiration (FNA) is the subject of diagnostic cytology. Diagnostic cytology is based on the fact that the exfoliated or collected cells reflect features of the tissue they arise from. The procedures are fast and simple, with the least morbidity, but usually yield only few cells. Techniques include FNA, brushings through an endoscope, tapping of fluid collections through a needle, and direct scrapings such as the Papanicolaou (Pap) smear. The most common specimens are from the cervix (Pap-test), breast (FNA or nipple aspiration), thyroid (FNA), lung (bronchial cytology), lymph nodes (FNA) and urinary bladder (urine cytology). Cytology is used for the initial approach to a patient with a yet undiagnosed tumour mass and for the follow-up of patients treated for a carcinoma, but its greater value is in cancer screening.

The major challenge that we are facing today is to control cancer by population-based screening. Most screening procedures aim at finding incidental, asymptomatic cancers, precancerous lesions associated with high risk of developing cancer and identifying individuals who can benefit most from specific prevention strategies. The most successful application of cytology is the early diagnosis of uterine cervical carcinoma through examination of cervical smears, a technique established by G. Papanicolaou. Today, the value of cervical smears (Pap-test) for the screening of cervical carcinoma is beyond doubt. The Pap-test has been responsible for the reduction in the incidence of invasive squamous cell carcinoma of the cervix, since mass cytology screening has led to the diagnosis of preclinical lesions. In this setting, screening intervenes in the development of advanced malignant tumours. Screening for other malignancies includes bronchial cytology, nipple aspiration and urine cytology, but their use is doubted. Exfoliative cytology is of little practical value in the initial evaluation of tumours of the urinary bladder, since they are usually accessible to biopsy and histological examination. It is useful in cases where, due to inflammation, diverticula, etc., the bladder biopsy may be negative because of sampling. In cancer-screening smears, the cytologist is called to identify subtle morphological deviations that confer the currently healthy individual a risk for future malignancy. The detection of the earliest changes of neoplastic transformation is very difficult. In cytology material, it is particularly difficult to differentially diagnose cytological *atypia*, which is used to denote alterations due to infection, trauma, physical or chemical stimuli, from true *dysplasia*. The latter is a constellation of abnormal features in cells, which include nuclear pleomorphism (i.e. variable appearance of nuclei, regarding shape and size), prominent nucleoli and increased nuclear-to-cytoplasmic ratio. The main objective in cytological diagnosis is to detect those cellular abnormalities that are the precursors of cancer.

6.4 Histopathology

The word Histopathology originates from the Greek words *histos* (tissue), *pathos* (suffering) and *logos* (study) and as its name implies it is a discipline devoted to the study of the cause, the pathogenesis, the morphological changes and functional derangement in cells, tissues and organs that underlie disease. Anatomic pathology originated in Europe three centuries ago and among the great pioneers are Morgagni, who encouraged the postmortem search for the cause and nature of disease, and B.C. Ruge and J. Veit from Berlin University who introduced surgical biopsy, with the application of the microscope, as an essential diagnostic tool. Since then, the histological techniques have been continuously improving and pathologists have been incorporating a variety of methods in their everyday practice, making diagnosis more refined and definite. They integrate data from gross and microscopic examination, cytological and molecular methods so that they can face common diseases such as cancer and inflammation.

Pathologists contribute to several steps in the work-up of a patient:

1. Before surgery: with the interpretation of needle biopsy material.

2. During surgery: with the use of frozen sections and rapid diagnosis.

3. After surgery: with the examination of the fixed specimen and final diagnosis.

4. In recurrence of disease;

5. Even after the patient's death by recognizing the actual nature and extend of disease.

In cancer today, the correct diagnosis is only the first step. The particular challenge is to discover the molecular abnormalities that dictate each malignant growth and, based on these data, to develop more rational and effective approaches for treatment. Pathology is the discipline that acts as a bridge between Clinical Medicine and Basic Sciences.

Tumours are classified into two broad categories: benign and malignant.

6.4.1 Benign tumours

Benign tumours can arise from many cell types. They can expand locally, but they do not invade nearby structures and they never metastasize. However, they can cause problems: cosmetic and through mass effect (e.g. adenoma of the pituitary gland). Benign tumours are designated with the suffix 'oma'. Thus, benign tumours of epithelial origin that arise in glands or form glandular structures are called adenomas (Figure 6.1, left) and those that form papillae (fibrovascular, finger-like stalks with epithelial lining) are called papillomas. Benign mesenchymal tumours, based on the latest Wold Heath Organization (WHO) classification, are generally named according to their line of differentiation, i.e. lipoma, fibroma, osteoma, leiomyoma (Figure 6.1, right).

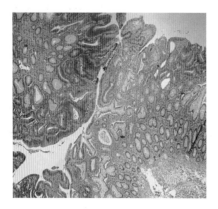 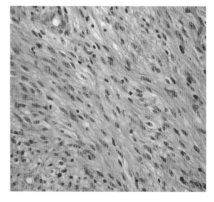

Figure 6.1 Left: tubular adenoma of the sigmoid colon; right: leiomyoma of the uterus

6.4.2 Malignant tumours

Malignant neoplasms are all called cancers and according to their cell of origin they are divided in carcinomas and sarcomas.

Carcinomas
Carcinomas arise from epithelial tissues derived from ectoderm or endoderm (skin, respiratory tract, gastrointestinal tract, urinary tract, breast, endocrine glands etc). Based on their architectural and cytological features, as well as their presumed cell of origin, carcinomas are further subdivided into several entities, e.g. squamous cell carcinoma (Figure 6.2, left), adenocarcinoma, renal cell carcinoma, hepatocellular carcinoma, etc. The term 'carcinoma *in situ*' refers to the malignant transformation of epithelial cells that is limited to the epithelium, without invasion of the basement membrane. When the tumour extends through the basement membrane it becomes invasive, and when it spreads beyond the primary site it is called metastatic (Figure 6.2, right).

Sarcomas
Sarcomas arise from mesenchymal tissues, derived from the mesoderm (bone, cartilage, fascia, adipose tissue, smooth or skeletal muscle, endothelial or mesothelial cells). Based on their line of differentiation they are characterized as osteosarcoma, chondrosarcoma (Figure 6.3, left), liposarcoma (Figure 6.3, right), leiomyosarcoma, etc.

Lymphomas
Lymphomas arise from haematopoietic cells and lymphoid tissues and have no benign counterpart. Melanomas arise from melanocytes (Figure 6.4, right) and their benign counterpart is the nevus (Figure 6.4, left).

Other neoplasms
Teratoma is a neoplasm derived from all three germ layers, the most common being the teratoma of the ovary (Figure 6.5, left). Neoplasms, which consist of more than one cell

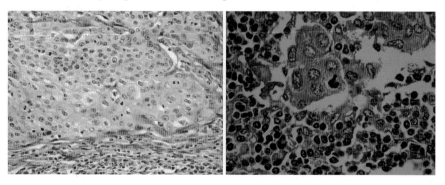

Figure 6.2 Left: invasive squamous cell carcinoma; right: metastatic squamous cell carcinoma in lymph node

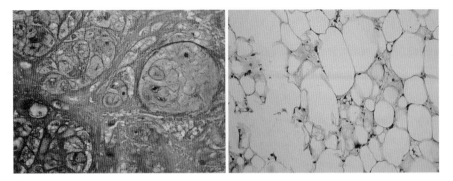

Figure 6.3   Left: chondrosarcoma; right: liposarcoma, with characteristic multivacuolated lipoblasts

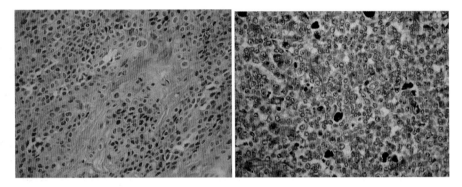

Figure 6.4   Left: nevus; right: melanoma

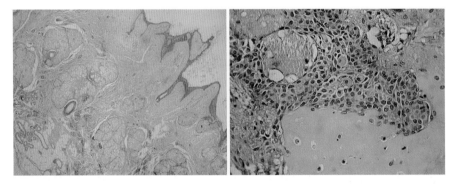

Figure 6.5   Left: teratoma of the ovary. Note the presence of skin, sebaceous glands and adipose tissue. Right: benign mixed tumour (pleomorphic adenoma) of the parotid gland. Note the presence of epithelial and stromal (chondroid) elements

type, but arise from only one germ layer, are called mixed tumours, the best example being the benign mixed tumour (pleomorphic adenoma) of the parotid gland (Figure 6.5, right). Hamartoma is a benign neoplasm which consists of haphazard growth of tissues normally presently at the site, while choristoma is the benign neoplasm composed of tissues not normally found at the site. The suffix '-blastoma' denotes neoplasms that resemble primitive embryonic tissues, e.g. medulloblastoma, neuroblastoma, retinoblastoma.

Recently, between the benign and malignant neoplasms, a third category, that of borderline tumours, has been added. This category is better exemplified by epithelial ovarian neoplasms, and denotes tumours of intermediate clinical behaviour between benign and malignant. In soft tissue tumours, the third category, between benign and malignant, is called intermediate and is further subdivided in locally aggressive and rarely metastasizing neoplasms.

6.4.3   Features of cancerous cells

Anaplasia, or loss of differentiation, is a characteristic feature of cancer cells. Malignant neoplasms also exhibit morphological and functional changes, such as variability in the size and shape of cells and their nuclei (pleomorphism, Figure 6.6, left), large nuclei, increased nuclear/cytoplasmic ratio, increase nuclear DNA content (hyperchromasia) and increased number of mitoses, many of which are atypical with tripolar, quadripolar or multipolar spindles (Figure 6.6, right). The level of differentiation of malignant tumour varies and the tumour is graded based on the extent of resemblance to the tissue of origin. Thus, well-differentiated neoplasms look very similar to the corresponding normal tissue and moderately differentiated resemble to some extend the normal tissue. Poorly differentiated and anaplastic neoplasms bear no similarity to normal tissue and it may be difficult to determine the cell of origin by light microscopy alone. In such cases, immunostaining (see below) and electron microscopy may provide valuable information.

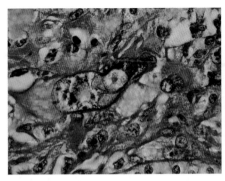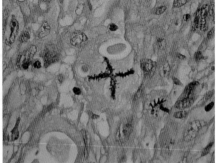

Figure 6.6   Sarcoma. Note the nuclear pleomorphism (left) and the atypical mitoses (right)

The regular every-day practice in surgical pathology is the gross examination of specimens, followed by fixation in formalin, submission of representative sections (max thickness 3 mm), embedding in paraffin, cutting in sections 4–5 μm thick, and staining with haematoxylin and eosin (H+E). With the H+E stain, the nuclei are stained purple–blue by the haematoxylin, whereas the cytoplasm and extracellular materials are counterstained by eosin. The H+E stain provides adequate information regarding morphology in most situations. Of further diagnostic utility are the 'special stains'. The most common are: PAS (periodic acid–Schiff) stain, that demonstrates glycogen, neutral mucosubstances, basement membranes, fungi and parasites; Ziehl–Neelsen for acid-fast microorganisms; Gram for bacteria; Congo red for amyloid; Reticulin stains for type III collagen and basement membranes, trichrome stains; Perls stain for hemosiderin, Fontana–Masson stain for melanin; von Kossa stain for calcium; Alcian blue stain for mucin, etc.

6.4.4   Immunohistochemistry

Immunohistochemistry, which was developed in the 1980s, is another widely used method for identifying antigens in tissue sections with the use of the appropriate antibodies, after exposing to antigenic epitopes. Today a large number of antibodies is available and are particularly useful for establishing the correct diagnosis. For example, in it known that in 3–5 per cent of all cancers, the patient may present a metastatic neoplasm of unknown primary site. As part of the work-up of the patient, a biopsy is taken for pathology examination. Morphology alone, as estimated by light microscopy examination of H+E stained slides leads to the identification of the tumour in 65 per cent of the cases. In such cases, for example, the presence of neoplastic glandular configurations leads to the diagnosis of adenocarcinoma (Figure 6.7, left), while the presence of solid neoplastic cell nests with distinct borders, intercellular bridges and keratin pearls indicates squamous cell carcinoma. If the morphologic

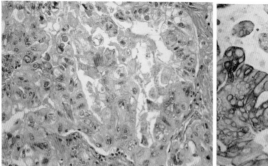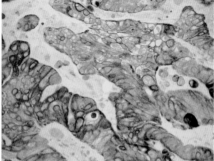

Figure 6.7   Adenocarcinoma of the colon. Left: with the haematoxylin and eosin stain neoplastic glandular configurations are noted. Right: with immunohistochemical stain for cytokeratin 20, the neoplastic cells are stained positive (brown chromogen is DAB)

features are not adequate for diagnosis, immunohistochemical identification of tumour-specific products or markers may be of extreme help. For example the expression of cytokeratins is a clue for carcinoma, of CLA (common leukocyte antigen) is a clue for lymphoma, of vimentin is a clue for sarcoma, of HMB-45 is a clue for melanoma etc. Furthermore, immunohistochemical markers can help to define the exact cell lineage. For example, there are more than twenty subtypes of cytokeratins with different molecular weights, and their pattern of expression can be used to further identify carcinomas according to their site of origin, e.g. an adenocarcinoma immunopositive for cytokeratin 20 and negative for cytokeratin 7 is most probably from the colorectum (Figure 6.7, right). An adenocarcinoma that exhibits positive immunoreactivity for PSA is from the prostate, while a carcinoma immunopositive to thyroglobulin is of a thyroid primary.

Immunohistochemistry is also useful for identifying the particular characteristics of each tumour with regard to responsiveness to targeted therapy and prognosis. In the last decade, the role of adhesion molecules, in particular of the epithelial-cadherin (E-cadherin) in diagnosis and prognosis of various types of cancers has been documented. It is a general phenomenon, that down-regulation of E-cadherin expression is associated with advanced stage of disease and poor prognosis.

The best example is the individualization in breast cancer treatment that has started approximately two decades ago with the discovery of the first oestrogen receptor, ERα, a member of the nuclear receptor superfamily of ligand-activated transcription factors. Its detection in breast carcinomas (mostly by immunohistochemical methods) influences decisions on whether to give or not adjuvant therapy with anti-oestrogens (Figure 6.8, left). The *Her2/neu* is an oncogene that encodes a transmembrane tyrosine kinase. It is the best example of utilization of laboratory-based data for the benefit of the patient, since it has been successfully used as a target for specific therapy. Overexpression of Her2/neu (c-erb-B2) protein arises from amplification of the *Her2/neu* gene, has been detected in 20–40 per cent of human breast carcinomas and is associated with poor prognosis. The vast majority of *Her2/neu* studies have been performed using immuno-histochemistry in archival pathology material (Figure 6.8, right).

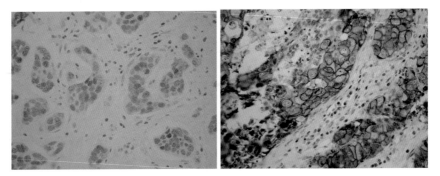

Figure 6.8 Invasive ductal carcinoma of the breast. Left: nuclear ERα immunoreactivity (brown chromogen is DAB). Right: complete membranous immunoreactivity for *Her2/neu* protein (brown chromogen is DAB)

The introduction of new molecular laboratory techniques, such as FISH (fluoresence in situ hybridization), allowed assessment of the level of *Her2/neu* gene amplification in histological sections. FISH has been proven valuable in the work-up of several neoplasms, by detecting chromosomal translocations, deletions or amplifications in tissue sections and cytological smears. More recently, a novel technology to detect DNA probes, CISH (chromogenic in situ hybridization), has been developed. Microarray-based expression profiling has been developing with increased pace and has the potential to revolutionize the practice of pathology. It can be generated from surgical cancer specimens and provides each tumour with its unique molecular 'signature' that can be used to predict chemotherapy responses and disease-free and overall survival. Aggregate patterns of gene expression (metagenes) have been identified that are capable of predicting outcomes in individual patients with great accuracy.

6.5   Summary

A number of assays are available for the diagnosis and prognosis of cancer. These include recognition of molecules in the blood and urine of patients, as well as cells and tissues that are analysed for malignancies. Tumours often produce secret molecules that are differentiated, mutated or overproduced compared to normal cells. Such molecules are recognized and identified in biological fluids, such as blood and urine, and can offer indications as to the potential for tumour development, or the presence and stage of cancer. These molecules, known as tumour markers, are not specific enough to offer tests that can unequivocally determine the presence and status of cancer. However, they are very valuable tools in conjunction with other techniques. Such other techniques include smear tests, such as the cervical smear that has been very effective in reducing the incidence of cervical carcinoma, and histopathological examinations that can detect abnormalities in cells removed from the affected tissue and can diagnose and differentiate malignant from benign tumours and normal tissue. The value of diagnostic assays is great and the number of tests available offers a significant tool in the prevention and treatment of cancer.

6.6   Self-assessment questions

Question: What are tumour markers?

Answer: Tumour markers are substances that may be found in blood, urine or body tissues and are associated with cancer. Their identification and quantification in biological media and tissue samples aids greatly in patients' diagnosis, management, and prognosis.

Question: What are the types of molecules that act as tumour markers in serum?

Answer: Tumour markers are usually proteins, and they can be tumour antigens, hormones, enzymes, immunoglobulins, adhesion molecules, but also smaller biochemical entities.

Question: Name some serum antigens used as diagnostics for cancer.

Answer: There are a number of tumour antigens present in serum. Some of them include the carcinoembryonic antigen (CEA), alpha-fetoprotein (AFP), CA19-9, CA125, CA15-3, CA72-4, CA27-29 and prostate specific antigen (PSA).

Question: What are smear tests measuring/trying to identify?

Answer: In cancer-screening smears, the cytologist is called to identify subtle morphological deviations that confer the currently healthy individual a risk for future malignancy.

Question: Describe the steps that a pathologist contributes in the work-up of a cancer patient.

Answer: Pathologists contribute to several steps in the work-up of a patient: 1. Before surgery: with the interpretation of needle biopsy material. 2. During surgery: with the use of frozen sections and rapid diagnosis. 3. After surgery: with the examination of the fixed specimen and final diagnosis. 4. In recurrence of disease. 5. Even after the patient's death by recognizing the actual nature and extend of disease.

6.7   Further reading and resources

Bassi P, De Marco V, De Lisa A, Macini M, Pinto F, Bartoloni R and Longo F. Non-invasive diagnostic tests for bladder cancer: a review of the literature. *Urol Int* 2005, **75**, 193–200.

Batistatou A, Scopa CD, Ravazoula P, Nakanishi Y, Peschos D, Agnantis NJ, Hirohashi S and Charalabopoulos KA. Involvement of dysadherin and E-cadherin in the development of testicular tumours. *Br J Cancer* 2005, **93**, 1382–1387.

Billous M, Dowsett M, Hanna W *et al*. Current perspectives on HER2 Testing: A review of National Testing Guidelines. *Mod Pathol* 2003, **16**, 173–182.

Dolled-Filhart M, Ryden L, Cregger M, Jirstrom K, Harigopal M, Camp RL and Rimm DL. Classification of breast cancer using genetic algorithms and tissue microarrays. *Clin Cancer Res* 2006, **12**, 6459–6468.

Kasper DL, Braunwald E, Fauci AL, Hauser SL, Longo DL and Jameson JL (eds) *Harrison's Principles of Internal Medicine*, sixteenth edition. McGraw-Hill, New York, 2005.

Kufe DW, Bast RC, Hait W, Hong VK, Pollock RE, Weichselbaum RR, Holland JF and Frei E III (eds) *Holland Frei – Cancer Medicine 7*, seventh edition. Elsevier, Edinburgh, 2006.

Kumar V, Abbas AK, Fausto N (eds) *Robbins and Cotran Pathologic Basis of Disease*, seventh edition. W.B. Saunders Company, Philadelphia, 2004.

Kyzas PA, Stefanou D, Batistatou A, Agnantis NJ, Nakanishi Y, Hirohashi S and Charalabopoulos K. Dysadherin expression in head and neck squamous cell carcinoma: association with lymphangiogenesis and prognostic significance. *Am J Surg Pathol* 2006, **30**, 185–193.

Lewis F, Jackson P, Lane S, Coast G and Hanby AM. Testing for HER2 in breast cancer. *Histopathology* 2004, **45**, 207–217.

Rosai J (ed.) *Rosai and Ackerman's Surgical Pathology*, eighth edition. Mosby-Year Book Inc, London, 2004.

Underwood JCE (ed.) *General and Systemic Pathology*. Churchill Livingstone, Edinburgh, 2004.

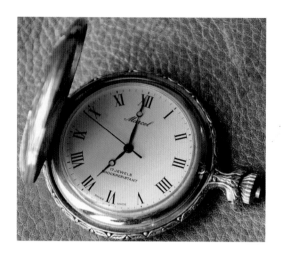

In the previous chapter we read about the various diagnostic methods that either precede or supersede the initial encounter with cancer. Some diagnostic assays, as we saw earlier, are used as regular testing methods to determine whether an individual is at risk of developing cancer (such as smear tests), whilst others are used for diagnosing whether a tumour is benign or malignant, follow the response to treatment, or determine the nature and stage of the disease. In this chapter we will follow tumour imaging, a technique that spreads through the realm of prognosis, diagnosis, imaging and therapy of cancer. Parts of this chapter, such as mammography, fall within the regular tests offered to the public to secure an early diagnosis of breast cancer and thus improve therapeutic outcome. On the other hand, imaging can be used to monitor the size and location of known tumours or facilitate the search for metastatic disease. Finally, nuclear medicine techniques used in imaging are now closely interlinked with radiotherapy, as the imaging part of the techniques assist on the clear definition of the tumour and direct the therapy on the location of the cancer. Thus, this chapter is also a transition between the diagnosis of the disease and its treatment, which will be dealt with in the next chapter.

7

Tumour imaging and therapy

Alan C Perkins

Academic Medical Physics, Medical School, University of Nottingham, UK

7.1   Introduction

Imaging investigations play an essential role in both the diagnosis and treatment of patients with cancer. From the moment a patient first visits the doctor, the patient journey relies on the use of medical imaging techniques. A fundamental principle of care for the cancer patient is that the earlier a diagnosis is made the greater is the likelihood of patient survival. Not only is imaging used for both the initial diagnosis and staging of disease, but it is used for monitoring the effectiveness of treatment and increasingly for early screening in order to pick up pre-clinical signs of disease. Modern imaging procedures are generally termed non-invasive, although it must be appreciated that the majority of imaging procedures involve the use of one form of radiation or another and also the administration of drugs and contrast agents. Table 7.1 gives a summary of the main imaging modalities discussed in this chapter. A fundamental aim of imaging procedures is to show fine structures within the patient without the need for surgical exploration. Equipment designers and manufacturers are all striving to produce high resolution imaging systems with the ultimate aim of providing as much information as possible to aid in the diagnosis of pathological conditions such as the growth and spread of tumours.

Medical imaging is a highly complex branch of medical science involving a range of specialized scientific staff including radiologists, radiographers, medical physicists and clinical technologists. The procedures undertaken in diagnostic medical oncology are usually carried out in specialized departments in cancer centres. Because of the different

The Cancer Clock   Edited by Sotiris Missailidis
© 2007 John Wiley & Sons Ltd

Table 7.1 The main techniques for cancer imaging

Modality	Brief outline of imaging technique
X-ray	X-rays generated in an X-ray tube are directed through a window towards the patient. The X-rays are attenuated by the body to form a shadow graph on a radiographic film, solid state detector or image intensifier.
X-ray CT	A fine beam of X-rays is produced by an X-ray generator mounted on a scanning gantry. The beam is repeatedly scanned across the patient from different angles. Interaction of the X-rays with an array of crystal-photodiode detectors provides the data for the scan. The images are then mathematically reconstructed using a computer.
Nuclear medicine	*Gamma scan*: The patient is injected with a tracer amount of radioactivity tagged on to a drug known as a radiopharmaceutical. The drug is chosen because of its ability to localize in tumours and specific tissues. Gamma rays emitted by the tracer are detected by a gamma camera and an image of the localized activity can be produced. In one form of imaging known as SPECT the gamma camera rotates around the patient and the image is reconstructed to produce image slices similar to a CT scan.
	PET scan: A particularly sensitive form of imaging known as PET scanning uses a positron emitting tracer that is injected into the patient. The positron is the antiparticle of the electron and when the two come together the two particles annihilate each other producing a pair of gamma rays that are detected by the scanner. The image is reconstructed by computer.
Ultrasound	A hand held scanning probe is used to generate high frequency pulses of sound that are scanned across the patient. The different tissues in the body reflect the sound back towards the probe. The returning echoes are detected by the same probe and displayed as a series of grey levels in the image, the brighter areas resulting from the stronger echoes. Automatic rapid pulse firing produces a real-time image capable of showing the movement of internal structures such as the heart. Where there is tissue movement or flowing blood a change in frequency of the reflected sound occurs due to the Doppler effect. The frequency information can be given a colour level that can be displayed as a colour Doppler image.

| MRI | The patient is placed in a large magnet. A strong magnetic field causes the nuclear protons in hydrogen atoms to spin parallel with the direction of the field. Radio waves are used to add energy to the protons causing them to flip out of line with the field. These then gradually give up this energy and emit a radio signal that is detected. Measuring the time delay, known as the relaxation time enables an image of the proton properties to be reconstructed. |

CT, computerized tomography; PET, positron emission tomography; MRI, magnetic resonance imaging; SPECT, single photon emission computerized tomography.

information obtained by each imaging modality, imaging investigations are often used in combination with each other or with other diagnostic tests. In order to diagnose different types of disease, a specific diagnostic pathway is used as an aid in selecting which investigations are carried out. This is necessary to determine the type and stage of tumour in individual patients. Only when this is known can the appropriate form of treatment be planned. In many cases the final diagnosis can only be confirmed when tissue samples are available for histological classification. Imaging procedures are often used to guide the insertion of needles for biopsy, to facilitate the retrieval of tissue samples for histological typing.

Many health care providers, including the NHS in the UK, use referral criteria that have to be met before an investigation can go ahead. This may be due to a legal requirement, because of the different forms of radiation used and the necessity for safe practice. In some cases, for example in nuclear medicine, there are prescribed levels of radiation that may be used for individual procedures. Many healthcare providers specify that referral criteria have to be met before authorizing financial reimbursement to the imaging service provider.

With the widespread availability of computer-based information technology, imaging departments are being linked together with computer networks for the display and storage of medical images. These networks for picture archiving and communications are known as PACS. The result is that the X-ray film will rapidly become a thing of the past. However, more importantly, the computer network will ensure that medical, nursing and paramedical staff will have immediate on-line access to diagnostic images and reports.

7.2 X-ray imaging

Diagnostic X-rays are carried out in purpose built rooms containing an X-ray generator, patient bed and image detector. Within an X-ray generator, electrons released by a heated filament are accelerated through an evacuated tube by means of a high voltage supply. These collide with a dense metal target such as tungsten, generating much heat and X-ray radiation. The original German term Wilhelm Roentgen used for this form of radiation created by electrons hitting a target was *bremsstrahlung*, which when translated means 'breaking radiation'. The voltage and current applied to the X-ray tube affect the energy and number of X-ray photons produced. X-ray energy is measured in electron volts and is normally expressed in thousands, i.e. keV. In general, radiographic procedures use energies of between 40 and 140 keV, with lower energies (around 40 keV) being used for soft tissue imaging such as mammography for the detection of breast tumours and higher energies around 100 keV used for abdominal imaging. The X-ray beam passes through aluminium filters before being directed into the patient to remove some of the low-energy X-rays that would only add unnecessary radiation dose to the skin and the first few centimetres of tissue. These low-energy X-rays would not have enough energy to penetrate the full depth of a patient and so would not contribute to the final image information.

In the basic radiographic technique, a beam of X-rays is directed from the generator through the patient and collected using a suitable detector or an image intensifier system (X-ray camera). Traditionally, radiographic films were placed in a light tight cassette and then processed in film processor. However, these have now largely been replaced with digital X-ray detectors. The physical basis of the imaging technique is the differential attenuation of X-rays from tissues having different density or, more correctly, having a different atomic number. The final image is essentially a shadow of the attenuation from the dense body structures. The more dense tissues, such as bones, attenuate the X-rays to a greater degree and therefore this area remains white on the image because there is little or no exposure. In a chest X-ray, the soft tissues and air in the lungs do not cause much attenuation and so the exposed areas appear black in the image.

As the X-rays pass through the patient they may be scattered away from their original direction due to interaction with electrons and atoms in the patient. These scattered X-rays may be detected randomly adding noise and degrading the image. Scatter grids are placed between the patient and the detector to remove some of this scatter.

7.2.1 Mammography

Breast cancer is among the most common of all cancers, occurring in nearly 1 in 10 women. Mammography is considered important since it is used to screen healthy women for small, curable, breast tumours. If these tumours are detected at an early stage, then there is a greater probability of complete cure. Mammographic screening is for women who have no previously known breast problems. Screening is not for women with implants, or women who have breast symptoms such as lumps or bloody nipple discharge. A mammogram is an examination that takes about 20 minutes and provides two views of each breast. The technique involves low-energy X-rays, since the thickness of tissue being imaged is small compared with the full thickness of the body. Since X-ray images depend on the difference in X-ray stopping power (attenuation) of different tissues, it is possible to detect small differences due to the presence of tumour tissue. In general, a clear separation between normal functioning tissue and abnormal cancerous tissues is not possible since their attenuation is very similar. When an apparent lesion is seen in only one view, it is referred to as a mammographic 'density' and additional views must be obtained to confirm or exclude the presence of a mass. Although the dense area may be a mass, it may be nothing more than several overlapping dense areas of tissue. However, when a mass is confirmed on two views, it is further characterized to determine if enough features are present to justify tissue biopsy or removal. In many cases, additional imaging using ultrasound will be performed to identify the nature of the lesion. Diagnosis often takes the form of shape analysis. Round and oval shapes are associated with benign processes, in part because they imply a well-circumscribed margin, whereas irregular, invasive structures are associated with malignancy. In older women, the functional glandular tissue diminishes, leaving only thin supporting tissues clearly outlined by fatty tissues (see Box 7.1). Mammography in these 'mature' breasts is very effective, since even small cancers are well outlined by fat. In addition, many cancers develop calcium deposits that strongly stop X-rays and are easily seen on mammograms.

Box 7.1 Mammogram

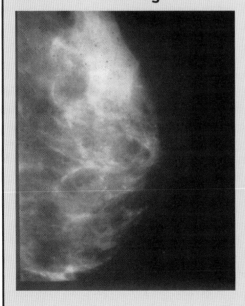

An example of an X-ray mammogram. Mammograms are commonly used every 2 years, for screening purposes in women between the ages of 50 and 69. Studies show that the regular use of mammograms in women of this age group has the potential to reduce deaths from breast cancer by up to 40 per cent. Studies have also looked at whether regular mammograms would be beneficial for women aged 40 to 50 years; however the evidence is not conclusive. There are also some concerns about the adverse effects of increased exposures to radiation from some screening programmes.

7.2.2 X-ray CT

Conventional X-ray images are two-dimensional and tissues of similar density can look the same in the images. In 1971 a British engineer, Godfrey Hounsfield, combined X-ray imaging with a computer by taking a number of X-ray images of the same area, but at

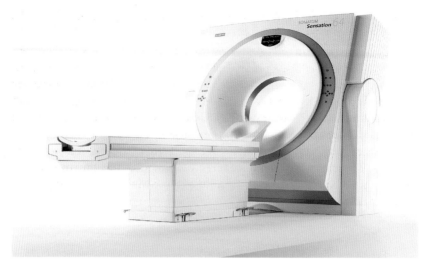

Figure 7.1   A 64 slice spiral CT scanner. Reproduced courtesy of Siemens Medical Solutions

slightly different angles. A cross-sectional image could then be reconstructed by computer. Hounsfield called this technology CT (computerized tomography), but it is also called a CAT scan (computerized axial tomography). CT scanners are basically measuring the attenuation of a fine beam of X-rays that is scanned across the patient from a number of angles. Because the X-ray beam is highly collimated and the detector will only accept X-rays travelling in the original line of fire, scatter is virtually eliminated and the quality of the image is vastly improved. Figure 7.1 shows a clinical CT scanner. The X-ray generator is mounted on a circular gantry and can rotate around the patient at rapid speeds, although from the outside no moving parts can be seen. A scanning sequence of translation and rotation is performed and the values are used to reconstruct a tomographic slice through the patient. As the patient bed moves through the rotating X-ray generator, the path of the beam represents corkscrew or spiral giving rise to the term spiral CT. The mathematical processes used to reconstruct the images are known as filtered back projection and require a computer to calculate the intensity values in the final reconstructed image. A more detailed description of the technique can be found elsewhere. The final image is shown as attenuation values, expressed in Hounsfield units and displayed in levels of grey between black and white. The upper and lower intensity levels in the image may be altered to give a viewing window more suited to either soft tissue or bone, depending upon the anatomical site of interest. One of the obvious advantages of this form of image display is the ability to visualize soft tissues, such as the liver and kidneys. This is especially valuable for the detection of tumours and metastatic deposits. Additional diagnostic information may be obtained by the administration of radiographic contrast agents. These are generally iodine based for cardiovascular studies and contain barium for gastrointestinal investigations.

Diagnostic X-rays are now used so extensively in medicine that they represent the largest man-made source of exposure of ionizing radiation to the population (approximately 1000 times that resulting from the routine discharge of radioactivity from the nuclear power industry). Whilst there is a high degree of confidence in the safe use of X-rays and radioactivity for nuclear medicine investigations, there is a continual need for the education of medical staff with regards to balancing the perceived benefit from the investigation against the relative hazards of radiation for all diagnostic imaging investigations. There has been some concern over increases in the number of X-ray CT examinations, which account for a large proportion of the radiation exposure to the general public.

7.3 Nuclear medicine

Nuclear imaging includes imaging with gamma cameras and positron emission tomography (PET) scanners and has an extremely important role in oncology. One aspect of nuclear imaging that should be understood is that this type of imaging demonstrates physiology rather than anatomy. For example, this may be the uptake of a receptor molecule, the result of a metabolic process or binding of an antibody to an antigen. The technique basically involves the administration of a tracer amount of an appropriately radiolabelled drug or compound, known as a radiopharmaceutical. This drug is selected for its ability to localize in a specific tumour or tissue type. The image is formed by detection of the gamma rays given off by the radioactive decay of the label. The images obtained provide a functional map of the whole body biodistribution and uptake. A list of the physical characteristics of the most commonly used radionuclides is given in Table 7.2.

Technetium-99m, with a physical half-life of 6 hours, is the most commonly administered radionuclide and is used for investigations such as bone scanning, lung perfusion imaging and cardiac imaging, as well as tumour imaging. Some other tumour-imaging radiopharmaceuticals are listed in Table 7.3.

Table 7.2 Gamma emitting radionuclides commonly used in nuclear imaging

Radionuclide	Principal photon energy (keV)	Physical half-life
Technetium-99m	140	6h
Indium-111	173, 247	2.8d
Iodine-123	160	13h
Iodine-131	360	8d
Thallium-201	78	73.1h

Table 7.3   Examples of tumour-detecting radiopharmaceuticals

Gamma emitters	Tc-99m-MDP bone imaging for skeletal metastases
	Tc-99m-Monoclonal antibody imaging (various tumours)
	In-111-monoclonal antibody imaging
	In-111-peptides (e.g. somatostatin receptor imaging)
	I-123-MIBG (metaiodobenzylguanidine of neuroectodermal tumours)
Positron emitters	Fluorine-18-fluorodeoxygyglucose (glucose utilization)
	Fluorine-18-fluorothymidine (cell proliferation)
	Carbon-11-methionine (cell proliferation)

7.3.1   The gamma camera

The main instrument for conventional nuclear imaging is the gamma camera (Figure 7.2). Gamma cameras generally have one or two large rectangular crystal detectors, approximately 1 cm thick and over 40 cm wide. The detector crystal is

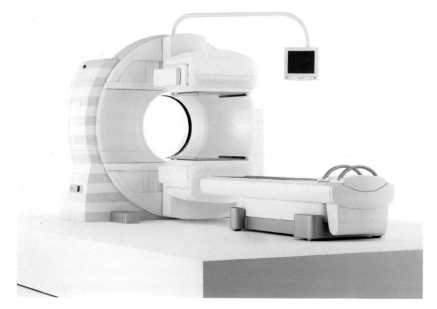

Figure 7.2   A dual-head gamma camera. Reproduced courtesy of Siemens Medical Solutions

backed by an array of tightly packed photomultiplier tubes. The gamma rays are channelled onto the crystal by a lead collimator. This is a lead plate with a large number of small holes to channel the gamma rays, thereby projecting them on to the detector crystal. Any gamma ray not following the direction of the holes will be absorbed or attenuated by the lead. Different types of collimator, with varying thicknesses of lead septa between the holes, are used for different energies of gamma rays, commonly referred to as low energy (140 keV maximum), medium energy (150–300 keV) and high energy (300–400 keV). On reaching the crystal, the gamma ray is absorbed and the energy is given off in the form of a light flash or scintillation. The photomultiplier tubes collect the light and the output is used to record the position of the event. By collecting thousands of these events over a short period of time, a planar image of the activity is produced. In addition to conventional imaging with a gamma camera, there are two other forms of imaging: SPECT and PET. Single photon emission computed tomography (SPECT) uses the conventional gamma-emitting radiopharmaceuticals and a gamma camera designed to rotate around the patient. The name signifies that, at any instant in time, a single gamma photon is being detected. The data are reconstructed to form cross-sectional images in the same way as with X-ray CT scanning. SPECT images may be recorded following conventional planar imaging without increasing the amount of radio-activity administered to the patient.

7.3.2 Positron emission tomography

PET is a technique of growing importance in oncology. This technique is based on the use of short-lived positron emitting radionuclides such as fluorine-18 and carbon-11. Positrons are positively charged antimatter to the negatively charged electrons. When emitted by radioactive decay, positrons rapidly combine with electrons annihilating each other and producing two gamma photons each with energy of 511 keV and travelling in opposite directions. Imaging is performed using dedicated equipment known as a PET scanner (see Figure 7.3). This contains a ring of detectors for detection of the paired gamma rays. PET scanning is normally carried out in combination with CT scanning, using hybrid systems. This produces a fused image of the uptake of the PET tracer with a CT image, allowing the accurate identification of the anatomical site of uptake of the tracer. The main tracer used in oncology is F-18-fluorodeoxyglucose (FDG). This tracer essentially follows glucose uptake of tissues. FDG is brought inside the cell by specific transporters. Inside the cell, FDG undergoes enzymatic transforma-tion to FDG-6 phosphate. Thus it is effectively trapped in the cells, allowing the measurement of tissue glucose metabolism. Malignant tumours replace oxygen respira-tion by a fermentation of sugar. The phosphorylation process accumulates FDG-6 phosphate inside tumour cells where it is impossible for it to transfer outside the cell membrane. Although there is a relatively high cost for the installation of a PET scanner and the need for medical cyclotrons to produce the short-lived tracers, this type of

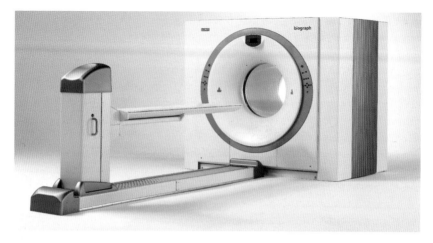

Figure 7.3   A PET CT scanner. Reproduced courtesy of Siemens Medical Solutions

imaging has proved to be cost effective in the management of many cancers such as lung, colon, head and neck and lymphoma.

7.3.3   Intra-operative probes

A further application that has proven to be of particular value in surgical oncology is the use of a sterile nuclear probe detector during surgery, to assist in the localization of tumours and certain other tissues prior to resection (Figure 7.4). Surgical intra-operative nuclear procedures include the use of the technetium-99m bone scanning agent (Tc-99m-HDP) for the intra-operative localization of osteoid osteoma and the use of Tc-99m-nanocolloid for the detection of sentinel nodes. This procedure is increasingly becoming a standard procedure in the management of patients with tumours of the breast and melanoma. The radiolabelled colloid is injected beneath the skin in close proximity to the tumour and will clear from the site through the lymphatic drainage system. The first lymph node the tracer accumulates in is the sentinel node. Once this has been identified using a combination of a blue dye and the probe detector, the node is removed and examined for evidence of tumour cells that may have been shed from the primary site. The presence or absence of tumour cells in this node will determine the nature of further treatment of the patient. In addition, a range of other radiopharmaceuticals for intra-operative tumour detection have been used, such as radiolabelled monoclonal antibodies.

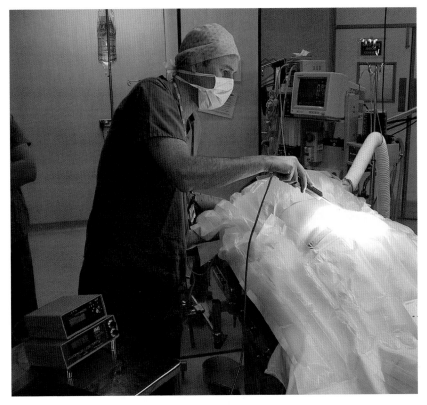

Figure 7.4 Use of a nuclear intra-operative probe to localize tumour uptake and so define the site for surgical excision prior to the start of surgery. Reproduced courtesy of Siemens Medical Solutions

7.4 Ultrasound imaging

Ultrasound imaging uses high frequency sound waves generally within the range of 1 to 20 megahertz (MHz). (The highest frequency of human hearing is around 20 000 Hz. Anything above this frequency is known as ultrasound.) The technique involves using a hand-held probe for scanning a focused beam of ultrasound into the body and then listening for reflected echoes. The principle is essentially the same as SONAR (sound navigation and ranging) used widely in sailing and ocean navigation.

A picture of an ultrasound scanner is given in Figure 7.5. The sound is generated by an array of transducer elements housed within the scanning probe (a transducer is a device that converts one form of energy to another). In the ultrasound probe, piezoelectric crystals are used that have the property of mechanically deforming when a voltage is placed across the opposite face of the crystal. In the scanning probe, the piezoelectric elements are used to convert electrical pulses to mechanical vibrations and vice versa. The probe is placed in contact with the skin and an acoustic coupling medium

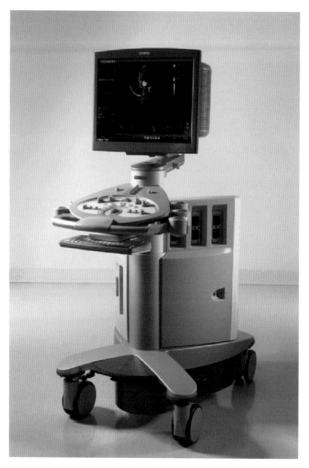

Figure 7.5   A real-time ultrasound scanner. Reproduced courtesy of Siemens Medical Solutions

(scanning jelly) is applied to aid the transmission of the sound from the probe to the patient. A pulse of sound is directed into the patient and reflections are generated at any change in acoustic impedance (Z), this being the product of the density (ρ) and the speed of sound (v) in the tissue, where $Z = \rho v$. The scanner measures the time taken for the returned pulse to be registered, assuming a mean value for the speed of sound in soft tissue of 1540 m/s. The position of the reflecting surface is registered as a bright spot on the display. After correcting for attenuation effects (energy losses), the final image is a map of sound echo levels in decibels (dB) displayed in a grey scale with the higher intensities displayed as brighter spots on the image. A real time image is produced by repeatedly scanning along the array of transducer elements to continually update the information. (In order to produce a smooth, flicker free image, the information has to be refreshed more frequently than 15 times per second.) Images are usually displayed as slices, but high quality three-dimensional displays are now widely available. Ultrasound is widely used for the examination of the breast and abdominal soft tissue masses, such as in the liver and kidneys. It is often the first line of investigation in the assessment of gynaecological tumours, since it is also widely used in obstetrics.

7.4.1 Colour doppler imaging

If the reflecting interface in the body is moving, a small change between the transmitted and reflected frequency of the sound is observed due to the Doppler effect. This effect has been used to identify information on blood flow and perfusion to tumours and is displayed as a colour image superimposed onto the grey scale image (Figure 7.6). Examples of equipment based on this principle include Duplex, Colour Doppler, Triplex and Power Doppler machines.

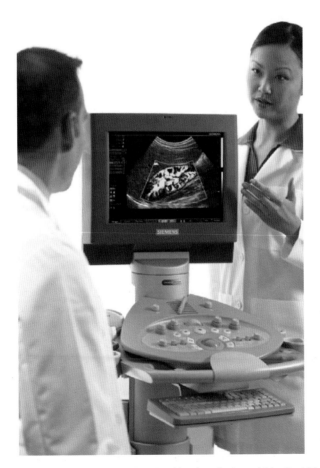

Figure 7.6 Colour Doppler image display showing blood perfusion within the kidney. Reproduced courtesy of Siemens Medical Solutions

Ultrasound equipment is relative inexpensive and mobile; however the accuracy of the diagnostic information depends upon the ability of the sonographer undertaking the examination. This type of investigation can easily be undertaken in the consulting room, intensive care unit or operating theatre. Ultrasound power levels are typically of the order of milliwatts per square cm (mW/cm^2). The main biological effect of ultrasound in tissues is one of mechanical vibration and heating. Mechanical effects include streaming and microbubble formation (cavitation). Virtually all experimental genetic studies undertaken in bacteria, yeast mammalian cells and laboratory animals have shown negative results. Despite the absence of adverse results from experimental studies it is still considered prudent to apply the basic principles of radiation protection to the medical use of ultrasound, with exposure being kept to a minimum, in relation to the clinical benefit. Guidelines for good practice have been established by bodies such as the American Institute for Ultrasound in Medicine (AIUM) and the European Federation of Societies of Ultrasound in Medicine and Biology (EFSUMB).

7.5   Magnetic resonance imaging

Magnetic resonance imaging (MRI) is one of the most recently introduced and possibly the most complex of imaging modalities. MR imaging was originally pioneered in the United Kingdom by Medical Physics researchers at the University of Nottingham and Aberdeen University. The basis of the technique is the magnetic dipole moment of protons within the nucleus of the hydrogen atoms. All charged atomic nuclei possess a magnetic moment. Protons are used for imaging because of the strong signal that can be generated due to the large amount of water in the body. Charged nuclei spin on an axis, in a circular path around the central direction of gravity. The motion of the axis about the direction of gravity is called precession. Protons are normally spinning with axes randomly orientated within the body. When the patient is placed in a strong magnetic field, they align either spin up or spin down, parallel with the magnetic field in a manner which could be likened to iron filings lining up on a sheet of paper above a bar magnet. By adding energy from a radio signal the protons can be raised to an excited state. After a period of time, they will give off this energy that can be detected as a radio signal. The time taken to give off this energy is called the relaxation time. Spatial information is obtained using a gradient magnetic field and scanning over the range of resonance frequencies for protons. A MRI system is shown in Figure 7.7. Most imaging systems use superconducting magnets with field strengths of between 0.5 to 7 Tesla, cooled with liquid helium to an operating temperature of about 4 K.

MRI excels in the examination of tumours of the brain and central nervous system as well as other lesions in bone and muscle. The use of ferromagnetic intravenous contrast media is an increasing component of diagnostic MRI investigations. The most commonly used agent is gadolinium-DTPA.

During the scan, the patient is exposed to static low frequency magnetic fields, time varying gradient magnetic fields and radio frequency waves. The entire body is placed in the magnet with no possibility for the screening of sensitive tissues. The scanning tunnel

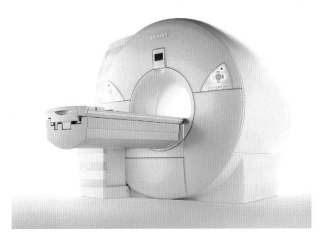

Figure 7.7 A 1.5 Tesla magnetic resonance imaging scanner. Reproduced courtesy of Siemens Medical Solutions

is relatively small and some patients can experience problems with claustrophobia, making the examination impossible in many cases. Some manufactures produce open magnet systems to reduce this problem and also to allow interventional procedures to be carried out during imaging. Experimental evidence indicates that acute human exposure to magnetic fields below 2.5 Tesla is unlikely to have any adverse effects on health. Nevertheless, exposure to such fields should only be undertaken with informed clinical guidance and some reservations still remain. Strong magnetic fields of up to 4 Tesla are known to exert a force on the flow of blood resulting in a reduction in blood flow and an increase in blood pressure. There have also been occasional reports of some subjects apparently experiencing vertigo, nausea and headache. Visual sensations due to magnetic phosphenes on movement of the head have also been described. Evaluation of the safety of the higher field strength systems is ongoing.

The magnitude of the magnetic field associated with magnetic resonance equipment is such that it is necessary to designate a controlled area around the magnet, normally to contain the 0.5 mTesla (5 Gauss) magnetic field contour. Access to this area by both patients and staff should be strictly controlled. Cardiac pacemakers are one the most well known contraindications for both patients and staff alike, since the field effects may cause malfunction of these devices. The presence of ferromagnetic objects and materials within patients in the form of implants and prostheses can also cause problems with MRI investigation. Ferromagnetic implants and clips are contraindicated because of the risk of rotational movement or displacement. Problems have also been encountered as a result of missile effects due to detachable objects carried by staff such as pins, scissors, keys, hairgrips and spectacles. These may be attracted towards the magnet causing both personal injury and damage to the equipment. These restrictions place particular constraints on anaesthesia and monitoring of patients whilst undergoing MRI investigations.

7.6   Radiation therapy

It is ironic that although exposure to ionizing radiation is known to have a direct link with the initiation and progression of cancer, it can also be used for its treatment. Within 3 years of the discovery of radioactivity in the form of radium by Marie Curie in 1898, early medical applications were being carried out. Initial radiation treatments were random and poorly conducted and there was evidence of much quackery and fraud. However, radium became widely used during the first half of the last century and, with the production of artificial radioactivity after the nuclear programmes of the 1950s, there was great enthusiasm for the clinical use of 'atoms for peace'. The basis of radiation therapy is the interaction of ionizing radiation (X-rays, gamma rays or electrons) with tissues at the intracellular level. This interaction depends on the energy created by the production of secondary charged particles, usually electrons, which can break chemical bonds and inflict molecular damage.

7.6.1   Therapeutic nuclear medicine

One of the main clinical applications for artificially produced radioactivity came with the production of iodine-131. In the body, iodine is virtually exclusively taken up by the thyroid gland in the neck. Administration of therapeutic amounts of iodine-131 is still widely used today as a major method for the treatment of thyroid cancer and thyrotoxicosis. Other forms of targeted radiotherapy are also widely used and many therapeutic radionuclides have been investigated as potential candidates for treatment purposes. These include beta-emitting radionuclides such as iodine-131, yttrium-90, samarium-153 and rhenium-186 and even alpha emitters such as astitine-211 and bismuth-212. For effective clinical use, it is essential that there is preferential uptake between tumour and normal tissue and that the tumour is radiosensitive. The use of therapeutic radiopharmaceuticals for targeting radioactivity to tumours is a particularly attractive approach since, for the more penetrating radiations, the radiopharmaceutical does not have to target every cell. Thus, beta emitters with a range of penetration of the order of millimetres in tissue offer the greatest potential for targeted therapy. Cell death may therefore be achieved along the path of the emitted radiation through a *bystander effect*.

The high uptake of bone seeking agents used in nuclear medicine has led to the widespread use of beta emitting agents for the palliation of painful bone metastases from carcinoma of the prostate and breast. The main radiopharmaceuticals available include Sm-153-EDTMP, Sr-89-chloride, and Re-186-HEDP. Radiopharmaceutical treatments generally provide effective pain relief with response rates of between 40 and 95 per cent. Pain relief starts at between 1 to 4 weeks after the initiation of treatment and continues for up to 18 months and reduces analgesic use in many patients. Mild and reversible thrombocytopenia and neutropenia are the most common toxic effects. Continued pain relief may be achieved in many patients by repeat administration.

One group of agents offering great potential as therapeutic radiopharmaceuticals are monoclonal antibodies. The specificity of the antibody–antigen interaction is indisputable and so antibodies represent powerful targeting molecules. Paul Ehrlich first suggested the concept of using antibodies to deliver substances to tumour cells in 1896 when he coined the term 'magic bullets'. A 'vehicle' with specificity for a receptor expressed solely on malignant cells serves as a carrier molecule for a cytotoxic agent. Delivery of the radionuclide to tumour cells causes specific cell killing while sparing normal cells the cytotoxic effects. One particularly promising product to be developed in recent years is Zevalin, an yttrium-90 labelled monoclonal antibody (ibritumomab) directed at non-Hodgkin's lymphoma. Some of the benefits of antibody therapy in non-Hodgkin's lymphoma (nHL) are:

- nHL is inherently sensitive to radiation.

- Radiotherapy can be curative in early stage nHL but is less easily applied to advanced stage disease.

- There is a synergistic activity between the antibody and the radionuclide.

- Yttrium-90 is suitable for outpatient administration without the need for patient isolation.

7.6.2   Brachytherapy

Although liquid forms of radioactivity can be administered both systemically and inserted into body cavities, one standard form of treatment involves inserting solid sources of radioactivity into body cavities and tissues. This type of therapy is known as brachytherapy; the term *brachy* comes from the Greek word for short distance. The radioactive sources act over a local short distance in tissues to treat the tumour whilst giving low doses to normal tissues. The most common uses of this type of therapy are found in gynaecological tumours and prostate cancer. For the treatment of gynaecological cancer, tubes are first inserted into the cervix and uterus and radioactive sources are then placed into the tubes. This is known as an after-loading technique. The patient is confined to the treatment room for the duration of the treatment. In prostate cancer a number of radioactive seeds (normally containing iodine-125) are implanted into the prostate gland to irradiate the tumour volume. Once inserted into the prostate gland the seeds are permanent, emitting low-level radiation, for approximately 1 year after implantation until they decay away to background levels.

7.6.3   External beam radiotherapy

The most common form of radiotherapy is external beam therapy. The process involves directing beams of radiation at tumour tissue with the minimal possible exposure to healthy tissue. Radiotherapy is often used in addition to surgery and chemotherapy. By delivering radiation from a number of different angles, a high dose can be deposited in the tumour whilst sparing normal tissues as much as possible. Radiotherapy is a complex procedure and requires the patient to make a number of hospital visits to complete a full course of treatment. The main stages in radiotherapy are:

- Positioning and immobilization of the patient.

- Localization of the tumour.

- Delineation of the target and critical tissue structures.

- Dose prescription and dose limitation.

- Treatment planning.

- Evaluation.

- Simulation and verification.

For precise therapy it is necessary to accurately locate the tumour and then immo-bilize the patient during each course of treatment. The full treatment is normally prescribed to be given in a series of sessions. This is known as dose fractionation. The treatment is then given over days or weeks to help the healthy tissue to recover from each episode of radiation exposure. Originally, this was undertaken using treatment units containing large sources of gamma radiation such as cobalt-60. However, external beam therapy is now undertaken using high energy medical linear accelerators (see Figure 7.8). The linear accelerator uses microwave technology to accelerate electrons along a 'wave guide'. The electrons then collide with a heavy metal target. As a result of the collisions, high-energy X-rays are scattered from the target. The X-rays are collected and shaped to form a beam that matches the patient's tumour. The beam emerges from a part of the accelerator called the gantry. The patient lies on a moveable treatment couch and lasers are used to make sure the patient is in the proper position. The gantry moves around the patient as radiation is delivered to the tumour. Linear accelerators normally produce either low-energy megavoltage X-rays (4–6 MeV), high-energy megavoltage X-rays (15–20 MeV) or electrons. Most patients are treated with X-rays because of the skin-sparing properties, good penetration and beam uniformity. Electron beams are useful for managing superficial tumours.

Advances in engineering, technology and computing, combined with an increased scientific understanding of radiobiology, have all contributed to advance the effective-ness of radiotherapeutic procedures. Linear accelerators now deliver a precise intensity modulated beam of radiation defined with multileaf collimators and offer the possibility for portal imaging for treatment verification. One particular problem in effective tumour therapy is in defining the volume of tumour to be treated. Imaging plays a major role in identifying the exact limits of tumour. Traditionally this has been

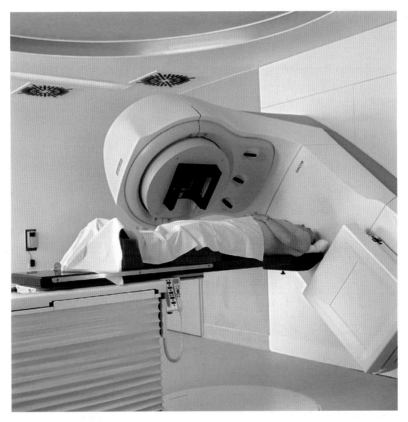

Figure 7.8 A linear accelerator in use for external beam radiotherapy. The gantry moves around the patient directing a prescribed dose of radiation to the tumour. Reproduced courtesy of Siemens Medical Solutions

undertaken with a treatment-planning simulator using a dedicated X-ray CT system, however the use of MRI and PET imaging is now widely practised. Cancer treatments often combine surgery and radiotherapy, since they complement one another very well. Surgery is good for the removal of large tumours. Radiotherapy is effective in treating microscopic disease. As a result, many diseases are treated with surgical intervention followed by a course of radiotherapy. As with any medical procedure, side effects can occur. The main side effect experienced by patients is a skin reaction to the radiation. This can be redness, itching, feeling of burning, soreness and possible peeling of the skin over the area being treated. In many ways this skin reaction is like sunburn, but this may be more in patches.

7.7 Conclusions

Imaging investigations provide essential information in the management of patients with cancer and play a major part in modern healthcare delivery. As can be seen, they not only aid in the initial diagnosis of the disease, but are also essential for assessing both the extent and stage of the disease. Diagnostic imaging systems all function by directing one or more forms of radiation into the patient. This may be ionizing radiation such as X or gamma rays, or other forms of radiation, such as sound or radio waves. The information received back is processed to produce the image. An experienced interpreter can assess the information contained in clinical images to help guide the oncologist to diagnose the disease and to help plan the best way to treat the patient. These images are also used to define the tumour for the delivery of radiation treatments. In this way imaging and radiotherapy are inextricably linked for the diagnosis, staging, planning, treatment and follow up of patients with malignant disease.

7.8 Acknowledgement

Thanks to Mark Hall and Andy Jeffery of Siemens Medical Solutions, Bracknell UK for supplying the equipment photographs and for giving permission for their publication in this chapter.

7.9 Self-assessment questions

Question:	Which are the main forms of radiation used in medical imaging and what are the main side effects?
Answer:	Ionizing radiations: X-rays in radiography, mammography and CT imaging, gamma rays in nuclear medicine, SPECT and PET imaging. Non-ionizing radiation: ultrasound, fluctuating magnetic radio waves in MRI. Risks associated with imaging: use of ionizing radiations include low radiation exposures and possible increased risk of cancer. Ultrasound can result in tissue heating and mechanical effects. MRI risks of rapidly changing field gradients, ferrous metal implants in the patient and projectiles in scanning rooms. Not suitable for patient with cardiac pacemakers. Some possibility of reaction to injected contrast agents.
Question:	How are imaging investigations used to help the management of patients with cancer?
Answer:	Imaging of patients enables non-invasive examination of internal organs and tissues and the assessment of abnormality. Imaging is used to diagnose primary tumours and metastatic involvement. It is also used in the assessment of the stage and grade of the disease.

Finally, imaging is used to determine the effect of treatment and to review any subsequent recurrence or progression of disease.

Question: What is the difference between an anatomical and functional imaging investigation? Give examples of each.

Answer: Imaging modalities used to outline anatomy, or structure includes radiography, mammography, X-ray CT, ultrasound and MRI. Use of contrast agents can add functional information to show movement and transit of the agent. Soft tissue detail is shown well by ultrasound. Real time ultrasound will show heart and vessel function with additional information given using Doppler imaging. Functional MRI will show neurological function. Nuclear medicine (SPECT and PET) is a physiological imaging modality and can show uptake, binding and metabolic activity.

Question: How are X-rays used in the diagnosis and treatment of cancer?

Answer: X-ray techniques include radiography, mammography and CT imaging. Radiography shows dense structure such as bone. Improved tissue contrast is achieved using CT imaging. Administration of contrast agents can aid diagnosis e.g. iodine contrast agents are used to demonstrate vascular abnormalities and barium enema to show colon tumours. High energy X-rays from linear accelerator are used for external beam radiotherapy.

Question: What are the three main types of radiation therapy used in cancer treatment?

Answer: (a) Therapeutic radiopharmaceuticals normally containing beta emitters, administered to the patient for *in vivo* targeted radiotherapy e.g. iodine-131 for treatment of thyroid cancer or use of yittrium-90-labelled antibody for non-Hodgkin's lymphoma.

(b) Brachytherapy, the insertion or implant of sources of radioactivity for local tumour therapy, e.g. iodine-125 seed for treatment of prostate cancer.

(c) Linear accelerator for external beam radiotherapy for deep or diffuse tumours. Planned treatment delivered from a gantry rotating through a number of different directions around the patient.

7.10 Further reading and resources

Administration of Radioactive Substances Advisory Committee. Notes for guidance on the clinical administration of radiopharmaceuticals and use of sealed radioactive sources. *Nucl Med Commun* 2000, **21**(Suppl), S1–93.

Brent RJ, Jensh RP and Beckman DA. Medical sonography: reproductive effects and risks. *Teratology* 1991, **44**, 123–146.

Curry TS, Dowey JE and Murry RC (eds) *Christensen's Physics of Radiology*, fourth edition. Lea and Febiger, Philadelphia, 1990.

Dawson LA and Sharpe MB. Image-guided radiotherapy: rationale, benefits, and limitations. *Lancet Oncol* 2006, **7**(10), 848–858.

Ferrari A, Rovera F, Dionigi P, *et al.* Sentinel lymph node biopsy as the new standard of care in the surgical treatment for breast cancer. *Exp Rev Anticancer Ther* 2006, **6**(10), 1503–1515.

Hailey D. Open magnetic resonance imaging (MRI) scanners. *Issues Emerg Health Technol* 2006, (92), 1–4.

ICRP Publication 52. *Protection of the patient in nuclear medicine*. Pergamon Press, Oxford, 1987.

ICRP Publication 53. *Radiation dose to patients from radiopharmaceuticals*. Pergamon Press, Oxford, 1988.

Kremkau FW. *Diagnostic Ultrasound*. WB Saunders, Philadelphia, 1998.

Marshall NW, Faulkner K, Busch HP, Marsh DM and Pfenning H. A comparison of radiation dose in examination of the abdomen using different radiological imaging techniques. *Br J Radiol* 1994, **67**, 478–484.

National Council on Radiation Protection and Measurement (NCRP). *Biological effects of ultrasound: mechanisms and clinical implications*. NCRP Report No 74, Bethesda MD, 1983.

Notes for guidance on the clinical administration of radiopharmaceuticals and use of sealed radioactive sources. Administration of Radioactive Substances Advisory Committee.

NRPB. *Protection of the patient in X-ray computed tomography*. Documents of the NRPB vol 3. no 4, 1992.

NRPB. *Board statement on clinical magnetic resonance diagnostic procedures*. Vol 2, No 1 HMSO, London, 1991.

Oriuchi N, Higuchi T, Ishikita T, Miyakubo M, Hanaoka H, Iida Y and Endo K. Present role and future prospects of positron emission tomography in clinical oncology. *Cancer Sci* 2006, **97**(12), 1291–1297.

Perkins AC and Hardy JG. Intraoperative nuclear medicine in surgical practice. *Nucl Med Commun* 1996, **17**, 1006–1015.

Perkins AC. *Nuclear Medicine Science and Safety*. John Libbey, London, 1995.

Royal College of Radiologists. *Making the best use of a department of radiology. Guidelines for doctors*, fifth edition. Royal College of Radiologists, London, 2003.

Samant R and Gooi AC. Radiotherapy basics for family physicians. Potent tool for symptom relief. *Can Fam Physician* 2005, **51**, 1496–1501.

Sanghani M and Mignano J. Intensity modulated radiation therapy: a review of current practice and future directions. *Technol Cancer Res Treat* 2006, **5**(5), 447–450.

Shrimpton P and Wall B. CT – An increasingly important slice of the medical exposure of patients. *Br J Radiol* 1993, **66**, 1067–1068.

Shrimpton P, Hart D, Hillier M, Wall B and Falkner. Survey of CT practice in the UK. Part 1: Aspects of examination frequency and quality assurance. NRPB-R248. HMSO, London, 1991.

Shrimpton PC, Wall BF and Hart D. Diagnostic medical exposures in the U.K. *Appl Radiat Isot* 1999, **50**, 261–269.

Silva AK, Silva EL, Egito ES and Carrico AS. Safety concerns related to magnetic field exposure. *Radiat Environ Biophys* 2006, **45**(4), 245–252.

Thacker J. Investigations into genetic effects and inherited changes produced by ultrasound. In: *Biological Effects of Ultrasound*. Nyborg WL and Ziskin MC, eds. Churchill Livingstone, Edinburgh, 1985.

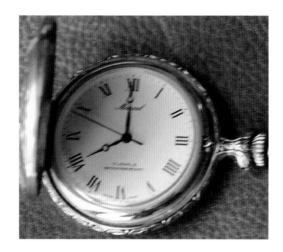

Surgery is one of the oldest procedures available for the cure of disease. The removal of diseased tissue to offer a cure to the individual has been applied since antiquity. Amputations or even cranial surgeries to relieve pressure and the use of implants have been identified in the remains found in excavation sites. Thus, it is not surprising that surgery for cancer was available much earlier than other cancer therapies were ever developed. However, during the last few years, surgery applied to cancer has developed into the specific discipline of surgical oncology, following the development of radiotherapy and chemotherapy as separate modalities. Furthermore, the surgeon, that in the past used to operate alone, is now a part of a big, multidisciplinary team.

Cancer therapy includes high degrees of specialization, with professionals even specializing in cancers of particular organs or types of tissues. In this respect, surgeons now specialize on particular organ-based groupings, such as dermatological, upper gastrointestinal, breast and colorectal cancers or even sub-specialities of hepato-pancreato-biliary, endocrine or vascular surgery. That has allowed specialized knowledge of both cancer biology and organ physiology, participation on research and clinical trials and integration in bigger, multidisciplinary teams in specialized cancer centres that offer the best care possible for the patients and the potential to result in the best outcome possible for the individual.

8

Surgery

Bassam Zeina

Milton Keynes General Hospital, UK and Teskreer Hospital, Damascus, SYRIA

8.1   Introduction

8.1.1   What is surgery?

Surgery is an operation to repair or remove part of the body, in order to diagnose or treat a condition.

8.1.2   What is cancer surgery?

Cancer surgery is basically removing cancer physically and is considered the foundation of cancer treatment.

8.1.3   Who deals with cancer surgery?

Modern oncology services take a team approach in the diagnosis and treatment of cancer. About 80 per cent of patients with suspected tumours are referred first to a surgeon.

It is essential that the surgical oncologist team requires a keen awareness of alternative, non-surgical treatment strategies, the role of adjuvant therapies, and maintain close collaboration in treatment protocols with oncology colleagues.

The Cancer Clock   Edited by Sotiris Missailidis
© 2007 John Wiley & Sons Ltd

8.1.4   Aims of cancer surgery

Cancer surgery may aim to achieve one or more of the following:

1. Diagnosing the cancer

2. Preventing the cancer

3. Treatment (removing the cancer)

4. Relieving the symptoms cancer may cause.

5. Cancer surgery may be the only treatment, or, more often, it may be supplemented with other treatments, such as chemotherapy and/or radiation.

8.2   Cancer surgery as a diagnostic procedure

It is often essential to study the growth under the microscope in order to determine whether the growth is malignant (cancerous) or benign (non-cancerous).

A form of cancer surgery is performed to recover a sample that can be studied or observed under the microscope to provide an accurate diagnosis, and this may include:

- A cytological diagnosis of malignancy following one of the following:

  o A smear

  o Fine needle aspirate

  o A needle core biopsy.

- Open surgical biopsy may be required before starting a treatment programme:

  o To remove a part (incisional biopsy)

  o To remove the entire tumour (excisional biopsy).

Important rules for cytological and tissue diagnostic procedures:

1. The tissues or cells should be representative of the whole lesion:

   a. When endoscopic or needle biopsies are used, multiple biopsies should be taken in order to avoid false negatives.

b. Areas of haemorrhage or necrosis should be avoided.

c. It is desirable to obtain adequate tissue at the first attempt.

2. When a deep as well as superficial lesion is biopsied, implantation of cells into deep and healthy tissues should be avoided.

3. Biopsies from skin and mucosal surfaces should include the interface between normal and abnormal tissue.

4. The diagnostic biopsy should not compromise any possible subsequent surgical or non-surgical treatment.

5. The histopathologist at the lab must be supplied with adequate clinical data.

6. The biopsy should be handled with care and it should not be crashed and traumatized during the procedure.

8.3   Cancer surgery as a preventive method against cancer

If it is suspected that cancer may develop in certain tissues or organs then a preventive operation may be applied to remove the tissue that is suspected to develop cancer. Thus, as a way of preventing cancer, it is recommended to consider removing those tissues or organs before cancer develops. For example, if a patient has a genetic condition called familial polyposis, cancer surgery may used to remove rectum and colon, because people with this condition have a considerable risk of developing colon cancer in the future. Similarly, women who have been identified bearing particular cancer related genes, such as *BRCA1* and *BRCA2,* and thus have high probability of developing breast cancer, are offered the possibility to have prophylactic surgery and remove their breast and ovaries, thus removing any possibility of such cancer ever developing. This may seem a very dramatic solution, especially for this particular cancer that has various psychosomatic implications, but it is often recommended and remains an acceptable choice within groups of women at high risk of developing the disease.

Other examples, where a pathology or even a tumour exists but is not yet malignant and is removed to avoid cancerous development, include the removal of the pancreas, total pancreatectomy, in patients with intraductal multifocal papillary mucinous tumour of the pancreas, or even liver transplantation for cases of advanced cirrhosis, in which small, undetectable hepatocellular carcinomas may develop, offering a means of preventing liver cancer. Some examples of prophylactic surgery for the prevention of cancer are shown in Table 8.1.

Table 8.1 Prophylactic surgery as a means of preventive cancers associated with a pathological condition or genetic predisposition (adapted from the IARC World Cancer Report)

Condition	Associated cancer	Prophylactic surgery
Cryptorchidism	Testicular	Orchidopexy
Familial colon cancer FAP, familial adenomatous polyposis or HNPCC, hereditary non-polyposis colorectal cancer	Colon	Colectomy
Ulcerative colitis	Colon	Colectomy
Multiple endocrine neoplasia MEN1, MEN2	Medullary cancer of the thyroid	Thyroidectomy
Familial breast cancer BRCA1, BRCA2	Breast	Radical mastectomy
Familial ovarian cancer BRCA1	Ovary	Oophorectomy
Intraductal multifocal papillary mucinous tumour of the pancreas	Pancreas	Total pancreatectomy
Liver cirrhosis	Liver	Liver transplantation

8.4 Cancer surgery as a treatment or part of the treatment

Common reasons for cancer surgery include one or more of the following:

8.4.1 Surgery as a primary treatment

Surgery gives the best chance for a cure for many tumours, especially if the cancer is localized and hasn't spread. In this case, the surgeon defines an area around the tumour and operates in this area in order to avoid cutting through the tumour or leaving remaining tumour mass that could subsequently spread or metastasize (see Figure 8.1).

Although the above defined method offers the best chances for success, it can often be mutilating and create a series of psychosomatic responses (see also Chapter 12). However, with the development of novel chemotherapeutic and radiotherapeutic approaches, a more conservative approach to surgery can be taken. This is often the case with mastectomy. Although radical mastectomy is very effective, it has been shown that in early stages of disease, where the size of invasive tumour is small due to early diagnosis through mammographic screening, conservative breast-conserving surgery following with postoperative radiotherapy and/or chemotherapy can offer similar results.

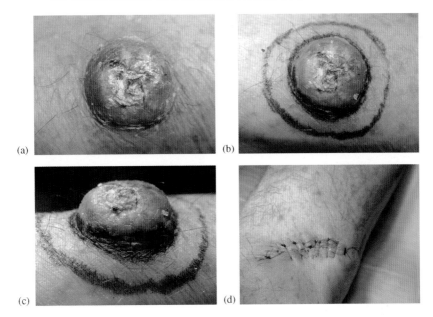

Figure 8.1 This man has a skin cancer on his left wrist (a); This was marked with a safety margin of normal looking skin (b,c); the skin cancer was removed and the skin was closed side to side using stitches (d)

8.4.2 Cancer staging

Staging defines how cancer is advanced. Surgery allows the doctor to evaluate the size of the tumour and determine whether it has travelled to the lymph nodes and other organs.

8.4.3 Debulking (cytoreductive) surgery

Debulking is used when it is not possible to remove all of a tumour, as doing so may harm an important organ severely. In this case, the surgeon may remove as much of the tumour as possible (debulking) in order to make chemotherapy or radiation therapy more effective. Cytoreductive surgery is often employed as the primary treatment of ovarian cancer as well as cancer of the biliary tract.

8.4.4 Palliative surgery (relieving symptoms or side effects)

Cancer surgery could also be used to improve quality of life rather than treat the cancer itself. When pain is caused by a tumour that is pressing on an organ, a nerve or bone, cancer surgery is used to relieve the pain caused. Another example might include removing tumours that are obstructing the lungs or intestine. For example, some cancers in the abdomen may grow large enough to obstruct the intestine. This may require surgery for effective relief.

Surgery is often combined with other cancer treatments, such as chemotherapy and radiation therapy. The choice of cancer treatment depends on the type of cancer and its stage and it is decided by the oncology team after consideration of the options.

8.5 Classic/traditional cancer surgery

The aim of cancer surgery is physically removing all of the cancerous cells from the body. The surgeon usually does this by cutting into the body and removing the cancer along with some surrounding healthy looking tissue, to ensure that all of the cancer is removed. In order to determine if the cancer has spread, some lymph nodes in the area may also be removed. Taking some regional lymph node helps to assess the chance of the patient being cured, as well as the need for any further treatment and the regime to be followed.

In classic/traditional cancer surgery a scalpel or other cutting instruments are used, aiming to completely remove the cancer and surrounding margin of tissue or nearby lymph nodes. For example, in the case of breast cancer, the surgeon may treat the breast cancer by removing the whole breast or by removing the cancer and some of the surrounding healthy looking tissue and some or all lymph nodes under the armpit.

8.6 Other common techniques in cancer surgery

Many other surgical techniques and methods for treating cancer and precancerous conditions exist, as instrumentation and practices have evolved over the years. Some common types of cancer surgery are now listed.

8.6.1 Electrosurgery

Electrosurgery is the use of high-frequency electrical currents to kill cancer cells, for example on the skin.

8.6.2 Cryosurgery

Cryosurgery is the use of very cold material, such as liquid nitrogen spray, or a cold probe to freeze and destroy cancer cells or cells that may become cancerous, such as lesions on the skin and irregular cells in the cervix that could change and form cervical cancer.

8.6.3   Laser surgery and photo dynamic therapy (PDT)

Laser uses beams of high-intensity light to vaporize cancer cells. In some cases, the heat of the laser accomplishes this. In other cases, the laser or non-laser light is used in photo-dynamic therapy to activate a previously administered chemical (dye) that cancer cells absorb. When the chemical is stimulated by light, the chemical generates very active species called free radicals (see Chapter 2) that kill the cancer cells.

8.6.4   Mohs' micrographic surgery

In Mohs' surgery, the cancer is removed piece by piece. Each piece removed is examined microscopically straight away. If examination under the microscope shows that some cancer might still be present, then more tissue is removed and examined. This process continues until there are no signs of any cancer cells left. This technique minimizes the removal of healthy tissue, while making sure that the cancer has all been taken away. It is useful for removing cancer from sensitive areas such as near the eye and for assessing how deep a cancer goes.

8.6.5   Laparoscopic surgery

A laparoscope is used to see inside the body without making large incisions. Instead, several small incisions are made and surgical tools and a tiny camera are inserted into the body. The surgeon watches a monitor that projects what the camera sees inside the body. Laparoscopic surgery is used in cancer diagnosis, treatment, staging and symptom relief.

8.6.6   Image-guided surgery

Many cancers can be treated using image-guided surgery, which is less invasive than traditional surgery. In this type of surgery the surgeon can rely on real-time images of the body for guidance when operating. For instance, rather than opening the skull to see inside the brain, the surgeon may use magnetic resonance imaging (MRI) to visualize the surgery site. MRI images allow the surgeon to be very precise and avoid critical sites. Other imaging techniques are used as well, including ultrasound and computerized tomography (CT).

   Cancer surgery continues to evolve. Researchers are investigating other surgical techniques with an eye toward less invasive and more efficient procedures.

8.7   Before and after cancer surgery

Preparation and healing from cancer surgery varies greatly based on the cancer and the organ affected, the surgical technique and the patient's health. But in general this includes three stages.

8.7.1   Preparation for the surgery

Most patients may undergo certain tests, such as blood tests, urine tests, X-rays and other imaging tests, in the days preceding the surgery. These tests will help the doctor assess the patient's surgical needs, such as the blood type in case a transfusion is needed, and identify potential risks, such as infections, that may influence the surgery.

8.7.2   Anaesthesia

When a patient is undergoing surgery, they will need some type of anaesthetic (a medication that blocks the sensation of pain). Options for anaesthesia will be based on the type of cancer surgery. This could be local or general anaesthesia.

8.7.3   Recovery

Recovery depends largely on the type of surgery. The patient may stay in the hospital for a significant amount of time before going home, or may be released in a very short time and additional home or outpatient support may be provided (see also Chapters 10 and 11).

8.8   Cancer surgery associated risks

The techniques used in cancer surgery have improved dramatically in recent years. However, everything from removing a mole to open heart surgery involves risk. A brief overview of these risks is given below:

- *Pain*   Pain is a common side effect of most operations. Some operations are more painful than others. Pain can be kept to a minimum by taking appropriate medication.

- *General anaesthesia risk*   Any time a patient go under general anaesthesia, he is at some risk, although the risks in modern units are extremely low and estimated at around one death in 200, 000 cases.

- *Bleeding*   All surgical procedures carry a risk of bleeding. Bleeding depends on the type of operation and the organ involved. Most patients may experience a small degree of bleeding under the dressing. But, this is not generally a problem. Excessive bleeding, during or after cancer surgery, depends on the organ involved, the type and size of cancer, and the operation technique used but in general it is rare. The patient may consider donating blood before surgery.

- *Infection* The surgical site may become infected. Infection can lengthen the recovery time after surgery. Wound infections are generally treated with antibiotics.

- *Partial or complete loss of an organ* The surgeon may need to remove a part or an entire organ, in order to the remove the cancer. Thus cancer surgery may leave the patient without a part of a limb, a kidney, a breast. This can have implications in the lifestyle and subsequent care of the patient.

- *Venous clots* This complication might happen while recovering from surgery and can be very serious. Blood clots most commonly occur in the lower legs. The clot can be very dangerous and even deadly if the blood clot breaks off and travels to the lung. Getting the patient up and out of bed as soon as possible after the operation will decrease this possible side effect.

- *Altered bladder and bowel function* Immediately after the surgery some patients may experience difficulty emptying the bladder and/or having a bowel movement. Typically this lasts for only few days and is dependent on the specific anaesthesia.

- *Problems with wound healing* include haematoma (an accumulation of blood in the wound) and seroma, an accumulation of clear fluid in the wound. Both usually respond readily to treatment.

- *Lymphoedema* Sometimes after surgery it may be harder than before for lymph fluid to drain from the surgical site. This can result in swelling in the limb after breast surgery, for example. There are many ways to prevent and manage lymphoedema (see Chapter 11).

- *Anxiety* Whatever cancer treatment is recommended, almost every one will feel some anxiety about the condition, the surgery and the treatment process. Knowing what to expect can help. Patients are encouraged to talk with their doctor and ask informed questions. Details of the psychological aspects related with cancer will be discussed in detail at a later chapter within this book (Chapter 12).

8.9 Informed consent

Before any surgery the patient is generally asked to sign a form called 'informed consent'. This means that the patient is agreeing to the surgery, fully understanding what is going to happen and what risks are accepted in the process. The patients are encouraged to have time to read and understand the process and risks before they sign their 'informed consent' form.

Informed consent forms are designed to make sure that:

1. The doctor has told the patient exactly the surgical plan.

2. The patient is aware of alternative treatment options.

3. The patient understands the plan for surgery and its associated risks.

Patients are advised to read over the form carefully. Be sure to sign a consent form only for the procedure that the patient and doctor have discussed and agreed upon in advance.

8.10   Summary

Surgery is the first method applied for the treatment of cancer and remains a cornerstone in the primary care of cancer patients. Oncology surgery constitutes the removal of all or part of the tumour for diagnosis or treatment of the disease. Surgical oncology has emerged as a specialist discipline and professionals that specialize on particular organs or tumours form part of a large, multidisciplinary group of professionals in dedicated cancer centres. Surgery can be either prophylactic, in the case that genetic or disease factors indicate high risk of cancer development to justify the removal or organs or tissue to prevent malignancy, diagnostic, when tissue is removed for observation to confirm is malignant or benign nature, or therapeutic, where all or part of the cancer is removed as part of a treatment regime. Surgery is often used as part of regime, together with pre and post-operative chemotherapy and radiotherapy. This, together with early diagnosis of the disease, has often led to less mutilating applications of surgery and reduced risks and side effects. Furthermore, technological developments have offered various alternatives to classic surgery that may be more efficient and/or less invasive for particular types of cancer and facilitate less hospital stay and faster rehabilitation.

8.11   Self-assessment questions

Questiogn: What is surgery and what is cancer surgery?

Answer: Surgery is an operation to repair or remove part of the body, in order to diagnose or treat a condition. Cancer surgery is the physical removal of cancer.

Question: What are the main aims of cancer surgery?

Answer: The main aims of cancer surgery are cancer prevention, diagnosis and treatment or the relief of symptoms associated with cancer.

Question: Name kinds of surgery related to cancer therapy.

Answer: Surgery in the treatment of cancer is used either as primary treatment, cancer staging, debulking or palliative care.

Question: Name some of the types of surgery used in the treatment of cancer.

Answer: Classical or traditional surgery, electrosurgery, cryosurgery, laser surgery and photodynamic therapy, Moh's micrographic surgery, laparoscopy, image-guided surgery.

Question: Describe image-guided surgery.

Answer: In this type of surgery the surgeon can rely on real-time images of the body for guidance when operating. For instance, rather than opening the skull to see inside the brain, the surgeon may use magnetic resonance imaging (MRI) to visualize the surgery site. MRI images allow the surgeon to be very precise and avoid critical sites. Other imaging techniques are used as well, including ultrasound and computerized tomography (CT).

Question: Name some potential risks associated with surgery.

Answer: Pain, general anaesthesia, bleeding, infection, partial or complete loss of an organ, venous clots, altered bladder or bowel function, wound healing, lymphedema, anxiety.

8.12 Further reading and resources

Barr L, Cowan R and Nicolson M. Managing patients with cancer. In: *Churchills's Pocketbook of Oncology*. Churchill Livingstone, Edinburgh, 1999, pp. 2–15.

Norman Coleman C. Diagnosis and treatment. In: *Understanding Cancer*. The Johns Hopkins University Press, Baltimore, 1998, pp. 10–27.

http://www.healthline.com/galecontent/surgical-oncology [accessed 26 April 2007] http://www.med.nyu.edu/mininvasive/surgeries/cancer/ [accessed 26 April 2007]

http://www.lef.org/protocols/prtcl-026.shtml [accessed 26 April 2007]

http://www.mayoclinic.com/health/cancer-surgery/CA00033 [accessed 26 April 2007]

World Cancer Report, World Health Organization, International Agency for Research on Cancer, Stewart B.W and Kleihues (eds), IARC Press, 2003.

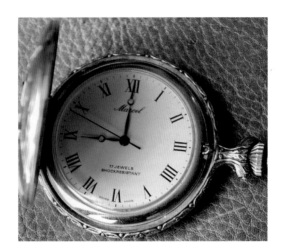

In the previous chapters we have already discussed two potential therapeutic approaches against cancer, radiotherapy and surgery. However, one of the front lines of dealing with cancer is cancer therapeutics. It is a vast area that covers the use of any molecular entities with potential therapeutic properties against the disease. Some of the first cancer chemotherapy agents were based on the nitrogen mustards, molecules used in chemical warfare during the Second World War. Probably the most widely used cancer therapy agents are based on the fact that cancer cells divide rapidly compared to normal cells. In fact, some of the kinds of cancer that are offering better therapeutic outcomes, such as various leukaemias, do so because they have a very short doubling time compared to the normal cells. Thus, they get more affected by the chemotherapy agents that target cellular DNA and block transcription and replication. On the other hand, cancers that multiply more slowly, in a matter of days or weeks, appear more resistant to such therapies because damage to normal cells becomes considerable and therapy has to stop before cure has been achieved.

Improved knowledge of cancer biology and the various cellular pathways has allowed the development of agents that target particular receptor proteins with promising results and reduced side effects. Furthermore, the development of immunotherapies and biologics, such as antibodies, has seen a bloom in the development of cancer therapeutics with more FDA approvals in the past 5 years than ever before. Finally, the complicated nature of the disease and the development of resistance warrant, more often than not, the use of multi-agent treatment regimes that can target cancer from various points simultaneously, increasing therapeutic potential. This is a dramatically changing arena with constant development and many compounds in the company pipelines.

9

Anticancer therapeutics

Teni Boulikas, Nassos Alevizopoulos, Angela Ladopoulou, Maria Belimezi, Alexandros Pantos, Petros Christofis and Michael Roberts

Regulon Inc. (USA), Athens, Greece

9.1 Introduction

Approximately 210 cancer types are present in the entries of the National Cancer Institute in USA (http://www.cancer.gov/cancertopics/alphalist [accessed 3 May 2007]). Overall, cancers of the lung, breast, bowel, stomach and prostate account for almost half of all cancer diagnosed worldwide. However, the types of cancer being diagnosed vary enormously across the world. For example, prostate cancer represents 16 per cent of all cancers in North America but only 8 per cent of cancers in southern Europe. Even more strikingly, gastric and liver cancers represent 19 per cent and 14 per cent, respectively, of all cancer cases in eastern Asia, whereas these two cancer forms have a very low incidence in North America and Europe and are not present in the four most frequent cancers. Total new cancer cases per 10 000 population per year also vary among geographical regions from the highest 331 in North America to 93 in western Africa. The cancer death rate per 10 000 population per year also varies among geographical regions from 133 in eastern Europe to 70 in South Central Asia (see http://info.cancerresearchuk.org/cancerstats/geographic/world/commoncancers/ [accessed 3 May 2007])

9.1.1 Problems in cancer

Problems in cancer biology that are crucial points for intervention to combat cancer include early detection, genotyping and identification of gene expression profiling that

The Cancer Clock Edited by Sotiris Missailidis
© 2007 John Wiley & Sons Ltd

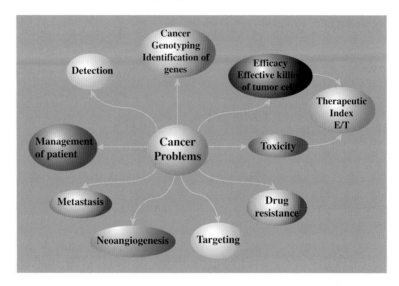

Figure 9.1 Summary of the unmet needs or problems in cancer

might determine which chemotherapy regimes to follow, the efficacy of a chemotherapy treatment and the side effects, killing chemoresistant tumours after failure of front-line chemotherapy, targeting solid tumours and metastases with minimal damage to normal tissue, arresting the process of neoangiogenesis responsible for sprouting of new vessels within growing tumours, preventing metastasis of malignant cells and the management of the cancer patient (Figure 9.1).

Major hurdles arise from toxicity of currently available chemotherapy regimes and inefficiency of cancer treatments, especially for advanced stage of the disease, chemoresistance of tumours and inability to cope with many sites of tumour progression after spreading of the disease. One additional obstacle in oncology is how to implement ingenious discoveries deciphering pathways of molecular carcinogenesis and ways to arrest tumour cell proliferation leading to new experimental molecules, targeting a plethora of cancer mechanisms, to the clinic. Although these studies often work in cell culture, the success rate of new drugs from inception to clinical application and marketing is 1 per cent. Unmet needs across the cancer market remain high, with most therapies conferring low levels of specificity and high toxicity.

9.1.2 Cancer treatments

Although chemotherapy, surgery and radiotherapy continue to be the mainstay treatments of cancer, a number of additional modalities are currently used or are expected to change the landscape of the anticancer drug market and the ways hospitals undertake management of cancer patients. Biological drugs and targeted therapies (Figure 9.2) are those that are aimed at specific cellular targets such as small molecules that inhibit a specific protein molecule that is a key player in signal transduction, in apoptosis, in the cell cycle or in other important cellular pathways. For example, Tarceva is a small molecule

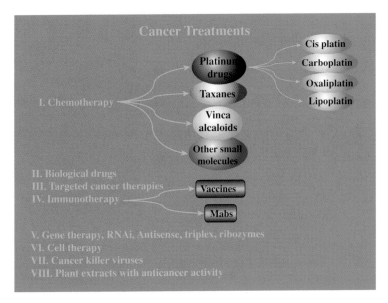

Figure 9.2 A glimpse of cancer treatments currently in use or expected to provide important drugs or approaches in the near future

(see below) that functions by inhibiting the epidermal growth factor receptor (EGFR) whose function is required by many cancer cells and as a result EGFR is overexpressed in several cancers. Drug discovery by screening of libraries of 10^{12} or more small molecules for a specific function is an effervescent field in anticancer drug discovery.

Proteins that play a key function in cellular processes of cancer cells might also be targets of gene therapy, of RNAi (inhibitory RNA also called small interfering RNA, siRNA), antisense, ribozymes, aptamers and triplex-forming oligodeoxyribonucleotides. Cell therapy, still at its infancy in the field of cancer, can become an important future player in cancer immunotherapy. Cancer cells can be removed from a patient, transduced *ex vivo* with genes such as for interleukin-2 (*IL-2*), and reintroduced under the skin of the patient to elicit an immune reaction against his/her tumour. Use of monoclonal antibodies aimed at a target such as Her2/neu (trastuzumab, commercial name: Herceptin), vascular endothelial cell growth factor (VEGF; bevacizumab) or EGFR (cetuximab, commercial name: Erbitux) made an important impact recently in the treatment of cancer. Herceptin is the first antibody to receive US Food and Drug Administration (FDA) approval whereas Avastin received FDA approval as first line treatment against non-small cell lung cancer (NSCLC) and is expected to become a blockbuster drug. A method older than Hippocrates has been used extensively by modern drug designers and pharmaceutical companies. We trust that nature has developed mechanisms in plants, marine organisms and others to keep proliferating cells under control. Our job then, is to test whole extracts, then fractions and finally individual components for anticancer activities in cell cultures or animals. We then try to come up with the identification of the compounds endowed with anticancer activity, the elucidation of their structure and methods for chemical synthesis to spare depletion or destruction of the plant or marine organism. Such an example of human ingenuity led to the development of taxanes and epothilones, whereas vinca alkaloids also owe their development to plants.

9.1.3 Classification of chemotherapy drugs

Chemotherapy drugs can be classified into six major groups (Figure 9.3). These are:

1. *Platinum co-ordination complex*: (a) cisplatin, (b) carboplatin, (c) oxaliplatin.

2. *Antimicrotubule agents*: (a) vinca alkaloids (vinblastine, vinorelbine), (b) taxanes (paclitaxel, docetaxel).

3. *Antimetabolites*: (a) methotrexate, (b) fluoropyrimidines (e.g. 5-fluorodeoxyuridine (5FU), capecitabine), (c) cyrocine arabinose (e.g. cytarabine), (d) gemcitabine.

4. *Antitumour antibiotics*: (a) actinomycin D, (b) mitomycin C, (c) bleomycin, (d) anthracyclines (doxorubicin, daunorubicin), (e) podophyllotoxins (etoposide, teniposide), (f) camptothecins (irinotecan, topotecan).

5. *Alkylating agents*: (a) cyclophosphamide, (b) nitrogen mustard- or L-phenylalanine mustard-based agents (mechlorethamine & melphalan, respectively), (c) nitrosoureas e.g. carmustine, (d) alkane sulfonates, e.g. busulfan.

6. *Others*, includes drugs that do not fall into any of these categories.

Since the scope of this review is to present emerging therapeutics in cancer, a number of drugs at the clinical level or preclinical stage will also be presented, though the list is not exhaustive.

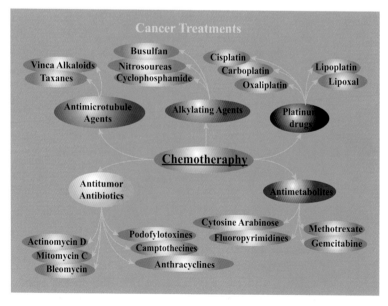

Figure 9.3 Classification of chemotherapy drugs

9.2 Platinum drugs

9.2.1 Cisplatin

Cisplatin (Figure 9.4), since its serendipitous discovery in 1965, its identification in 1969 and its clinical application in the early 1970s, continues to be a cornerstone of modern

(a) **Cisplatin, Carboplatin and Nedaplatin and their adducts in DNA.**

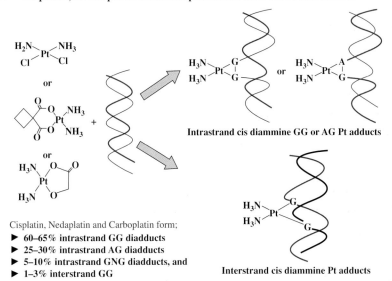

Cisplatin, Nedaplatin and Carboplatin form;
▶ **60–65% intrastrand GG diadducts**
▶ **25–30% intrastrand AG diadducts**
▶ **5–10% intrastrand GNG diadducts, and**
▶ **1–3% interstrand GG**

Intrastrand cis diammine GG or AG Pt adducts

Interstrand cis diammine Pt adducts

(b) **Oxaliplatin and its adducts in DNA.**

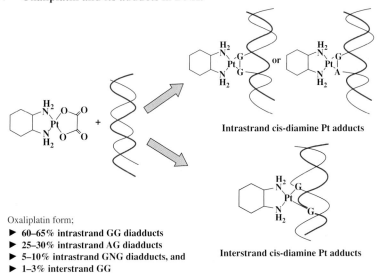

Oxaliplatin form;
▶ **60–65% intrastrand GG diadducts**
▶ **25–30% intrastrand AG diadducts**
▶ **5–10% intrastrand GNG diadducts, and**
▶ **1–3% interstrand GG**

Intrastrand cis-diamine Pt adducts

Interstrand cis-diamine Pt adducts

Figure 9.4 Differences in DNA adduct formation between platinum compounds with two amino groups on the Pt atom (a) and those of oxaliplatin (b)

chemotherapy playing an important role among cytotoxic agents in the treatment of epithelial malignancies. Cisplatin, usually in combination with other drugs, is being used as first line chemotherapy against cancers of the lung, head-and-neck, oesophagus, stomach, colon, bladder, testis, ovaries, cervix, uterus, and as second line treatment against most other advanced cancers such as cancers of the breast, pancreas, liver, kidney, prostate as well as against glioblastomas, metastatic melanomas, and peritoneal or pleural mesotheliomas. The clinical use of cisplatin has been impeded by severe adverse reactions including renal toxicity, gastrointestinal toxicity, peripheral neuropathy, asthenia, and ototoxicity.

Cisplatin reacts directly with sulfur groups (such as glutathione) and intracellular levels of glutathione have been linked to cisplatin detoxification. The antitumour properties of cisplatin are attributed to the kinetics of its chloride ligand displacement reactions leading to DNA crosslinking activities (Figure 9.4). DNA crosslinks inhibit replication, transcription and other nuclear functions and arrest cancer cell proliferation and tumour growth. A number of additional properties of cisplatin are now emerging including activation of signal transduction pathways leading to apoptosis. Firing of such pathways may originate at the level of the cell membrane after damage of receptor or lipid molecules by cisplatin, in the cytoplasm by modulation of proteins via interaction of their thiol groups with cisplatin, for example involving kinases and other enzymes, or finally from DNA damage via activation of the DNA repair pathways.

Cisplatin, when combined with other cytotoxic agents, has shown an improved response rate and survival in a moderate to high number of patients suffering from a number of malignancies. Furthermore, a number of agents have been shown to ameliorate experimental cisplatin nephrotoxicity; these include antioxidants (e.g. melatonin, vitamin E, selenium, and many others), modulators of nitric oxide (e.g. zinc histidine complex), agents interfering with metabolic pathways of cisplatin (e.g. procaine HCl), diuretics (e.g. furosemide (frusemide) and mannitol), and cytoprotective and antiapoptotic agents (e.g. amifostine and erythropoietin). On the contrary, nitric oxide synthase inhibitors, spironolactone and gemcitabine augment cisplatin nephrotoxicity. Various pathways can also lead to cisplatin resistance. Thus, the discovery of novel platinum molecules could lead to novel advancements in bypassing cisplatin resistance. Some of the next generation platinum compounds will be presented below.

9.2.2 Lipoplatin™

The Lipoplatin™ formulation is based on the formation of reverse micelles between cisplatin and 1,2-dipalmitoylphosphatidylglycerol (DPPG) under special conditions of pH, ethanol, ionic strength and other parameters. Cisplatin-DPPG reverse micelles are subsequently converted into liposomes by interaction with neutral lipids. Lipoplatin and the platform encapsulation technology applied to its manufacturing procedure adds a strong tool in molecular oncology to wrap up preexisting anticancer drugs into nanoparticle formulations that alter their biodistribution, lower their side effects, minimize the toxic exposure to normal tissues while maximizing tumour uptake and

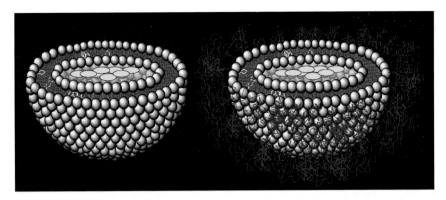

Figure 9.5 Section through a nanoparticle showing the lipid bilayer and the cisplatin molecules in its lumen (yellow spheres) (left) and that of Lipoplatin nanoparticle (right) showing the PEG molecules on its surface (red hair-like structures) coating the particle with a hydrophilic inert polymer giving the ability to escape detection from macrophages and evade immune surveillance. From Boulikas T, Pantos A, Christofis P, *et al. Cancer Ther* 2007, **5**, in press, with kind permission

penetration of the drug. The shell of the liposome in the Lipoplatin formulation has a number of patented features that differentiates it from previous drug formulations. The negatively charged DPPG molecule on the surface gives to the nanoparticles their fusogenic properties, an important feature for cell entry across the nuclear membrane barrier (Figure 9.5). In addition, their small size results in passive extravasation to tumours, whereas a more avid phagocytosis characteristic of tumour cells further enhances the intracellular and nuclear uptake of the drug. A polyethylene glycol-coating also gives to the particles long circulation properties in body fluids, essential for tumour accumulation. For example, Phase I studies have shown a half-life of 120 h for Lipoplatin at 100 mg/m^2 compared to 6 h for cisplatin.

One important issue contributing to the therapeutic efficacy of Lipoplatin^{TM} results from its ability to target primary tumours and metastases and to cause a greater damage to tumour tissue compared to normal tissue. During tumour growth, neo-angiogenesis is needed to develop tumour vasculature to enable supply with nutrients for growth and expansion in a process known as neoangiogenesis. The tumour uptake of Lipoplatin^{TM} results from the preferential extravasation of the 100-nm liposome nanoparticles through the leaky vasculature of tumours. Indeed, the endothelium of the vascular walls during angiogenesis has imperfections that need a certain period for maturation. During angiogenesis, Lipoplatin^{TM} particles with long circulation properties evade immune surveillance and are able to pass through the leaky vasculature and concentrate in the tumour at about 2- to 40-fold higher concentrations compared to the adjacent normal tissue in human studies. One additional mechanism for the higher accumulation of Lipoplatin^{TM} in tumour tissue, compared to normal tissue, arises from the higher uptake of Lipoplatin^{TM} nanoparticles by tumours presumably arising from a more avid phagocytosis by tumour cells. The second mechanism results to a average of 5- to 10-fold higher uptake of Lipoplatin by tumour cells, compared to normal cells in human studies giving an overall 10 to 400-fold higher tumour cell uptake and binding to macromolecules.

The introduction of Lipoplatin[TM] has been an advancement in the field of platinum drugs mainly because of its ability to circulate with a half-life of ~100 h compared to 6 h for cisplatin, to have substantially reduced the nephrotoxicity, ototoxicity and neurotoxicity and to concentrate in tumours. Lipoplatin[TM] is currently under several Phase III evaluations in combination with gemcitabine or paclitaxel as first line treatment against NSCLC and is being compared to cisplatin plus gemcitabine or paclitaxel respectively. A third Phase III trial uses Lipoplatin[TM] in combination with 5 FU as first line treatment against head and neck cancers and is being compared to cisplatin plus 5 FU. All three trials have shown very promising results and Lipoplatin has shown the ability to preferentially concentrate in malignant tissue both of primary and metastatic origin following intravenous infusion to patients and reduce the side effects observed with cisplatin. In this respect, Lipoplatin emerges as a very promising drug in the arsenal of chemotherapeutics.

9.2.3   Carboplatin

Over 20 years of intensive work toward improvement of cisplatin, and with hundreds of platinum drugs tested, has resulted in the introduction of the drugs carboplatin and oxaliplatin, used only for a narrow spectrum of cancers. The inception and promotion to the clinic of platinum drugs have been milestone achievements in clinical oncology.

Cisplatin analogues have been marketed (carboplatin, oxaliplatin) but none as yet has achieved a similar broad-spectrum effectiveness. Carboplatin proved markedly less toxic to the kidneys and nervous system than cisplatin and caused less nausea and vomiting, while generally (and certainly for ovarian cancer) retaining equivalent anti-tumour activity. Carboplatin constitutes a reasonable alternative to cisplatin in a combination with gemcitabine, since it shows synergy with gemcitabine *in vitro*, is easier to use in ambulatory patients, and has a better nonhaematologic toxicity profile. The combination of carboplatin with gemcitabine (Gemzar), initially hampered by unacceptable platelet toxicity, has gained increasing acceptance against NSCLC. Combinations of carboplatin with paclitaxel or docetaxel are also used against NSCLC, and carboplatin was shown to be a safe and effective first-line treatment for women with advanced ovarian cancer. Furthermore, carboplatin has been used in combination with other drugs for the treatment of prostate cancer, children with Wilm's tumour, anaplastic astrocytomas and glioblastomas.

9.2.4   Oxaliplatin

Oxaliplatin, produces the same type of inter- and 1,2-GG intrastrand cross-links as cisplatin (see Figure 9.4B) but has a spectrum of activity and mechanisms of action and resistance different from those of cisplatin and carboplatin. The cellular and molecular aspects of the mechanism of action of oxaliplatin have not yet been fully elucidated. However, oxaliplatin presents lack of cross-resistance with cisplatin and carboplatin. The anticancer effects of oxaliplatin are optimized when it is administered in combination with other anticancer agents, such as 5 FU, gemcitabine, cisplatin, carboplatin, topoisomerase I inhibitors, and taxanes. Oxaliplatin has a unique pattern of side effects and besides neurotoxicity they include haematological toxicity and gastrointestinal tract toxicity. Nausea and vomiting is usually mild to moderate and readily controlled with standard antiemetics. Sporadically, severe side effects may be observed such as tubular necrosis. Oxaliplatin, in combination with 5 FU, has been recently approved in Europe, Asia, Latin America and later in the USA (2003) for the treatment of metastatic colorectal cancer and has improved the response rate, progression-free and overall survival of patients with advanced colorectal cancer.

Recently, oxaliplatin has been used in a liposomal formulation achieved using Regulon's platform technology, Lipoxal. The drug finished stability test and preclinical studies and was approved for Phase I evaluation in patients with advanced disease of the gastrointestinal system (stage IV gastrointestinal cancers including colorectal, gastric and pancreatic) who had failed previous standard chemotherapy. Liposomal oxaliplatin (lipoxal) is a well-tolerated agent. Whereas the main adverse reactions of oxaliplatin are neurotoxicity, haematological and gastrointestinal toxicity; its liposomal encapsulation (Lipoxal) has reduced the haematological and gastrointestinal toxicity without reducing its effectiveness. Future studies are aimed at demonstrating the tumour targeting properties of the drug which are expected based on the fact that the liposome shell is similar to that of Lipoplatin (see above).

9.2.5 New platinum compounds

The success of cisplatin has triggered intensive work for discovery of new platinum-based anticancer drugs. However, from over 3000 compounds tested *in vitro* only about 30 have entered into clinical trials (1 per cent). Considering that less than 10 per cent of these will make it to registration, the success in new platinum drug design is less than 1 in 1000 compounds.

The medicinal use and application of metals and metal complexes are of increasing clinical and commercial importance. Specifically metal-based drugs, imaging agents and radionuclides have over the years claimed for an increased portion of an annual US$5 billion budget for the whole field. The clinical success of cisplatin [*cis*-diamminedichloroplatinum(II)] has been the main impetus for the evolution of the family of platinum compounds, which currently holds a vital role in metal-based cancer chemotherapy. Despite this success, there is still a limited range of tumours sensitive to cisplatin intervention, due to inherent as well as acquired resistance after treatment. Furthermore the side-effects of cisplatin treatment are severe and include the dose-limiting nephrotoxicity, neurotoxicity, ototoxicity and emetogenesis.

The elucidation of the molecular mechanisms that mediate cisplatin mode of action, resistance and sensitivity provided the necessary background for the design and synthesis of new platinum compounds with improved toxicity profile, circumvention of

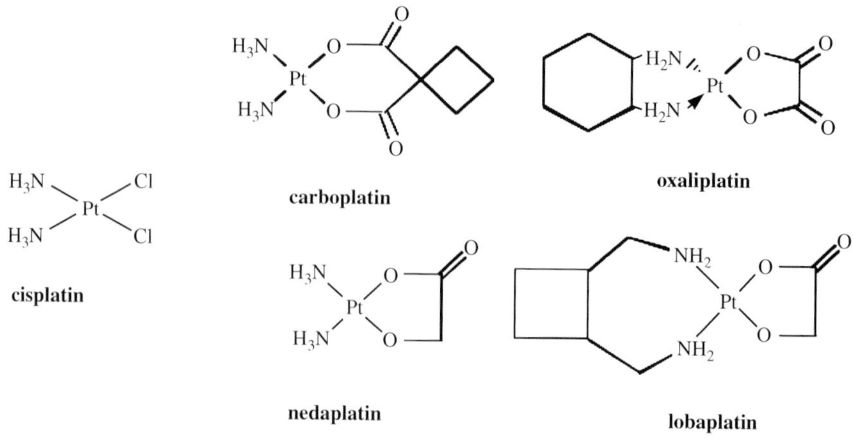

Figure 9.6 Structures of the clinically used platinum anticancer drugs

resistance and expansions of tumour panel. However after more than 30 years of intensive research, no more than 30 compounds have exhibited adequate pharmacological advantages relative to cisplatin, in order to be tested in clinical trials and only four registered for clinical use (Figure 9.6), thus proving that the search for novel platinum compounds remains a difficult task. From a mechanistic DNA-binding point of view, it is not too surprising that the introduction of these new platinum antitumour drugs did not represent a fundamental breakthrough in the treatment of cancer with platinum agents, due to the similarity in their mode of action.

Over the years alternative strategies for the design of new class of platinum anti-tumour compounds include the *trans* geometry, platinum complexes with different oxidation states (Pt(IV); picoplatin), polynuclear compounds that sufficiently deviate from the cisplatin structure, as well as conjugate compounds of platin derivatives with other anticancer agents or polymers and their encapsulation in liposomal formulations. These compounds have resulted in molecules with interesting results in terms of anticancer activity and reduced resistance and side effects.

9.3 Antimicrotubule agents

9.3.1 Taxanes

The advent of taxanes stabilizing tubulin, molecules that can inhibit signalling and a number of new approaches such as those targeting apoptosis or DNA topoisomerases is revolutionizing cancer chemotherapy. A plethora of clinical trials in progress optimizes the different ways drugs can be administered; for example, the addition of cisplatin or carboplatin to paclitaxel results in higher response rates than for each of the drugs as single agents.

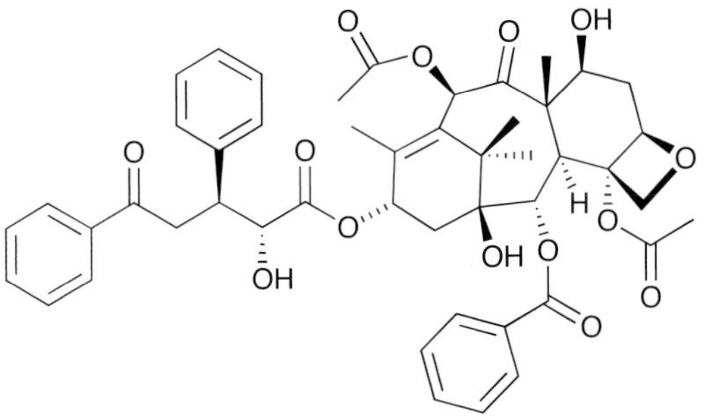

Figure 9.7 Chemical structure of paclitaxel

Paclitaxel (Taxol)

Paclitaxel (Figure 9.7; Taxol, Onxol) is a naturally occurring taxane molecule that inhibits depolymerization of tubulin in the spindle apparatus, thus inducing apoptosis in dividing cells. It is FDA approved for salvage therapy in ovarian cancer and in both metastatic and adjuvant setting in breast cancer. It is also used in lung, head and neck and bladder cancers. The dose-limiting effect is myelosuppression – mostly neutropenia – that can be reduced with shorter infusions of the same dose. Other common side effects are: mucositis – especially after longer infusions; peripheral neuropathy – usually mild that increases with cumulative dose; acute neuromyopathy that occurs for several days after infusion and could require opiate analgesics in order to control pain; cardiovascular side effects, including hypertension, hypotension, premature contractions, bradyarrhythmias – that do not usually require intervention; and hypersensitivity reactions to the drug including chest pain, dyspnoea, urticaria, wheezing, hypotension – that can be reduced by premedication with corticosteroids and H1, H2 histamine receptor blockers. Alopecia is one of the expected side effects, whereas nausea, vomiting, diarrhoea, liver toxicity and interstitial pneumonitis are uncommon.

Docetaxel (Taxotere)

Docetaxel (Figure 9.8; Taxotere) is a semisynthetic taxane, a class of compounds that inhibit the mitotic spindle apparatus by stabilizing tubulin polymers, leading to death of mitotic cells. It is approved by FDA for metastatic breast cancer and first and second line treatment for NSCLC, but clinical experience is increasing in ovarian cancer and other epithelial neoplasms.

Myelosuppression and alopecia are universal side effects with myelosuppression being the dose-limiting effect. Oedema and fluid accumulation, including pleural effusions and ascites are common and can be dose limiting. Fluid accumulation can be partially prevented with corticosteroid treatment before and after each cycle of docetaxel. Mild sensory or sensorimotor neuropathy is common. Mucositis and diarrhoea are common and usually mild. Hypersensitivity reactions are uncommon and can be prevented through premedication with corticosteroids and antihistamines. Rash and elevated liver function tests are uncommon.

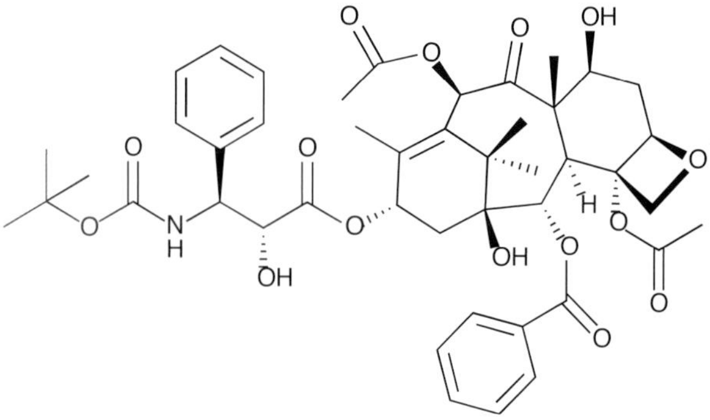

Figure 9.8 Chemical structure of docetaxel

Other taxane-like anti-microtubule agents
Ixabepilone (BMS-247550), a synthetic analogue of epothilone B, belongs to a new class of chemotherapeutic agents that disrupt microtubule function and induce cytotoxicity in a similar way to that seen with the taxanes paclitaxel and docetaxel. While its target is similar to that of taxanes, this novel agent has demonstrated significant activity in patients with prostate cancer refractory to taxane-based therapy. The predominant toxicities in the patients treated with ixabepilone alone or in combination with estramustine phosphate included neutropenia, neuropathy, and fatigue.

9.3.2　Vinca alkaloids

The vinca alkaloids are a subset of drugs that are derived from the periwinkle plant *Catharanthus roseus* (also *Vinca rosea*, *Lochnera rosea*, and *Ammocallis rosea*). While it has been historically used to treat numerous diseases, it has most recently been employed for its anti-cancer properties. All vinca alkaloids are administered intravenously (i.v.). After injection, they are eventually metabolized by the liver and excreted. They work in a cell-cycle specific manner, halting mitosis of affected cells and causing cell death. The mechanism of action involves binding to the tubulin monomers and keeping the microtubules (spindle fibres) from forming. These alkaloids also seem to interfere with cells' ability to synthesize DNA and RNA. Although the plant has medical uses, it can produce many serious side effects if smoked or ingested. There are four major vinca alkaloids in clinical use. These are vinblastine (Figure 9.9), vinorelbine, vincristine and vindesine. Their chemical structures have identical features (shown in red).

Vinblastine
Vinblastine (Velban, Velsar) acts as an inhibitor of tubulin polymerization and mitosis. This contrasts the stabilization of tubulin polymers by taxanes, a more recently developed class of anticancers. It also seems to fight cancer by interfering with glutamic acid metabolism (specifically, the pathways leading from glutamic acid to the Krebs' cycle

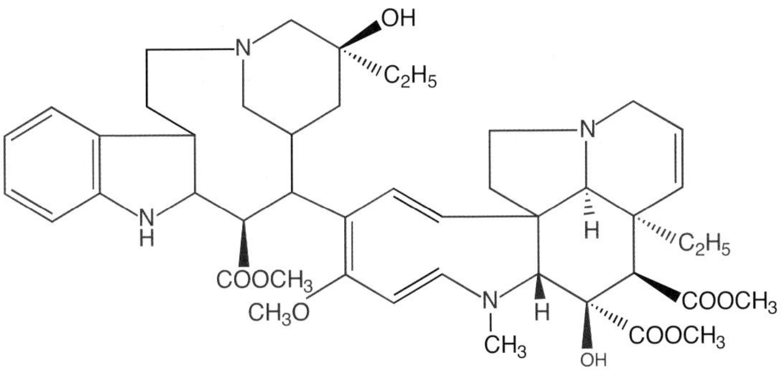

Figure 9.9 Structure of vinblastine

and to urea formation). Vinblastine is administrated i.v. It is approved by FDA for multiple haematological and solid tumours. It is most often used in Hodgkin's disease, non-Hodgkin's lymphoma, breast cancer, and germ cell tumours.

The major adverse effect of vinblastine is haematological toxicity which occurs much more frequently than with vincristine therapy. Leukopenia (granulocytopenia) occurs most commonly and is usually the dose-limiting factor in vinblastine therapy. Other side effects include nausea, vomiting and constipation, dyspnoea, chest or tumour pain, wheezing and fever during administration. Some rare cases of syndrome of inappropriate antidiuretic hormone secretion as well as angina pectoris have been reported.

Vinorelbine
Vinorelbine (Navelbine) is a semisynthetic vinca alkaloid that acts the same way as vinblastine. It is approved from the FDA for the treatment of relapsed metastatic breast cancer and for NSCLC either as a single agent or combined with a platinating agent. It is a mild vesicant, requiring extravasation precautions. Myelosuppression –mostly leukopenia – is the dose-limiting effect. Not significant nausea and vomiting are reported as well as neuropathy – but milder than it is observed with vinblastine – and tumour pain during administration. Acute reaction, such as dyspnoea, chest pain and wheezing has been reported during administration but can be prevented in some cases by premedication with corticosteroids.

Vincristine
Vincristine (Oncovin, Vincasar) is another vinca alkaloid FDA approved to treat acute leukaemia, rhabdomyosarcoma, neuroblastoma, Wilm's tumour, Hodgkin's disease and other lymphomas. Vincristine is administrated i.v. Peripheral neuropathy is the dose-limiting side effect, making it unsuitable for patients with neuromuscular disorders. Likewise, people with some forms of Charcot–Marie–Tooth syndrome should avoid vincristine. Other side effects include mild myelosuppression, constipation – rather commonly – autonomic neuropathy, CNS toxicity, nausea and vomiting. There have been reported a few cases of acute cardiopulmonary or pain symptoms during administration as well as transient elevation of liver function tests.

Vindesine

Vindesine has a serum half-life of about 24 hours and is administered at a dose of 3 mg/m^2 per of body surface. Its toxicity and side effects are similar to those of vinblastine. Vindesine is used mainly to treat melanoma and lung cancers (carcinomas) and, with other drugs, to treat uterine cancers.

9.4   Antimetabolites

9.4.1   5-Fluorouracil

5-Fluorouracil (Figure 9.10; Adrucil, Efudex) is a pyrimidine antimetabolite that inhibits the enzyme thymidylate synthase and is available in solution. 5-Fluorouracil is approved by FDA for colon, rectum, gastric, pancreas and breast cancer but is used in a wide range of other neoplasms in combination regimes. It is used for intrahepatic arterial infusion of liver metastases from gastrointestinal (GI) tumours and also used topically for various cutaneous neoplasms and disorders.

The dose-limiting side effect is GI toxicities (primarily mucositis for bolus injection and diarrhoea for prolonged infusions). Rare patients with dihydropyrimidine dehydrogenase deficiency have excessive GI toxicity. Myelosuppression is generally less with continuous infusion schedules. Nausea and vomiting are quite uncommon and mild. Dermatitis and other cutaneous toxicities including hand–foot syndrome are common. Cerebellar ataxia and myocardial ischaemia are rare.

9.4.2   Xeloda (capecitabine)

Capecitabine (Figure 9.11; Xeloda) is an oral antimetabolite prodrug. It is readily absorbed by the gastrointestinal tract, metabolized *in vivo* to fluorouracil in the liver by carboxylesterase and cytidine deaminase and then in turn in the peripheral tissues and tumour tissue by thymidine phosphorylase (Figure 9.11). Thymidine phosphorylase is expressed at higher levels in most tumour tissues, so capecitabine produces higher levels of fluorouracil in tumour tissue. It is FDA approved for metastatic breast cancer and metastatic colorectal cancer, but it is also used in head and neck squamous cell cancer. The dose-limiting side effects include myelosuppression and palmar-plantar erythrodysaesthesia. Other side effects include nausea, vomiting, rash, diarrhoea, fatigue, stomatitis and hyperbilirubinaemia.

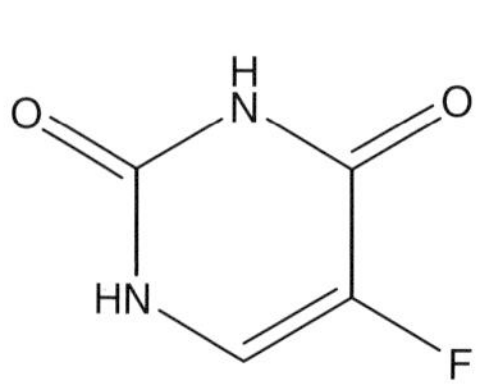

Figure 9.10   Structure of 5-fluorouracil

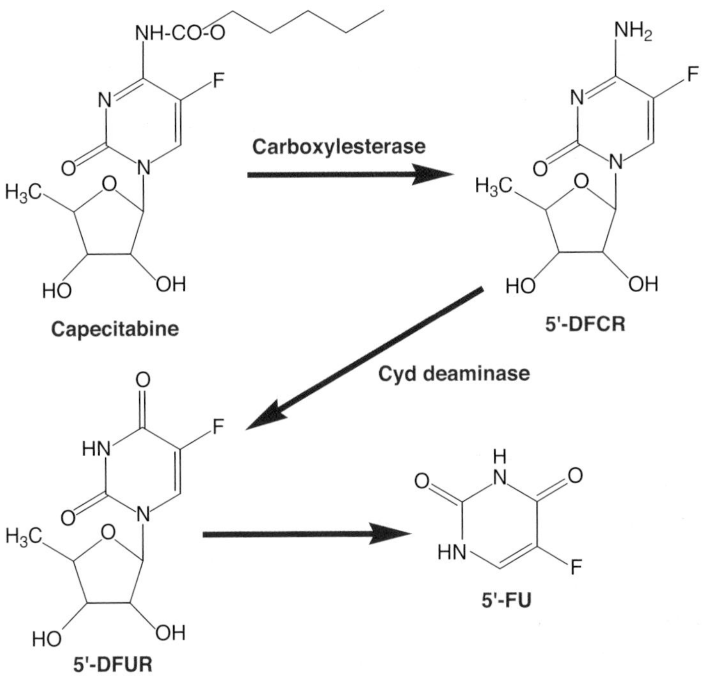

Figure 9.11 Structure and mechanism of capecitabine

9.4.3 Structure of gemcitabine

Gemcitabine (Figure 9.12; Gemzar) is a nucleoside analogue that exhibits cell cycle-dependent and S-phase-specific cytotoxicity, likely due to inhibition of DNA synthesis. Gemcitabine is approved by FDA for advanced pancreatic adenocarcinoma, NCSLC and metastatic breast cancer, but it is broadly used in bladder cancer as well. The dose-limiting effect is myelosuppression although it is mild. Other common side effects

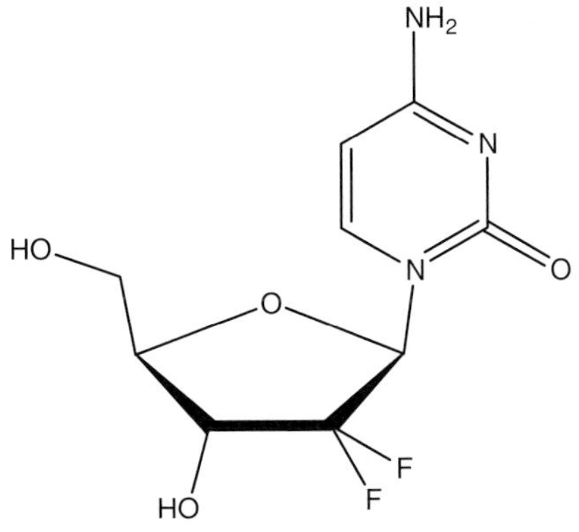

Figure 9.12 Structure of gemcitabine

include mild nausea and vomiting, elevated transaminases and fever. There have also been reported a few cases of haematuria, proteinuria, acute dyspnoea, rash, paresthaesias and CNS depression.

9.5   Antitumour antibiotics

9.5.1   Actinomycin D

Actinomycin D (Figure 9.13) is an antitumour antibiotic that inhibits transcription. The major side effect is haematological toxicity and is dose-limiting. It is primarily manifested by leukopenia and thrombocytopenia. Other side effects like anaemia, pancytopenia, reticulopenia, agranulocytosis, and aplastic anaemia may also occur. Nausea and vomiting are usual side effects. Actinomycin D is approved for the treatment of Ewing's sarcoma, Wilm's tumour, rhabdomyosarcoma, germ cell tumours but is also being used against gestational trophoblastic tumours, melanoma, ovarian cancer and other type of malignancies.

Standard therapy for Wilms' tumour is the combination of vincristine and actinomycin D with a survival of about 85 per cent. Actinomycin D is used for the treatment of trophoblastic tumours either as a single agent or in combination with methotrexate, cyclophosphamide and vincristine (EMA-CO) depending on the type of the tumour (non-metastatic, low risk and high risk metastatic).

9.5.2   Mitomycin C

Mitomycin C (Figure 9.14; Mutamycin) is an antitumour antibiotic that inhibits DNA and RNA synthesis. It is FDA approved for the treatment of adenocarcinomas of the

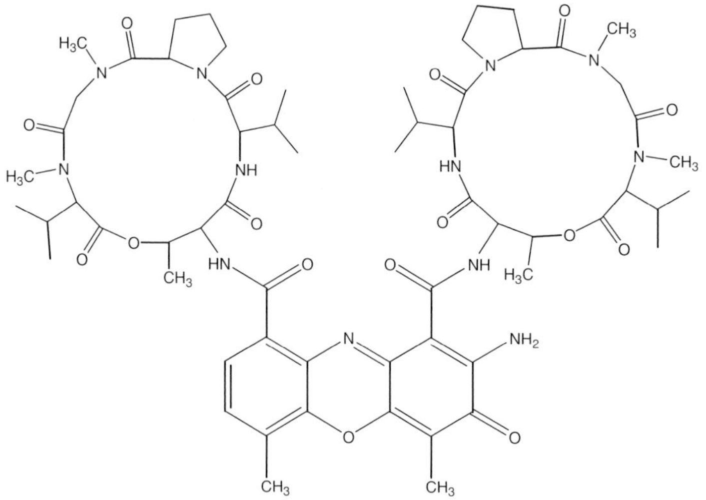

Figure 9.13   Structure of actinomycin D

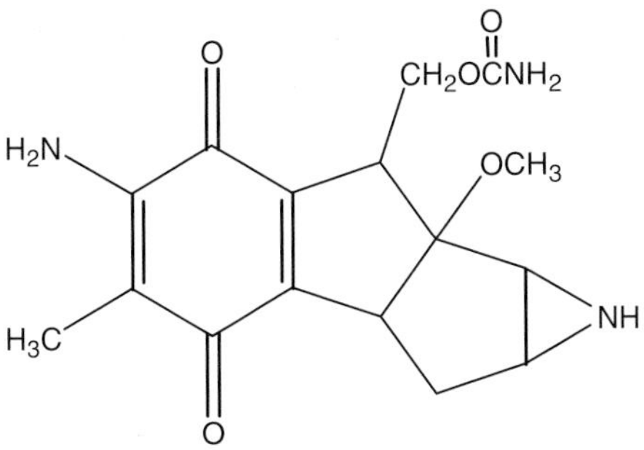

Figure 9.14 Structure of mitomycin C

stomach and pancreas but is also used in breast and lung cancer. Myelosuppression is the most serious and frequent toxic effect of mitomycin and is usually manifested by thrombocytopenia and/or leukopenia. Nausea, vomiting, anorexia and fatigue are common while diarrhoea, stomatitis, renal insufficiency, rash and fever are uncommon. Veno-occlusive disease of the liver, haemolytic-uraemic syndrome and interstitial pneumonitis have been rarely observed.

9.5.3 Bleomycin

Bleomycin (Figure 9.15) is an antitumour antibiotic and is administered i.v. It is usually used in germ cell tumours, Hodgkin's disease and squamous cell cancers. It is also used

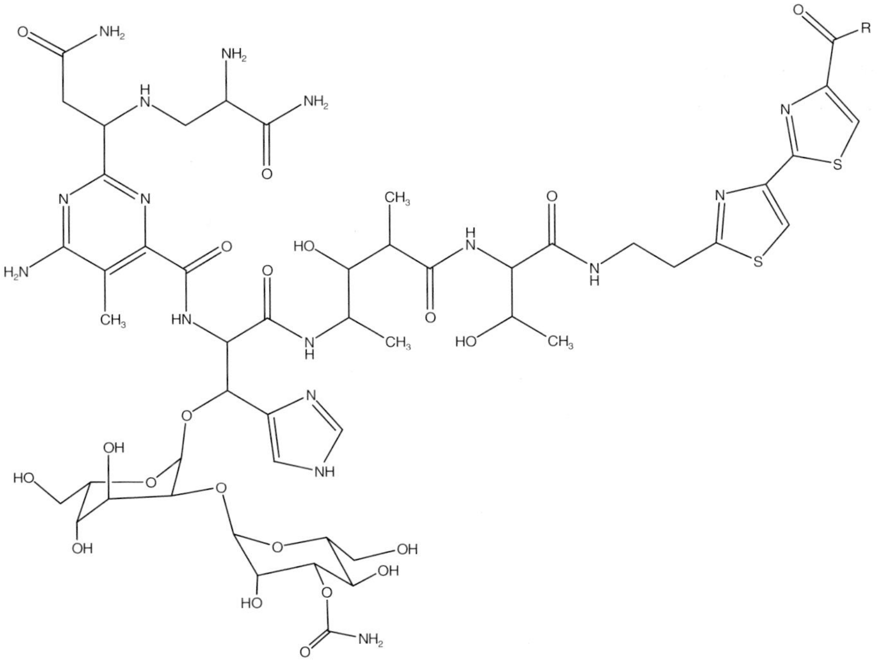

Figure 9.15 Structure of bleomycin

off-label for melanoma, ovarian cancer and Kaposi's sarcoma as well as a sclerosing agent for malignant pleural or pericardial effusions. The dose-limiting side effect of bleomycin is pulmonary toxicity. Other common toxicities include fever, chills, rash, exfoliation and anorexia. Nausea, vomiting, myelosuppression, anaphylaxis and mucositis are rarely reported.

9.5.4 Anthracyclines

Anthracyclines, also known as the anthraquinones, are antibiotics originally isolated from *Streptomyces peucetius*. They are known for their binding to DNA through intercalation (binding between the DNA bases) due to the planar anthracycline chromophore. Furthermore, they inhibit the action of DNA topoisomerases, resulting in permanent DNA cleavage.

Doxorubicin
Doxorubicin (Figure 9.16; Adriamycin) is an anthracycline glycoside antineoplastic antibiotic. Leukopenia (principally granulocytopenia) is the predominant manifestation of haematological toxicity, the severity of which depends on the dose of the drug and on the regenerative capacity of the bone marrow. Thrombocytopenia and anaemia may also occur. Cardiotoxicity is another common effect that can be dose limiting. Acute anthracycline-induced cardiotoxicity usually is uncommon. Chronic cardiotoxicity, resulting in cardiomyopathy, usually occurs within 1 year after discontinuance of anthracycline therapy, is more common than acute cardiotoxicity, and is considered clinically the most important anthracycline-associated toxicity. Nausea, vomiting, diarrhoea and stomatitis as well as alopecia, rash and hyperpigmentation are also common. It is FDA approved for a variety of cancers but is most commonly used for breast carcinoma, adult carcinomas, paediatric solid tumours, Hodgkin's disease, non-Hodgkin's lymphomas and ovarian cancer.

Daunorubicin
Daunorubicin (Figure 9.17) is an anthracycline glycoside antineoplastic antibiotic produced by *Streptomyces coeruleorubidus*. Myelosuppression is the dose-limiting side effect

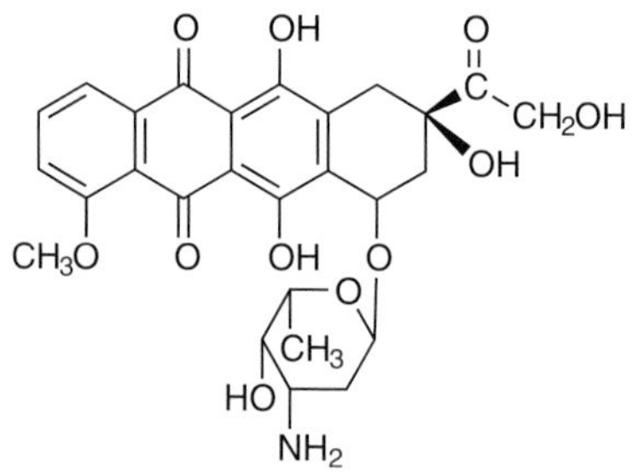

Figure 9.16 Structure of doxorubicin

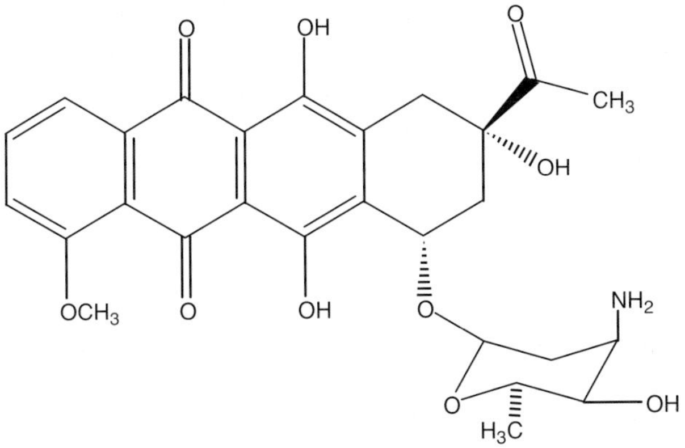

Figure 9.17 Structure of daunorubicin

and is primarily manifested by leukopenia, which is usually severe, and thrombocytopenia; anaemia may also occur. Alopecia, nausea, vomiting and stomatitis are common while elevated liver function, diarrhoea, rash and transient arrhythmias are uncommon.

Daunorubicin hydrochloride is used in combination with other antineoplastic agents for the treatment of acute myeloid (myelogenous, non-lymphocytic) leukaemia (AML, ANLL) in adults as well as a component of combination chemotherapeutic regimens for the induction of remissions of childhood or adult acute lymphocytic (lymphoblastic) leukaemia (ALL).

Liposomal doxorubicin
Liposomal doxorubicin (Doxil) is the liposomal preparation of doxorubicin. It is approved for recurrent metastatic ovarian cancer and acquired immune deficiency syndrome (AIDS)-related Kaposi's sarcoma but it is also used in metastatic breast cancer and multiple myeloma. The principal dose-limiting toxicity of PEG-stabilized liposomal doxorubicin in patients with AIDS-related Kaposi's sarcoma has been myelosuppression, commonly manifested by leukopenia and neutropenia; anaemia and thrombocytopenia also occur frequently. In patients with ovarian cancer, myelosuppression has generally been moderate and reversible. Anaemia was the most common adverse haematological effect in patients with ovarian cancer. Palmar–plantar erythrodysaesthesia (PPE), characterized by swelling, pain, erythema, and occasionally desquamation of the hands and feet, has been reported in patients receiving liposomal doxorubicin. Nausea and stomatitis are common but mild, while alopecia and acute infusion reactions (chest pain, back pain, dyspnoea and wheezing) can occur uncommonly. The drug is given i.v. with promising results.

9.5.5 Podophyllotoxins

Etoposide
Etoposide (Figure 9.18; Vespid) is a plant alkaloid that inhibits topoisomerase II activity. It comes both in an oral and parenteral form. It has been approved by FDA

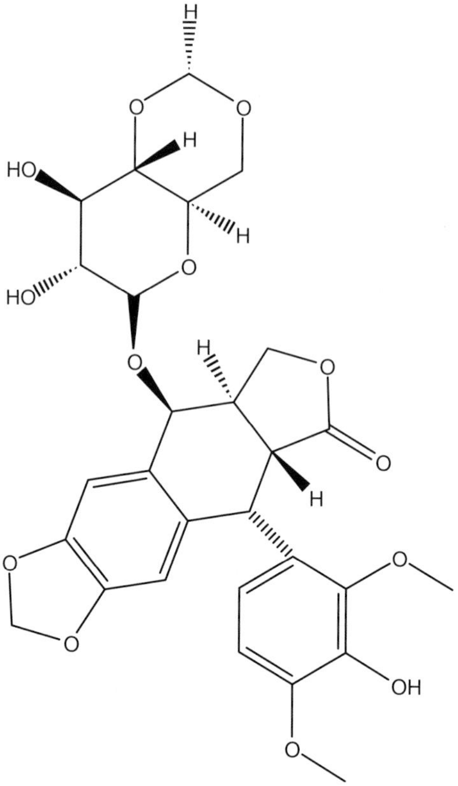

Figure 9.18 Structure of etoposide

for germ cell tumours and SCLC, but it is also used for lymphomas, AML, and NSCLC. Etoposide is also used as a high-dose therapy in the transplant setting for breast and ovarian cancer and lymphomas. Myelosuppression – primarily leukopenia – is universal and is the dose-limiting effect. Nausea and vomiting depend on administration. Stomatitis and diarrhoea are common only at high doses and alopecia is absent or mild. Other rare symptoms include hepatic toxicity, peripheral neuropathy and CNS changes. Rapid infusion of etoposide – shorter than 5 minutes – may also cause hypertension. Reports have also been made of the appearance of secondary AML.

Teniposide

Teniposide (Figure 9.19; Vumon) is also an inhibitor of topoisomerase II and acts in a similar way as etoposide. It is approved by the FDA for childhood ALL but it is also active against SCLC. The major and dose-limiting adverse effect of teniposide is myelosuppression manifested mainly by neutropenia. Nausea, vomiting, diarrhoea, stomatitis and anorexia are not very common and alopecia is generally mild. Other side effects like hypotension, fatigue, somnolence, allergic reactions, renal insufficiency and secondary leukaemia are rare.

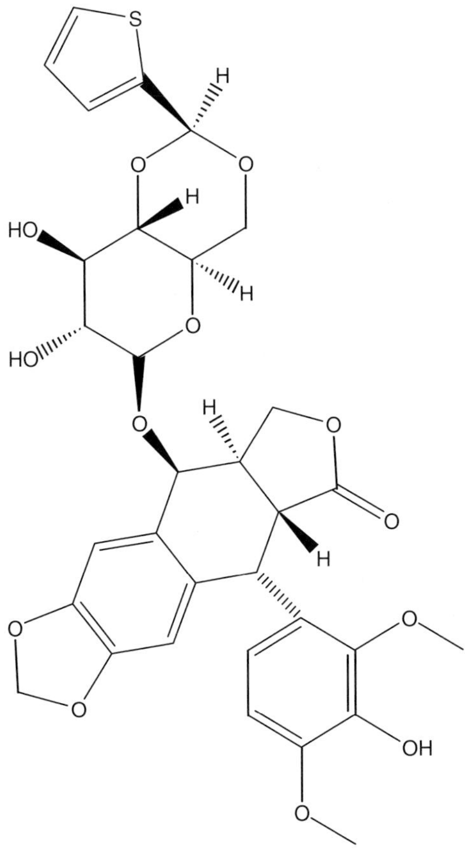

Figure 9.19 Structure of teniposide

9.5.6 Camptothecins

Irinotecan
Irinotecan (Figure 9.20; Camptosar) (CPT-11), a type I DNA topoisomerase inhibitor, is an antineoplastic agent. Myelosuppression – mainly in the form of neutropenia – and diarrhoea are common side effects and can be dose limiting. Flushing, alopecia and rash

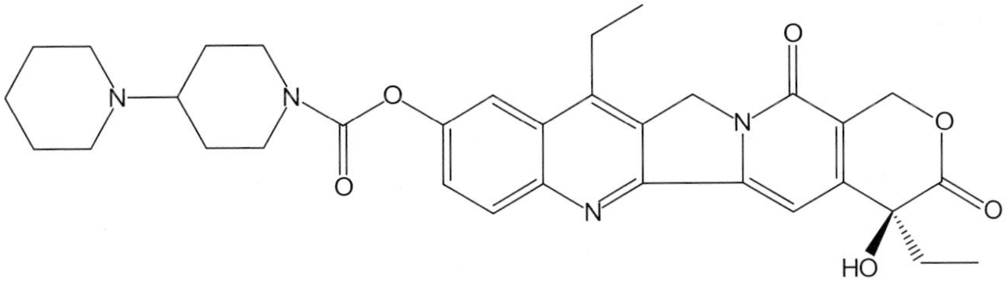

Figure 9.20 Structure of irinotecan

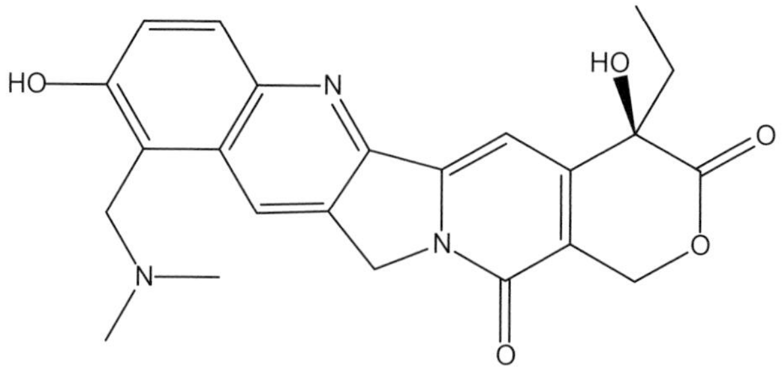

Figure 9.21   Structure of topotecan

are commonly manifested side effects whereas significant renal, hepatic, neurological and pulmonary toxicities are rare. It is approved by the FDA for refractory or recurrent metastatic colon cancer, but it is also used for the treatment of other malignancies including lung and ovarian cancer and lymphoma.

Topotecan
Topotecan (Figure 9.21; Hycamtin) is a semisynthetic camptothecin molecule that acts as an inhibitor of topoisomerase I, which is required for transcription and replication of the cells. It is FDA approved for the treatment of refractory, relapsed, ovarian carcinoma and for relapsed small cell lung cancer as well as post-menopausal or oestrogen receptor-positive metastatic breast cancer and myeloid leukaemias. The dose-limiting effect is myelosuppression – especially leucopenia. Thrombocytopenia, anaemia, nausea, diarrhoea, vomiting, while common, are not severe. Other common side effects include headache, fever, fatigue, anorexia, malaise and elevated liver function tests, whereas hypertension, tachycardia, urticaria, renal insufficiency, haematuria, neuropathy and mucositis are quite uncommon.

9.6   Alkylating agents

Alkylating agents are molecules that attack DNA by positioning themselves within the major groove of G-C rich regions of DNA. They form covalent bonds, usually with the N7 atom of guanine base, and depending on the molecule can establish a further link with DNA.

9.6.1   Cyclophosphamide

Cyclophosphamide (Figure 9.22; Cytoxan) is a prototypical alkylator drug that can be administered either orally or intravenously. The main effect of cyclophosphamide is due to its metabolite phosphoramide mustard. This metabolite is only formed in cells which have low levels of ALDH. Phosphoramide mustard forms DNA crosslinks between and within DNA strands, leading to cell death.

Cyclophosphamide has relatively little typical chemotherapy toxicity as ALDHs are present in relatively large concentrations in bone marrow stem cells, liver and intestinal

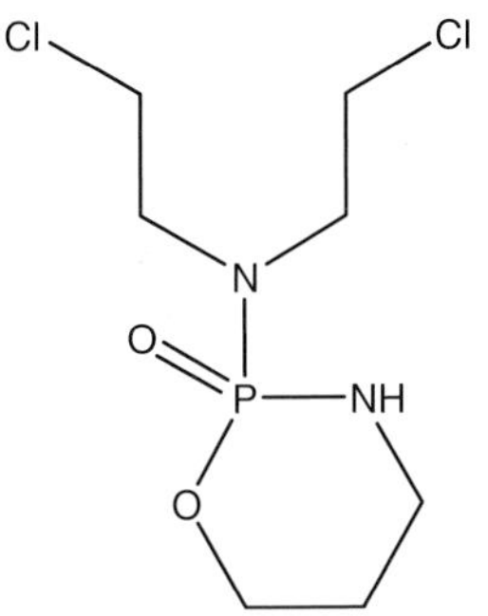

Figure 9.22 Structure of cyclophosphamide

epithelium. ALDHs protect these actively proliferating tissues against toxic effects of phosphoramide mustard and acrolein by converting aldophosphamide to carboxyphosphamide that does not give rise to the toxic metabolites (phosphoramide mustard and acrolein). It is FDA approved for many malignancies, and it is most commonly used in breast carcinoma, non-Hodgkin's lymphoma, ovarian carcinoma and testicular cancer. The dose-limiting side effect is myelosuppression with leucopenia being the most significant. Nausea and vomiting are common while haemorrhagic cystitis is uncommon with standard doses but common with higher doses. Other toxicities of high-dose therapy include syndrome of inappropriate secretion of antidiuretic hormone, pulmonary fibrosis and haemorrhagic myocarditis.

9.6.2 Ifosfamide

Ifosfamide (Figure 9.23; Ifex) is an alkylating agent. Ifosfamide is approved by FDA for recurrent germ cell tumours but also used in adult sarcomas, lymphoma, Hodgkin's disease, breast cancer and ovarian cancer. Administration of the drug usually causes myelosuppression, haemorrhagic cystitis and CNS toxicity that can be dose limiting – haemorrhagic cystitis can be largely prevented by co-administration of the unprotective agent mesna and nausea–vomiting can be minimized with modern antiemetic regimens. The CNS toxicity, including lethargy, stupor, coma, myoclonus and seizures is usually mild and reversible. Renal dysfunction has been reported but is usually reversible, while hepatic toxicity, diarrhoea and rash are rare side effects.

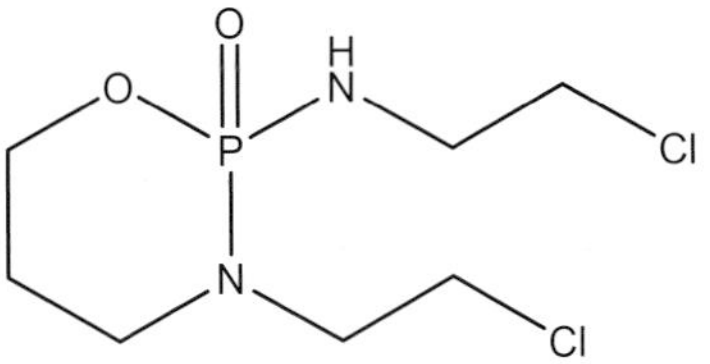

Figure 9.23 Structure of ifosfamide

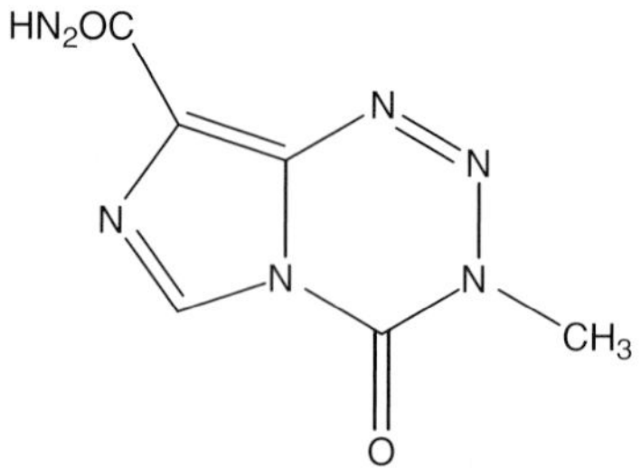

Figure 9.24   Structure of Temodal

9.6.3   Temozolomide (Temodal)

Temozolomide (Figure 9.24) is an alkylating agent developed in the UK by the Cancer Research UK and marketed by Schering. It is used for the treatment of brain tumours (glioblastomas) and is orally available in tablets of 5, 20, 100 and 250 mg.

Common side effects include fatigue and temporary effects to the bone marrow that are related to increased risk of infections, anaemia and bruising. Other side effects can include nausea, loss of appetite, altered taste, diarrhoea, loss of fertility and damage to the embryo.

9.7   Other antitumour agents

9.7.1   Tamoxifen

Tamoxifen (Figure 9.25; Nolvadex) is a non-steroidal antioestrogen with cytostatic effects on oestrogen-dependent and non-dependent malignant cells. It is FDA approved for breast cancer in postmenopausal patients or those with estrogen receptor-positive tumours. It is also used as chemoprevention for breast cancer in high risk patients and as

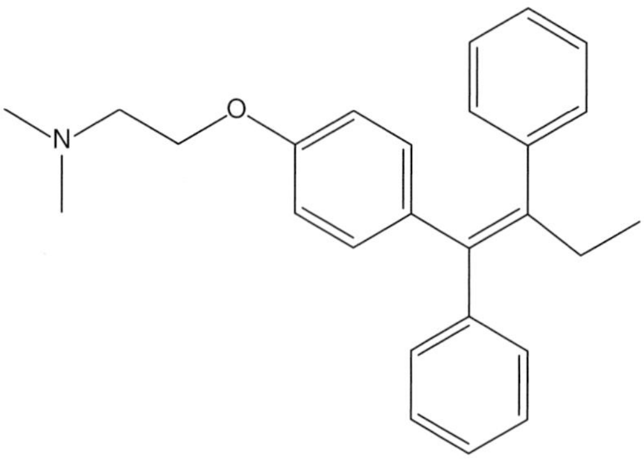

Figure 9.25   Structure of tamoxifen

treatment for melanoma and pancreatic cancer. Most common side effects include hot flushes, sweating, mood changes, weight loss or gain and stomach upset. Less common side effects are nausea, vomiting, constipation, diarrhoea, menstrual changes – including significant vaginal bleeding – venous thromboembolism, myelosuppression and retinopathy.

9.8 Combination chemotherapy

Combination chemotherapy is important in most cancer treatment regimes (see Box 9.1 for combination chemotherapy regimes) to exploit synergy between chemotherapy drugs. Similarly, concurrent chemotherapy and radiation has shown improved survival compared to radiation alone. The molecular mechanisms of chemotherapeutic drugs may differ; thus their combination will combat tumour cells more effectively. For example, the advantage of using combinations of gemcitabine, topotecan, liposomal doxorubicin, and prolonged oral etoposide with platinum has been attributed to inhibition of DNA synthetic pathways involved in the repair of platinum–DNA adducts. Gemcitabine and cisplatin act synergistically, increase platinum–DNA adduct formation and induce concentration and combination dependent changes in ribonucleotide and deoxyribonucleotide pools in ovarian cancer cell lines. The combination of nedaplatin and irinotecan, a topoisomerase I inhibitor, offers synergistic interaction in cell cultures by concurrent exposure to both drugs; on the other hand, sequential exposure to the two drugs led only to additivity. Many drug combinations involving platinum complexes have been explored, but those with taxanes are particularly noteworthy. Paclitaxel in combination with a platinum agent is now accepted as a standard component of first-line treatment for ovarian cancer, and produces improved survival.

Box 9.1 Chemotherapy regimes

EMA-CO	etoposide, high-dose methotrexate with folinic acid, actinomycin D, cyclophosphamide and vincristine
VAC	vincristine, dactinomycin, and cyclophosphamide
BEP	bleomycin, etoposide and cisplatin,
VIP	vindesine–ifosfamide–cisplatin
VAB-6	vinblastine, dactinomycin, bleomycin, cyclophosphamide, and cisplatin
BAP	bleomycin, actinomycin-D and cisplatin
CHOP-Bleo	cyclophosphamide, doxorubicin, vincristine, prednisone, bleomycin
OPEC	vincristine, cisplatin, teniposide, and cyclophosphamide
ADE	cytosine arabinoside, daunorubicin, and etoposide
G-FLIP	gemcitabine, 5-fluorouracil, leucovorin and cisplatin

FOLFIRI.3	a new regimen combining 5-fluorouracil, folinic acid and irinotecan
MOPPEBVCAD	mechlorethamine, vincristine, procarbazine, prednisone, epidoxorubicin, bleomycin, vinblastine, lomustine, doxorubicin and vindesine
ABVD	doxorubicin, bleomycin, vinblastine, and dacarbazine
ACVBP	doxorubicin, cyclophosphamide, vindesine, bleomycin, prednisone
CAV	cisplatin, Adriamycin, vindesine
DC	docetaxel plus cisplatin
MVP	mitomycin C, vindesine, and cisplatin
VCAP	vindesine. doxorubicin, cyclophosphamide and prednisone
VC	vinorelbine and cisplatin
VECP-Bleo	vindesine, epirubicin, cyclophosphamide, prednisone, and bleomycin
MOPP	mechlorethamine, vincristine, procarbazine and prednisone
ABV	doxorubicin, bleomycin and vinblastine
BEACOPP	bleomycin, etoposide, doxorubicin, cyclophosphamide, vincristine, procarbazine, prednisolone
VAD	vincristine, doxorubicin, and dexamethasone
PCV	procarbazine, lomustine, and vincristine
CEV	carboplatin, etoposide phosphate and vincristine
CHVP	cyclophosphamide, doxorubicin, teniposide, and prednisone
OPEC	of vincristine, cisplatin, teniposide, and cyclophosphamide
ProMACE-MOPP	methotrexate, doxorubicin, cyclophosphamide, etoposide, mechlorethamide, vincristine, procarbazine and prednisone

9.9 Growth factor signalling

Cancer can be described as a disease where cellular communication has broken down, allowing transformed cells to escape tight regulatory signals and replicate autonomously and continuously, ultimately invading and interfering with the functions of normal tissues. Under physiological conditions cells communicate with one another by activating receptors at the cell surface, which convey the signal through pathways of proteins located in the cytoplasm and subsequently through networks of transcription factors in the nucleus which control the expression of genes that mediate the cell's response. Typically, cancer develops as a result of aberrant growth factor signalling, where a pathway that instructs a cell to grow and divide becomes constitutively active. This could arise through mutations in a growth factor receptor, or through mutations in components of cell signalling pathways (see Figure 9.27).

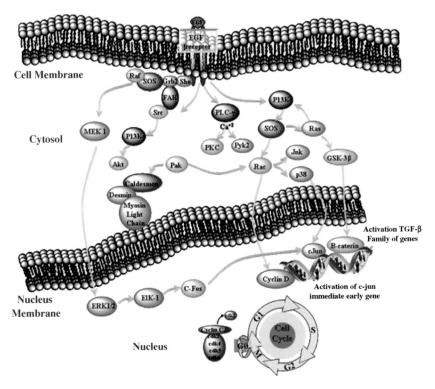

Figure 9.26 The EGFR signalling pathway

Collectively, genes that encode for mutated cellular proteins involved in promoting cell growth are termed oncogenes. A mutation in any one of the cell-signalling complex components illustrated in Figure 9.26 could generate an oncogene, e.g. mutations in the EGFR, Ras, Raf, and Akt, etc.

Therefore, an intense amount of research has been conducted in an effort to identify small molecules or antibodies that interfere with cell signalling and hence reverse the constitutive cellular growth that is mediated by oncogenes. One success story in this field has been the identification of Tarceva (erlotinib) as an efficient chemotherapeutic compound.

9.9.1 Tarceva

Tarceva (Figure 9.27) functions by inhibiting the EGFR, HER1, by competing with ATP for binding to the active site in the intracellular tyrosine kinase domain. This results in the blockade of downstream signalling pathways that mediate cell growth. Tarceva has shown particular efficacy against NSCLC and is often prescribed as a second line treatment in this indication, being comparable to docetaxel and in a similar patient population. Noted adverse reactions included severe rash, diarrhoea, hepatotoxicity,

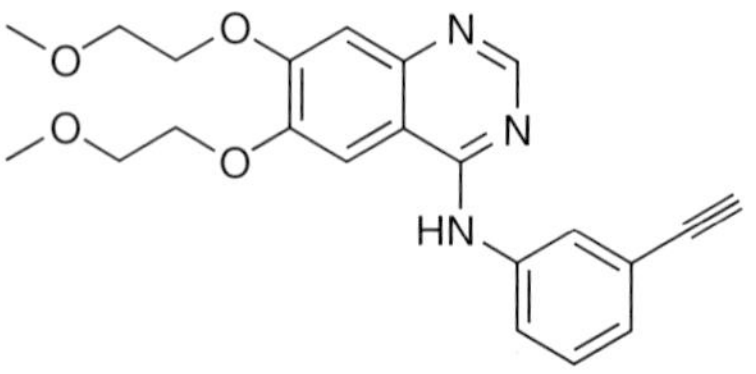

Figure 9.27   The structure of Tarceva

gastrointestinal bleed, corneal ulcers, myocardial ischemia/infarction, stroke and hae-molytic anaemia with thrombocytopenia. Nonetheless, in patients bearing a mutation in the EGFR, Tarceva can greatly increase survival time and leads to an overall improvement in the quality of life.

9.9.2   Other signal transduction inhibitors

A number of other signal transduction inhibitors (STI) are being tested in the clinic for a variety of indications. Table 9.1 illustrates a collection of some of these compounds that are currently in clinical trials.

Table 9.1   Compounds used in current clinical trials

Intracellular target	Drug	Target indication
EGFR	Gefitinib (Iressa)	NSCLC (FDA Approved), Unknown Primary (Phase III), Bladder (Phase III), Breast (Phase II), Adrenocortical (Phase II), Leukaemia (Phase II), Liver (Phase II), Skin (Phase II), Gastric (Phase II), Brain (Phase II), Ovarian (Phase II), Head and Neck (Phase II), Esophageal (Phase II)
EGFR	Erlotinib (Tarceva)	NSCLC (FDA Approved), Colorectal (Phase III), Breast (Phase II), Head and Neck (Phase II), Mesothelioma (Phase II), Brain (Phase II), Bladder (Phase II), Kidney (Phase II), Prostate (Phase II), Pancreatic (Phase II), Liver (Phase II), Unknown Primary (Phase I)
EGFR	EKB-569	Colorectal Cancer (Phase II), NSCLC (Phase II)
EGFR/HER-2	Lapatinib (GW572016)	Breast (Phase III), Head and Neck (Phase III), Prostate (Phase II), Esophagus (Phase II), Brain (Phase I/II), Ovarian (Phase I/II), Solid Tumours (Phase I)
EGFR/HER-2	AEE-788	Advanced Cancer (Phase I)
Pan-erbB	Canaternib (CI-1033)	Phase II MBC
Farnesyltransferase (Ras GTPases)	Tipifarnib (Zarnestra)	Breast (Phase II), Brain (Phase II), Multiple Myeloma (Phase II), Neurofibromatosis Type 1 (Phase II), Leukaemia (Phase I), Solid Tumour (Phase I), Pancreatic (Phase I), NSCLC (Phase I)

(Continued)

Table 9.1 (*Continued*)

Intracellular target	Drug	Target indication
Farnesyltransferase (Ras GTPases)	Lonafarnib (Sarasar)	Myelodysplastic Disease (Phase III), Breast , (Phase II) Progeria (Phase II), Brain (Phase I), Advanced Cancer (Phase I)
mTOR	Everolimus (RAD-001)	Pancreatic (Phase III), Breast (Phase III), Small Cell Lung (Phase II), Refractory Tumours (phase II), NSCLC (phase II), Kidney (Phase II), Melanoma (Phase II), Brain (Phase II), Endometrial (Phase II), Colon (Phase II), Advanced Cancer (Phase I), Lymphoma (Phase I), Head and Neck (Phase I), Solid Tumour (Phase I)
mTOR	Temsirolimus (CCI-779)	Breast (Phase II), Liver (Phase II), Melanoma (Phase II), Brain (Phase II), Kidney (Phase II), Leukaemia (Phase I), Multiple Myeloma (Phase I), Solid Tumour (Phase I)
Raf	Sorafenib (BAY-43-9006)	NSCLC (Phase II), Leukaemia (Phase II), Colorectal (Phase II), Melanoma (Phase II), Kidney (Phase II), Prostate (Phase II), Breast (Phase II), Brain (Phase II), Sarcoma (Phase II), Ovarian (Phase II), Head and Neck (Phase II), Bladder (Phase II), Gastro-Intestinal (Phase II), Lymphoma (Phase I), Pancreatic (Phase I)
MEK 1/2	PD-0325901	NSCLC (Phase II), Breast (Phase II)
MEK 1/2	AZD6244	Melanoma (Phase II), NSCLC (Phase II), Pancreatic (Phase II), Breast (Phase I)
Src	AZD0530	Breast (Phase I)Colorectal (Phase II)Pancreatic (Phase II)
Cyclin-dependent kinase	AZD5438	Advanced Cancer (Phase I)
NFκB	Bortezomib (Velcade)	Multiple Myeloma (FDA Approved), NSCLC (Phase III), Lymphoma (Phase III), Breast (Phase II), Head and Neck (Phase II), (Phase II), Kidney (Phase II), Pancreatic (Phase II), Liver (Phase II), Gastric (Phase II), Leukaemia (Phase I), Colorectal (Phase I), Brain (Phase I)

Gefitinib (Figure 9.28) was the first approved selective inhibitor of EGF's tyrosine kinase domain, working in a similar fashion to Tarceva, and was approved for the clinic in 2003 as a treatment for NSCLC. Gefitinib is currently only indicated for the treatment of locally advanced or metastatic NSCLC in patients who have previously received this chemotherapy. In 2004, AstraZeneca informed the FDA that a large randomized study failed to demonstrate a survival advantage for gefitinib in the treatment of NSCLC. It is

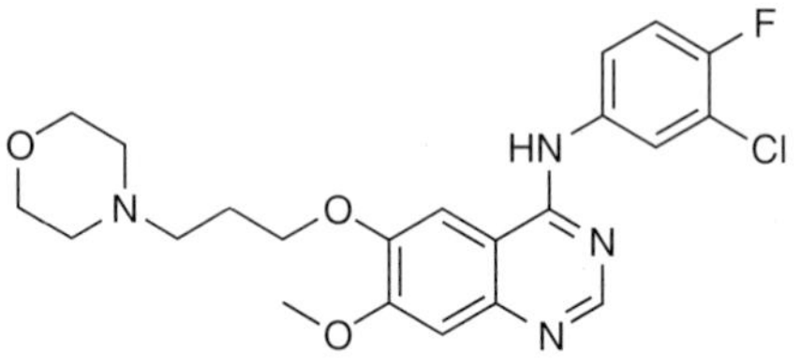

Figure 9.28   Structure of gefitinib

for this reason that Tarceva has replaced gefitinib in the US (except in patients with proven response).

In 2005 the FDA approved another STI drug, Sorafenib, to be used in the treatment of advanced renal cell cancer. This drug acts by inhibiting RAF kinase, platelet-derived growth factor (PDGF) and VEGF, thus preventing both cell proliferation and angiogenesis. Noted adverse reactions include skin rash, hand-foot skin reactions, diarrhoea and hypertension.

9.10   Cell cycling and cancer

Mutations in tumour suppressor genes (e.g. p53) that negatively regulate cell growth can also generate cancer by allowing cells to escape important growth checkpoints. Typically, tumour suppressor genes are involved in regulating the cell cycle, the process that a cell undergoes during its division into two daughter cells. Various molecules are under development, aimed at targeting different points at the cell cycle. Some of those are briefly presented below.

- Flavopiridol is a synthetic flavonoid inhibitor, which is under development by Sanofi Aventis in collaboration with the National Cancer Institute (NCI). Flavopiridol is a small molecule derivative of the alkaloid rohitukine, which inhibits cyclin-dependent kinases causing a halt to the cell cycle. At the same time it decreases the expression of a number of proteins that regulate the cell cycle.

- P276-00 is another rohitukine-derived small molecule drug that acts as a selective Cdk4-D1 and Cdk1-B inhibitor and is being developed by Nicholas Piramal India Limited. It is currently in phase I/II trials in Canada and India for the treatment of advanced refractory neoplasms.

- Ispinesib is a novel small molecule drug candidate that inhibits cell proliferation and promotes cancer cell death by specifically disrupting the function of a cytoskeletal protein known as kinesin spindle protein, or KSP. KSP is essential for cell proliferation. Ispinesib is being studied in a broad clinical trials program that consists of nine Phase II trials and five Phase I/Ib trials. The Phase II trials are evaluating ispinesib as monotherapy in each of NSCLC, ovarian cancer, breast cancer, colorectal cancer, hepatocellular cancer, melanoma, head and neck cancer, prostate cancer and renal cell cancer. The Phase I trials are evaluating ispinesib in solid tumours or acute leukaemia, chronic myelogenous leukaemia and advanced myelodysplastic syndromes. Additionally, three Phase Ib trials are being conducted to study ispinesib in combination with each of carboplatin, capecitabine or docetaxel.

- BI 2536 is a novel inhibitor of Polo-like kinase 1 (Plk-1), a cell cycle switch essential for cell proliferation, and is being developed by Boehringer Ingelheim. BI 2536 inhibits mitosis, resulting in cancer cell death by apoptosis. It is the first Plk-1 inhibitor being tested in clinical trials and is at phase I in the treatment of advanced non-Hodgkin's lymphoma and phase II in both advanced NSCLC and SCLC.

- SNS-032 is a novel amino thiazole small molecule cell-cycle modulator that targets CDK2, CDK7 and CDK9 that is being developed by Sunesis Pharmaceuticals. Pre-clinical studies have shown that SNS-032 induces cell-cycle arrest and apoptosis (or cell death) across multiple cell lines. SNS-032 is a small molecule that is currently administered by i.v. infusion, but also has the potential to be developed as an oral formulation. It is currently undergoing phase I clinical trials for the treatment of a variety of advanced solid tumours. Sunesis are also developing SNS-595 as a novel naphthyridine analogue that induces a G2 cell cycle arrest. This drug is currently in phase I trials for the treatment of a variety of haematological malignancies and phase II clinical trials for both ovarian and small cell lung cancers.

- AT7519 is Astex Therapeutic's most progressed drug candidate and is currently in phase I clinical trials for advanced solid tumours and for refractory non-Hodgkin's lymphoma. AT7519 is a potent cell cycle inhibitor that targets the cyclin dependent kinases.

- MKC-1 is a novel, orally active cell cycle inhibitor that is being developed by EntreMed and is currently in Phase II clinical trials for the treatment of breast cancer and NSCLC. MKC-1 inhibits mitotic spindle formation by binding to tubulin and the importin β proteins, thus preventing chromosome segregation during mitosis, and inducing apoptosis.

9.11   Apoptosis and cancer

Defects in the apoptotic process can lead to the onset of cancer by allowing cells to grow unchecked when an oncogenic signal is present. Thus, activating the apoptotic machinery is an ideal way to reduce tumour volume. Figure 9.29 illustrates the large number of proteins that are involved in apoptosis and that are a potential target for candidate small molecular drugs.

Obatoclax is currently the only small molecule inhibitor that targets apoptosis-regulating proteins in clinical trials and is being developed by GeminX Biotechnologies.

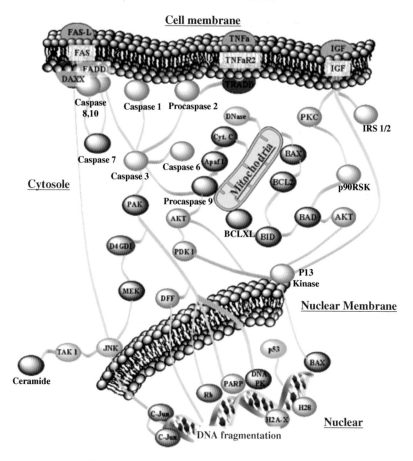

Figure 9.29   The cell death (apoptotic) pathway

It is designed to restore apoptosis through inhibition of the Bcl-2 family of proteins, thereby reinstating the natural process of cell death that is often inhibited in cancer cells. It is in Phase I clinical trials for use against mantle-cell lymphoma and Phase II trials for the treatment of myelodysplastic syndromes, NSCLC, follicular lymphoma, myelofibrosis and Hodgkin's lymphoma.

9.12   Angiogenesis and cancer

With the success of Avastin, the monoclonal antibody that prevents tumour blood vessel formation by blocking VEGF signalling, a number of small molecular drugs have been developed that also target this pathway. As of writing, none of these compounds have made it to the market; however there are several being developed and which are in different stages of clinical testing (see Table 9.2).

Table 9.2 New compounds under development

Molecular target	Drug	Company	Target indication
VEGF R1 EGF R1 RET TK	Vandetanib	AstraZeneca	NSCLC (Phase III), Thyroid (Phase II), Brain (Phase II), Head and Neck (Phase I)
VEGF R1, R2 PDGFβ R1	AG-013736	Pfizer	NSCLC (Phase II), Thyroid (Phase II), Pancreatic (Phase II)
VEGF	AVE0005 (VEGF trap)	Sanofi-Aventis Regeneron	Ovarian (Phase III), Lung (Phase II), Kidney (Phase II)
VEGF R1 PDGFβ R1 c-KIT	AMG 706	Amgen	NSCLC (Phase II), Breast (Phase II), Gastro-Intestinal (Phase II), Colon (Phase I), Bladder (Phase I), Ovarian (Phase I), Leukaemia (Phase I), Lymphoma (Phase I)
VEGF R1	PTK787/ZK22 2584	Novartis Schering	Sarcoma (Phase II), Pancreatic (Phase II), Prostate (Phase II), Kidney (Phase II), Multiple Myeloma Breast (Phase II), Brain (Phase I), Ovarian (Phase I)
Alpha-2 Integrin	E7820	Eisai Med Res	Solid Tumours (Phase II), Lymphoma (Phase I)
VEGF R2 Raf (A-, B-, C-)	RAF265	Novartis	Melanoma (Phase I)
VEGF R1, R2, R3	GW786034	Glaxo SmithKline	Kidney (Phase III), Breast (Phase II), Sarcoma (Phase II), Ovarian (Phase II), NSCLC (Phase II), Brain (Phase I/II), Liver (Phase I), Solid Tumours (Phase I), Colon (Phase I)

9.13 Cancer immunotherapy

Classical surgery, radiotherapy and chemotherapy constitute, without doubt, the forefront regarding the efficient therapeutic options in the treatment of cancer. Still, the need to develop new therapeutic approaches and protocols is urgent, in order to handle aggressive malignancies that do not respond to the anti-cancer approaches currently used in the clinic and to improve on the life span and the quality of life of cancer patients. Triggering the host's antitumour immunity using gene therapy strategies in combination with cytokines, costimulatory molecules, sensitized lymphocytes and antibodies is a very promising approach according to the outcome of many clinical trials.

Increasing the immunogenicity of tumours by causing local cytokine production can lead to local antitumour effects. Also, isolation of T cells from peripheral blood of patients and subsequent *ex-vivo* activation of T cells with cytokines followed by reintroduction to the patient would elicit an immune response against the tumour carrying the tumour antigen used.

Cells undergoing malignant transformation are believed to be eliminated from the body by white blood cells including natural killer cells (NK), lymphokine-activated killer cells (LAK), cytotoxic T lymphocytes (CTL), tumour-infiltrating lymphocytes (TIL), and activated macrophages; since established cancers in the human body may escape this potential defence mechanism of immunological surveillance, cancer patients have been treated with IL-2 to stimulate their cellular immune mechanisms to kill cancer cells; lengthy and complete remissions, however, were at a low rate and complications were encountered by the toxicity caused from the systemic administration of IL-2. Transfection of the *IL-2* gene into human melanoma cells increased cellular immune response. This and similar approaches have established the foundation of the *ex-vivo* cancer immunotherapy by transfer of autologous (cancer patient's) cells after transduction *in vitro* with cytokine genes. The ultimate goal is the activation of tumour-specific T lymphocytes capable of rejecting tumour cells from patients.

Ex-vivo approaches in immunotherapy have been aimed at isolating T cells directly from tumours (known as tumour infiltrating lymphocytes or TILs), stimulate TILs to proliferate in cell culture with IL-2 followed by their reintroduction into the blood stream of advanced cancer patients. IL-2 stimulates the differentiation of precursor lymphocytes into LAK cells and further stimulates LAK cell proliferation; LAK cells are probably produced by activation of NK cells or from activated T cells by IL-2. Administration of IL-2 plus amplified LAK cells into mouse models led to marked regression of disseminated cancers and leukaemia. LAK cells are able to destroy tumour cells that express histocompatibility antigens only weakly. IL-2, however, has several pleiotropic effects: stimulation of B-cell proliferation; activation of HLA class II antigen expression on endothelial cells, TILs, and melanoma cells; and enhanced production and release of TNF-α, and IFN-γ. TILs, which could potentially kill tumour cells, are found in many tumours but remain suppressed or anergic; this anergy may arise from the absence of lymphokines which provide signals for TIL cell activation and stimulation to proliferation, although ligands may be bound to the variable region of the T-cell receptor; indeed, nonimmunogenic tumours are rejected by syngeneic mice upon transfection by *IL-2* or *IL-4* genes; IL-2 lymphokine production by the tumour cells bypasses T helper function in the generation of an antitumour response rendering the tumour cells immunogenic. *Ex-vivo* gene therapy trials using cytokine gene transfer circumvent the problem of toxicity of IL-2 administration, providing a safer alternative to IL-12 protein therapy for cancer treatment.

9.13.1 Monoclonal antibodies as anticancer drugs

Ten years ago there were only two monoclonal antibody drugs on the world market, now there are nineteen FDA approved therapies including six blockbuster drugs. The market in 2005 was worth over $13bn, worldwide, representing an astounding growth of 37 per cent. Biotech pipelines are overflowing with over 160 monoclonal antibody based drugs.

The efficiency of antibodies in the treatment of cancer resulted in the approval by the FDA of more than five antibodies for therapeutic use since 1995. Among them are the humanized murine monoclonal antibody trastuzumab (Herceptin) that targets Her2/neu receptor and the chimeric monoclonal antibody cetuximab (Erbitux) against EGFR (ErbB1) receptor. Herceptin is the first antibody that received FDA approval for the treatment of solid tumours that overexpress Her2/neu, while another humanized monoclonal antibody, pertuzumab (Omnitarg) that inhibits Her2/neu heterodimerization, is now found in Phase II clinical trials. More than 20 monoclonal antibodies for cancer treatment are currently found in the clinical trial stages. Apart from the ErbB proteins, some of the most common cancer antigens used as targets are the cancer embryonic antigen (CEA), that is involved in cancers of the intestine, the MUC1 that is related with breast and lung cancers and is involved in the ErbB network and the CD20 in the B cells, that is a biological marker in the non-Hodgkin's lymphomas.

Antibodies can act either through activation of the host's immune system, inducing complement dependent cytotoxicity or antibody-dependent cytotoxicity, through inhibition of ligand binding to receptors and signalling activation or through conjugation to radioactive moieties and toxins.

Rituximab: a monoclonal antibody against CD20

Rituximab, (Rituxan® and MabThera®), is a monoclonal chimeric antibody against the B-cell surface antigen CD20 which is present in 95 per cent of non-Hodgkin's lymphoma (NHL) cells. Rituximab is the first monoclonal antibody approved by FDA in 1997 for relapsed or refractory low-grade or follicular CD20-positive, B-cell lymphomas. Marketed as Mabthera by Roche it was the top selling drug against cancer in 2005 with sales of 2.7 billion USD. Although originally developed against B-cell lymphoma it has found applications in other diseases such as rheumatoid arthritis and systemic lupus erythematosus. The antibody binds to CD20 molecules on the B-cell membrane through its murine anti-human CD20 portion, and targeting them for destruction by the body's own immune system. The actual mechanism for Rituximab is to eliminate B cells inducing the antibody-dependent cell-mediated cytotoxicity (ADCC) and complement-dependent cytotoxicity (CDC) responses and apoptosis through the human IgG1 portion of the antibody and especially the Fc fragment. This result is the elimination of B cells (including the cancerous ones) from the body, allowing a new population of healthy B cells to develop from lymphoid stem cells. Rituximab is efficiently used in bone marrow transplantation and in the management of renal transplant recipients due to its property to kill lymphoma cells that cause rejection of grafts to the recipient. It is especially useful in transplants involving incompatible blood groups and is also used as induction therapy in highly sensitized patients going for renal transplantation.

The most common side effects include fever, chills and malaise even though premedication with acetaminophen (paracetamol) and diphenhydramine is being administered. Nausea, vomiting, flushing, urticaria, angioedema, hypotension, dyspnoea, bronchospasm, fatigue, headache, rhinitis and pain at disease sites are other infusion-related side effects. These symptoms are self-limited and are generally improved with longer infusions. Other uncommon symptoms include short-lived myelosuppression, abdominal pain, myalgia, arrhythmias and angina pectoris.

Bevacizumab: a monoclonal antibody against VEGF

Angiogenesis is a critical step in tumour cell proliferation, growth, and metastasis. VEGF plays an integral role in tumour neovascularization and has been shown to be highly expressed in several cancer patients. Bevacizumab (Avastin®) is a humanized monoclonal antibody that targets the VEGF signalling pathway and was the first commercially available angiogenesis inhibitor. Bevacizumab stops tumour growth by preventing the formation of new blood vessels through targeting and inhibiting the function of VEGF that stimulates new blood vessel formation. The drug was first developed as a genetically engineered version of a mouse antibody that contains both human and mouse components. The US FDA approved bevacizumab for use in colon cancer in 2004. It was developed by Genentech and is marketed, in the US by Genentech and elsewhere by Roche. It is used in combination with standard chemotherapy drugs in patients with metastatic colorectal cancer and offers improved clinical outcomes when combined with other regimes in colon, lung, and breast cancers. Avastin is the third top selling anticancer drug (sales $2.2 billion in 2005) after rituximab and imatinib.

Trastuzumab: a monoclonal antibody against HER2/neu

Trastuzumab (Herceptin®) is a humanized monoclonal antibody against the extracellular domain of HER2/neu (erbB2) receptor. The Her2/neu receptor is overexpressed in 25–30 per cent of breast cancers with metastatic aggressiveness and poor prognosis. Her2/neu encodes a transmembrane tyrosine kinase glycoprotein and is part of a signalling cascade that involves the activation of PI3K/Akt and MAPK pathways and the promotion of invasion, survival and angiogenesis of cells. Herceptin is used against breast cancer in patients whose tumours overexpress HER2/neu with a response rate of ∼11 per cent, although it resulted in stabilization of tumours in many cases. It was the fourth top selling anticancer drug in 2005 with sales of ∼$2.2 billion.

Herceptin acts through its Fc domain, thus inducing an ADCC immune response and cancer cell lysis. It also inhibits the proteolytic cleavage of the Her2/neu extracellular domain, which causes the constitutive activation of the receptor and loss of cell proliferation control. Herceptin is administrated in combination with chemotherapy such as Adriamycin, cisplatin and taxanes.

Cetuximab: a monoclonal antibody against EGFR

Cetuximab (Erbitux®) is a chimeric monoclonal antibody against the ligand binding site in the extracellular domain of EGFR for treatment of metastatic colorectal cancer and head and neck cancer. EGFR activation results in phosphorylation of several downstream intracellular substrates that induce cell proliferation, angiogenesis, and inhibition of apoptosis. Cetuximab competes with ligands for receptor binding, causing receptor internalization and preventing ligand-mediated receptor tyrosine kinase phosphorylation. Cetuximab has 10-fold greater affinity for EGFR than the natural ligand. Cetuximab was approved by the FDA for use in metastatic colorectal in February 2004. It is the 13th best selling anticancer drug with sales of $686 million in 2005. Cetuximab was approved by FDA in March 2006 for use in combination with radiation therapy for treating squamous cell carcinoma of the head and neck (SCCHN) or as a single agent in patients who have had prior platinum-based therapy. In locally advanced head and neck carcinoma, cetuximab in combination with radiotherapy significantly improved survival compared with radiotherapy alone. Patients treated with cetuximab, occasionally develop a magnesium wasting syndrome with aberrant urinary excretion. There were cases of patients reporting fatigue and symptomatic hypocalcaemia and hypomagnesaemia while on cetuximab plus irinotecan therapy.

Panitumumab: a fully human monoclonal antibody against EGFR

Panitumumab (ABX-EGF) (Vectibix™) is the first fully human monoclonal antibody that has received its license from the FDA in September 2006 for clinical use on humans for patients suffering with non-curable colorectal cancer. It is an IgG2 antibody, produced by immunization of transgenic mice that carry human genes and produce human immunoglobulin light and heavy chains. It targets the extracellular ligand-binding domain of the receptor and acts in the same manner as Cetuximab, resulting in blockade of essential downstream signalling pathways that control apoptosis, proliferation and differentiation. Panitumumab is efficient in the treatment of a wide variety of cancer types, including NSCLC, renal, and colorectal cancer (CRC) as monotherapy and in combination with standard chemotherapeutic agents. Unlike Cetuximab it does not induce any immune response and there was no observation of unfavorable drug-drug interactions or any effect on the pharmacokinetics of other cytotoxic chemotherapeutic agents with which it is combined. A mild to moderate rash has been observed, which is a common reaction among drugs targeting the EGFR.

Ibritumomab tiuxetan: a monoclonal antibody against anti-CD20 for radioimmunotherapy

Ibritumomab tiuxetan (Zevalin®) is a monoclonal antibody radioimmunotherapy treatment for some forms of B-cell non-Hodgkin's lymphoma, a myeloproliferative disorder of the lymphatic system. The drug uses the monoclonal mouse IgG1 antibody ibritumomab in conjunction with the chelator tiuxetan, to which a radioactive isotope (either yttrium-90 or indium-111) is added. Zevalin was the first radioimmuno-agent to be approved by the FDA. As Rituximab, Zevalin binds to the CD20 antigen found on the surface of normal and malignant B cells (but not B-cell precursors), and triggers cell death via ADCC, CDC and apoptosis. Additionally, releases radiation from the attached isotope (mostly beta emission), killing the target cell as well as some neighboring cells. The combination of the above properties eliminate B cells from the body, allowing a new population of healthy B cells to develop from lymphoid stem cells with higher efficiency than Rituximab ($\sim$24 per cent).

Tositumomab: a monoclonal antibody against CD20 covalently bound to iodine-131

Tositumomab (Bexxar®) is a monoclonal antibody derived from immortalized mouse cells. It is a IgG2a anti-CD20 antibody and is covalently bound to iodine-131. It was approved by the FDA in 2003 and used to treat CD20 expressing lymphomas that were refractory to Rituximab. Its mechanism of action is similar to Zevalin radioimmunotherapy. Iodine-131 emits both beta and gamma radiation, and is broken down rapidly in the body. Bexxar advantage over conventional radiotherapy is the targeted delivery of radiation to the target that significantly reduces toxicity to other organs. Toxicities in general are short-term, predictable, and manageable, although unlike Bexxar, radioimmunoconjugates cause myelosuppression which is reversible after treatment.

Alemtuzumab: a monoclonal antibody against CD52

Alemtuzumab (Campath$^{\circledR}$) is a chimeric humanized monoclonal antibody (Campath-1H) against the 21–28 kDa cell surface glycoprotein, CD52. It is an IgG1 kappa with human variable framework and constant regions, and complementarity-determining regions from a murine (rat) monoclonal antibody (Campath-1G). CD52 is widely expressed on the surface of all mature (normal and malignant B and T) lymphocytes, and Campath is indicated for the treatment of B-cell chronic lymphocytic leukaemia (B-CLL). It was been approved by FDA in 2001 after exhibiting a 33 per cent response in patients with relapse cases of CLL as a single agent in patients who have been treated with alkylating agents and who have failed fludarabine therapy. Campath has also been used in combination with Rituximab and showed a 63 per cent response in patients with CLL that were resistant to conventional chemotherapy.

Gemtuzumab ozogamicin: a monoclonal antibody against CD33 linked to a cytotoxic agent

Gemtuzumab ozogamicin (Mylotarg$^{\circledR}$) is a monoclonal antibody used to treat acute myelogenous leukaemia. It is a monoclonal antibody to CD33 linked to a cytotoxic agent, calicheamicin. CD33 is expressed in most leukemic blast cells but is not found on normal haematopoietic stem cells.

Other antibodies with FDA approval for the treatment of cancer are shown in Table 9.3.

9.13.2 Cancer Vaccines

Anticancer vaccination embodies an ideal non-toxic treatment capable of evoking tumour-specific immune responses that can ultimately recognize and kill cancer cells. Cancer vaccines offer an attractive therapeutic addition, delivering treatment of high specificity, low toxicity and prolonged activity. No vaccination regime has achieved sufficient therapeutic efficacy necessary for clinical implementation and a reproducible survival benefit has proved elusive. Nevertheless, several immunological advances have opened new avenues of research to decipher the biological code governing tumour immune responsiveness, and this is leading to the design of potentially more effective immunotherapeutic protocols. One hundred and five different pipeline cancer vaccines have been identified of which 14 are in late-phase development. These candidates have a forecast sales potential of up to $3.1 billion in the pharmaceutical market by 2015.

Table 9.3 FDA approved monoclonal antibodies for the treatment of cancer

Antibody generic/trade name	Type	Target	Company	Approval date	Cancer type
Alemtuzumab/ Campath-1H	Humanized	CD52	Millenium AndILEX Partners	2001	B-cell chronic lymphocytic leukaemia
Bevacizumab/ Avastin	Humanized	VEGF	Roche/ Genentech	2004	Metastatic colorectal cancer
Cetuximab/ Erbitux	Chimeric	EGFR	Merck KgGA	2004 2006	Colorectal cancer Head and neck
Gemtuzumab ozogamicin/ Mylotarg	Humanized conjugated to calicheamicin	CD33	Wyeth	2000	Acute myelogenous leukaemia
Panitumumab/ Vectibix	Human	EGFR	Amgen/ Abgenix	2006	Colorectal cancer
Rituximab/ Rituxan Mab Thera	Chimeric	CD20	Roche/ Genentech	1997	Non-Hodgkin's lymphoma
Ibritumomab tiuxetan/Zevalin	Murine conjugated to ^{90}Yt	CD20	Biogen IDEC	2002	B-cell non-Hodgkin's lymphoma
Tositumomab/ Bexxar	Murine conjugated to ^{131}I	CD20	Corixa	2003	Non-Hodgkin's lymphoma
Trastuzumab/ Herceptin	Humanized	Her2/neu	Roche/ Genentech	1998	Breast cancer

Cancer vaccines have been developed based on a number of strategies. These include synthetic tumour peptide vaccines, DNA vaccines and the use of dendritic cells. The synthetic tumour peptides are based on the immunization with short antigenic peptide epitopes that are expressed on the surface of cancer cells, so that a protective antitumour immune response is elicited. DNA vaccines are one of the first successful applications of foreign genes into mammalian cells. The method consists in introducing the gene of a viral or bacterial antigen, which is taken up and expressed by the host's cells, to elicit an antigen-specific immune response. Dendritic cells from patients with cancer are deficient in number and functional activity, leading to inadequate tumour immunosurveillance. Loaded dendritic cell therapy is a vaccination strategy aimed at eliciting tumour antigen-specific, T-cell immune responses.

9.14 Gene therapy

Gene therapy is a revolutionary field of biomedical research aimed at introducing therapeutically important genes into somatic cells of patients to alleviate disease symptoms. Monumental progress in several fields including DNA replication, transcription factors and gene expression, repair, recombination, signal transduction, oncogenes and tumour suppressor genes, genome mapping and sequencing, and on the molecular basis of human disease are providing the foundation of gene therapy. Disease targets include AIDS, cystic fibrosis, adenosine deaminase deficiency, cardiovascular diseases (restenosis, familial hypercholesterolaemia, peripheral artery disease), Gaucher disease, α1-antitrypsin deficiency, rheumatoid arthritis and a few others. The main emphasis of gene therapy has been cancer.

Cancers tested in clinical trials for gene transfer include the cancers of breast, head and neck, ovarian, prostate, brain, non-small and small cell lung, colorectal, as well as melanoma, lymphoma, chronic myelogenous leukaemia, neuroblastoma, glioma, glioblastoma, astrocytoma, and others. A wide variety of delivery vehicles for genes have been tested including murine retroviruses, recombinant adenoviral vectors, adenoassociated virus, herpes simplex virus (HSV), Epstein–Barr virus, human immunodeficiency virus vectors, and baculovirus. Non-viral gene delivery methods use cationic or neutral liposomes, direct injection of plasmid DNA, and polymers. Various strategies to enhance efficiency of gene transfer have been tested such as fusogenic peptides in combination with liposomes, or polymers, to enhance the release of plasmid DNA from endosomes. Recombinant retroviruses stably integrate into the DNA and require host DNA synthesis; adenoviruses can infect non-dividing cells but cause immune reactions leading to the elimination of therapeutically transduced cells. Adeno-associated virus (AAV) is not pathogenic, does not elicit immune responses but new strategies are required to obtain high AAV titers for preclinical and clinical studies. Wild-type AAVs integrate into chromosome 19 whereas recombinant AAVs are deprived of site-specific integration and may also persist episomally; HSV vectors can infect non-replicating cells such as neuron cells, have a high payload capacity for foreign DNA but inflict cytotoxic effects. It seems that each delivery system will be developed independently of the others and that each will prove its strengths for specific applications.

A number of anticancer genes are being tested in preclinical or clinical cancer trials including: p53, RB, BRCA1, E1A, bcl-2, MDR-1, HER2, p21, p16, bax, bcl-xs, E2F, antisense IGF-I, antisense c-fos, antisense c-myc, antisense K-ras, and the cytokine genes GM-CSF, IL-12, IL-2, IL-4, IL-7, IFN-γ, and TNF-α. A promising approach is transfer of the HSV thymidine kinase (HSV-tk) gene (suicide gene) and systemic treatment with the prodrug ganciclovir which is converted by HSV-tk into a toxic drug killing dividing cells. Theoretically, expression of therapeutic genes preferentially in cancer cells could be achieved by regulatory elements from tumour-specific genes such as carcinoembryonic antigen.

Gene therapy approaches have suffered from the inadequate transduction efficiencies of replication-defective vectors. Replication-competent vectors, particularly adenoviruses that cause cytolysis as part of their natural life cycle, represent an emerging technology that shows considerable promise as a novel treatment option, particularly for locally advanced or recurrent cancer. Especially promising are adenoviruses that selectively replicate in tumour cells that have shown promising preliminary results in clinical trials, especially in combination with chemotherapy. Liposomal formulations of genes may overcome significant hurdles in gene therapy applications in a clinical setting. Many of those are in preclinical or cell culture studies and very few have surfaced to human clinical trials.

Combinations of gene therapy regimes with chemotherapy have synergistic antitumour effects. IFN-β inhibits cell cycle progression as an S phase block; pretreatment of tumour cells with IFN-β could significantly potentiate the cytotoxicity of cisplatin, 5-FU, paclitaxel and gemcitabine in cell cultures. Platinum-based chemotherapy enhances mutations in the p53 in the heterogenous cell population; transfer of the wild type p53 gene enhanced the sensitivity of chemoresistant cells to cisplatin and cisplatin-induced apoptosis.

9.15   RNAi (siRNA)

Small interfering RNAs (siRNA) are small double-stranded RNA molecules that mediate specific and highly potent post-transcriptional gene knockdown. siRNA-mediated knockdown of relevant genes resulted in tumour growth inhibition in a variety of human cancer cell types. However, clinical applicability of this technology has been hindered by the lack of an optimal delivery platform.

9.16   Antisense

The use of antisense RNA to knockdown gene expression has also had some success in the clinic. Indeed, antisense drugs to a number of different target molecules for different target indications have been developed and are currently undergoing clinical evaluation

Table 9.4 Current antisense therapies in clinical trials

Drug name	Target gene	Indication	Developer	Phase
Affinitac	Protein kinase C	Lymphoma	Eli Lilly	II
AVI-4126	C-Myc	Lymphoma	AVI Biopharma	I
Genasense	Bcl-2	Lymphoma	Genta and Aventis	III
		solid tumours	Genta and Aventis	II
MG98	DNA methyltransferase	Multiple myeloma	MethylGene	I
GTI-2501	Ribonucleotide reductase	Prostate	Lorus Therapeutics	II
GEM 231	Protein kinase A	Solid tumours	Hybridon	I
GTI-2040	Ribonucleotide reductase	Solid tumours	Lorus Therapeutics	II
Oncomyc-NG	C-Myc	Solid tumours	AVI Biopharma	I
ISIS 2503	Ha-Ras	Pancreatic cancer	ISIS Pharmaceuticals	II

Table 9.5 Current oncolytic viral therapy clinical trials

Drug name	Mode of action	Indication	Developer	Phase
ONYX-015	Oncolytic virus	SCCHN	Onyx Pharmaceutics	III
		Lung cancer	Onyx Pharmaceutics	III
G207	Oncolytic Herpes	Brain cancer	MediGene	I
Oncolytic HSV	Oncolytic virus	Liver cancer	Medigene	II
CG7870	Oncolytic virus	Prostate cancer	Cell Genesys	I

(see Table 9.4). However, with the advent of RNA interference, it is not clear how successful drugs based on antisense technology will be.

9.17   Viruses able to kill cancer cells

A novel class of targeted anticancer agents endowed with unique mechanisms of action has emerged from the study of therapeutic oncolytic viruses creating the field of virotherapeutics. Despite their promising preclinical data, however, corresponding clinical trials have been disappointed. Hurdles may arise from low penetration of viruses into the tumour cell mass, usually the lack of a systemic delivery method, lack of targeting to primary tumours and metastases without expression in normal tissue, their destruction by the immune system within the tumour once the previous problems are solved. Understanding the field of virotherapeutics necessitates consideration of innate immune defenses in human tumour cells. A number of oncolytic adenoviruses designed to replicate selectively in tumour cells by targeting molecular lesions inherent in cancer, or by incorporation of tissue-specific promoters driving the early genes that initiate viral replication, are currently under clinical evaluation (see Table 9.5).

9.18   Aptamers

Aptamers are small RNA or DNA oligonucleotides that are selected from vast combinatorial libraries for their ability to bind to almost any target of interest. Aptamers act in a way similar to that of antibodies, in that they aim to either block critical pathways and antigen-receptor interactions, or act as carriers for radionuclides and toxins. Aptamers offer smaller molecular weight, faster clearance, improved tumour penetration and reduced immunogenicity. They are quick to synthesize *in vitro*, but they are in early stages of development and they remain expensive to synthesize and prone to degradation by natural enzymes. A number of aptamers against both intracellular (ERK-2, Ras, Raf-1) and extracellular (PSMA, Tenascin-c, MUC1, nucleolin, PDGF and tyrosine kinase) cancer related targets have been developed. The anti-VEGF receptor aptamer has reached clinical trials for cancer and has received FDA approval for the treatment of macular degeneration.

9.19 Summary

A number of agents are currently available for the treatment of various forms of cancer, based on their properties to block different pathways within the cell. Earlier chemotherapy drugs were basing their action on the fact that cancer cells were fast replicating, and platinum complexes, alkylating agents and many antibiotics have been developed for their ability to target DNA and block transcription and replication processes with great success. Later developed, targeted therapeutics and biologic treatments have found their way to the market, with many more in clinical trials. These aim to target particular points in crucial pathways for tumour development and receptors that are mutated or overexpressed in cancer cells compared to normal tissue. Monoclonal antibodies have been the greatest blockbuster drugs of the latest years with many more in pipeline. Other novel therapies, including vaccines, gene therapies, antisense, aptamers, silencing RNAs and delivery systems are making rapid progress in this developing field.

9.20 Self-assessment questions

Question: What combination chemotherapies can make headlines in the next decade?

Answer: Gene therapy, cancer vaccines, monoclonal antibodies, targeting of signal transduction pathway with small molecules, and viruses able to kill preferentially tumours. Especially important are new methods of drug delivery leading to wrapping of preexisting drugs into liposomes, polymers, dendrimers, or other nanoparticles.

Question: Can advancements in the cancer field progress our knowledge in other disciplines?

Answer: Yes, in prevention of aging and prediction of genes. The use of gene therapy regimes against cancer will advance the gene therapy of cardiovascular disease, haemophilia, hypertension, sickle cell anaemia, arthritis, autoimmune diseases and others.

Question: Which ones of the new platinum-based anticancer drugs are more likely to become the blockbusters of the next decade?

Answer: Carboplatin and oxaliplatin are safer versions of cisplatin but have not shown a better therapeutic efficacy compared to cisplatin. There are ample opportunities in development of novel platinum compounds with improved therapeutic index. Also, formulations of pre-existing drugs such as liposomal formulations with tumour targeting abilities can enhance the therapeutic index of the active ingredient.

Question: What are the advantages of liposomal delivery of drugs?

Answer: The drug develops a different profile. Acquires lower and altered side effects, has an altered tissue biodistribution, its half-life increases and circulates for longer periods in body fluids. The PEGylation of the surface of liposomes gives to the particles their 'stealth' properties in the sense that they remain undetected by the macrophages and proteins of the serum after intravenous administration. A liposomal drug is no longer a small molecule but a nanoparticle able to extravasate preferentially through the compromised and leaky tumour vasculature during angiogenesis. Furthermore, such nanoparticles, because of their lipid shell, are taken up more avidly by tumour cells from their tendency for phagocytosis to satisfy their increased metabolic rate.

Question: Which are the main mechanisms of monoclonal antibodies for the direct destruction of cancer cells?

Answer: Monoclonal antibodies induce the following responses through their Fc fragments: (a) an antibody-dependent cellular cytotoxicity (ADCC), (b) complement-dependent cytotoxicity (CDC), (c) antigen binding.

Question: What was the aim of using IL-12 in cancer treatment?

Answer: IL-12 was used as a mediator in order to induce the production of cytokines (IFN-γ) and a strong T_H1 response that results in proliferation of cytotoxic lymphocytes and of IgG specific molecules from B cells that result in tumour phagocytosis and lysis.

Question: Name some antibodies that have been approved by FDA and their targets?

Answer: Trastuzumab (Herceptin) that targets Her2/neu receptor is used in breast cancer patients whose tumours overexpress the Her2/neu gene. Cetuximab (Erbitux) is a chimeric monoclonal antibody against EGFR (ErbB1) receptor. Bevacizumab is a humanized monoclonal antibody that targets the VEGF signalling pathway.

9.21 Further reading and resources

Ajani JA. Evolving chemotherapy for advanced gastric cancer. *Oncologist* 2005, **10**, S3:49–58.

Astsaturov I, Cohen RB and Harari PM. EGFR-targeting monoclonal antibodies in head and neck cancer. *Curr Cancer Drug Targets* 2006, **6**(8), 691–710.

Baselga J, Albanell J, Molina MA and Arribas J. Mechanism of action of trastuzumab and scientific update. *Semin Oncol* 2001, **28**(5 Suppl 16), 4–11.

Bhoola S and Hoskins WJ. Diagnosis and management of epithelial ovarian cancer. *Obstet Gynecol* 2006, **107**(6), 1399–1410.

Boulikas T and Vougiouka M. Cisplatin and platinum drugs at the molecular level. *Oncol Rep* 2003, **10**, 1663–1682.

Boulikas T and Vougiouka M. Recent clinical trials using cisplatin, carboplatin and their combination chemotherapy drugs. *Oncol Rep* 2004, **11**, 559–595.

Boulikas T. Status of gene therapy in 1997: molecular mechanisms, disease targets, and clinical applications. *Gene Ther Mol Biol* 1998, **1**, 1–172.

Brand TC and Tolcher AW. Management of high risk metastatic prostate cancer: the case for novel therapies. *J Urol* 2006, **176**(6 Pt 2), S76–80; discussion S81–82.

Di Francesco AM, Ruggiero A and Riccardi R. Cellular and molecular aspects of drugs of the future: oxaliplatin. *Cell Mol Life Sci* 2002, **59**, 1914–1927.

Evans DB, Wolff RA, Crane CH and Pisters PW. *UICC (International Union Against Cancer) Manual of Clinical Oncology*, eighth edition. Pollock RE, Doroshow JH, Khayat D, Nakao A and O'Sullivan B (eds). Wiley-Liss, NJ, USA, 2004.

Hill JM and Speer RJ. Organo-platinum complexes as antitumor agents (review). *Anticancer Res* 1982, **2**, 173–186.

Judson I and Kelland LR. New developments and approaches in the platinum arena. *Drugs* 2000, **59**(Suppl 4), 29–36; discussion 37–38.

Lin AM, Hershberg RM and Small EJ. Immunotherapy for prostate cancer using prostatic acid phosphatase loaded antigen presenting cells. *Urol Oncol* 2006, **24**(5), 434–441.

Martin F and Boulikas T. The challenge of liposomes in gene therapy. *Gene Ther Mol Biol* 1998, **1**, 173–214.

Nahta R, Hortobagyi GN and Esteva FJ. Novel pharmacological approaches in the treatment of breast cancer. *Exp Opin Investig Drugs* 2003, **12**(6), 909–921.

Ranson M and Thatcher N. Paclitaxel: a hope for advanced non-small cell lung cancer? *Exp Opin Investig Drugs* 1999, **8**(6), 837–848.

Raymond E, Faivre S, Chaney S, Woynarowski J and Cvitkovic E. Cellular and molecular pharmacology of oxaliplatin. *Mol Cancer Ther* 2002, **1**, 227–235.

Rosenberg B. Noble metal complexes in cancer chemotherapy. *Adv Exp Med Biol* 1977, **91**, 129–150.

Saunders M and Iveson T. Management of advanced colorectal cancer: state of the art. *Br J Cancer* 2006, **95**(2), 131–138.

Schrag D, Chung KY, Flombaum C and Saltz L. Cetuximab therapy and symptomatic hypomagnesemia. *J Natl Cancer Inst* 2005, **97**(16), 1221–1224.

Stinchcombe TE, Fried D, Morris DE and Socinski MA. Combined modality therapy for stage III non-small cell lung cancer. *Oncologist* 2006, **11**(7), 809–823. Erratum in *Oncologist* 2006, **11**(8), 958.

Thomson BN, Banting SW and Gibbs P. Pancreatic cancer – current management. *Aust Fam Physician* 2006, **35**(4), 212–217.

Wagner AD, Grothe W, Haerting J, Kleber G, Grothey A and Fleig WE. Chemotherapy in advanced gastric cancer: a systematic review and meta-analysis based on aggregate data, *J Clin Oncol* 2006, **24**(18), 2903–2909.

Wahl RL. Tositumomab and (131)I therapy in non-Hodgkin's lymphoma. *J Nucl Med* 2005, **46**(Suppl 1), 128S–140S.

Wu AM and Senter PD. Arming antibodies: prospects and challenges for immunoconjugates. *Nat Biotechnol* 2005, **23**(9), 1137–1146.

Wu J, Wu GY and Zern MA. The prospects of hepatic drug delivery and gene therapy. *Exp Opin Investig Drugs* 1998, **7**(11), 1795–1817.

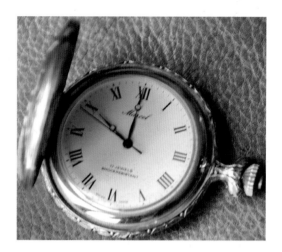

In the previous chapter we have discussed the various treatments available for the control of cancer in the aim to provide a therapeutic effect and increase the life expectancy of the patient or, ideally, provide a cure and allow the patient to return to their normal life. When discussing some of the therapeutics available, we saw the various side effects that these molecules can cause, effects such as diarrhoea, nausea and vomiting, hair loss, loss of appetite, fatigue, as well as depression and anxiety associated both with the disease and the side effects of the therapy. Appropriate measures need to be taken into consideration for the control of these symptoms and often medication is provided together with the anticancer therapeutic to control or minimise these side effects. However, it is often the case with a life-threatening disease like cancer that the therapeutic regimes may fail to achieve their ultimate aim of cure and the patient, sooner or later, may have to deal with the end-of-life experience. Whilst more and more cancers are now becoming curable, or disease can be controlled and life prolonged almost indefinitely, giving them the characteristics of a chronic disorder, a number of patients have to face that they are not responding any longer to therapy. At this stage, the professional health care providers have to make the difficult decision to let go of any attempts towards extending life and turn their attention to ease patient suffering and help them preserve their dignity at the final stages of life through control of their symptoms with palliative care.

10

Palliative care in oncology

Silvana dos Santos Barreto,[1] **Mariângela Freitas Lavor,**[2] **Maria da Glória Nunes dos Santos,**[3] **Marcelle Miranda da Silva,**[4] **Benedita Maria Rego Deusdará Rodrigues**[5] **and Maria Therezinha Nóbrega da Silva**[5]

1. Brazil Oncology Nursing Society, Rio de Janeiro, Brazil
2. Rio de Janeiro Action and Health Service Secretariat, Rio de Janeiro, Brazil
3. Palliative Care Hospital of the National Cancer Institute, Rio de Janeiro, Brazil
4. Specialist Oncology Nurse, Rio de Janeiro, Brazil
5. Rio de Janeiro State University School of Nursing, Rio de Janeiro, Brazil

10.1   Palliative care: concept and brief history

Cancer patients begin their treatment aiming at a cure. However, for some of them this aim is not achieved and they have to face the reality of a terminal illness. As the disease progresses, its symptoms are accentuated and concerns about quality of life become urgent. The pressing need arises for the existence of a differentiated care system to cater for the needs of patients and their families.

In medieval times, when such procedures were symptomatic and naturalistic, physicians had often only palliation to offer. Religious thought ruled concepts of health and illness; accordingly, their respective medical practices sought to treat bodies and souls. The therapist had fundamental obligations, which consisted of helping people to heal or smoothing the signs of impending death, when there were no more resources to prolong life. Importantly, death was certain and natural.

Since the eighteenth century, the development of a body of technical knowledge has supported the development of a medical market that offers drug interventions. With the development of medical science and prophylactic and curative drug discoveries,

The Cancer Clock   Edited by Sotiris Missailidis
© 2007 John Wiley & Sons Ltd

medical intentions have shifted from people to body and illness. Bodies have achieved the status of objects of scientific curiosity, and it has become more difficult to provide medicine tailored to the family and delivered at home. Patients are now hospitalized and their families are even more excluded from the process of caring for the diseased. The perception of impending death excludes the sick from family life at what consists in the life's final phase. In 1893 St. Lukes Hospice was founded in England to receive incurable patients, reinforcing the idea of the dying reclusion, hospitalizing death, keeping it away from social life.

From the Industrial Revolution onwards, technological advances fostered the perception that it is possible to heal all illnesses of the population, contributing to put aside the idea of death. However, in the twentieth century, this perception was altered by an understanding that it is not always possible to cure, as suggested by the increase of prevalence and incidence of non-transmissible chronic diseases, such as cancer. The consequent increase of costs of insistent curative and diagnostic measures, aiming at prolonging life, brought palliation back into focus. The Hospice movement, headed by Dr Cicely Saunders, landmarks the concept of palliative care used today.

Saunders' concern was increased quality of life for patients who fought against terminal diseases. The model she proposed defines 'palliative care' as a group of actions that enable a holistic approach to an incurable disease patient. These actions are carried out by a multi-professional team, combining clinical care, research and teaching for the effective control of symptoms and total control of pain (provided in hospital or home care), family support for caring for the patient during disease process and death, as well as support for the just-after-death period.

For the World Health Organization (WHO), 'palliative care' is defined as an approach that aims at promoting quality life for patients and families who face problems associated with life-threatening diseases, through prevention and suffering relief by early identification, correct evaluation, pain treatment and other physical, psychosocial and spiritual problems. According to the WHO, palliative care has as its philosophy neither the advancing nor the retarding of death, considering it as a natural event. It aims at relieving pain and other symptoms that provoke suffering, integrating psychological and spiritual aspects in caring for the patients, and offering support to help patients live as actively as possible, helping their families to deal with the patients' disease and their own grief. It can be used in the earliest stages of the disease, in association with other therapies used with the intention of prolonging life, as chemotherapy and radiotherapy, and include necessary investigations for a better comprehension and handling of suffering related to clinical complications that may occur during treatment.

10.2   Cancer epidemiology and palliative care around the world

According to the WHO, cancer is one of the main causes of mortality and morbidity in the world. There are around 25 million people with cancer nowadays; 10 million new cases of cancer are diagnosed every year in the world, but two-thirds occur in developing countries and more than 6 million deaths by this disease are registered.

The increasing rates of incidence and mortality by cancer observed in world population are related to aging, life style (obesity, diet, etc.), exposure to carcinogenic agents such as tobacco, and socio-economic factors (see also Chapter 1). In developing countries, high rates of incidence of infectious diseases directly connected to poverty still persist, and it is observed that these lead to the progressive increase of chronic degenerative disease occurrence, as cancer.

This poses a great challenge for governmental policy implementations in health. In general, what is observed in all sectors of health care is the population's difficulty in accessing information, associated to social inequalities, and insufficient health basic care networks. This situation makes effective implementation of curative and diagnostic measures difficult, which may contribute to late disease diagnosis, at a stage when the chances of successful implementation of treatments which aim at the cure and increase of the patient's disease-free life are decreased.

It is known that investments in early cancer diagnosis and prevention areas result in more social and economical benefits than advanced levels of disease treatment. In the USA in 2004 costs related to cancer have been estimated to almost 190 billion dollars, but half of this figure is related to productive loss owing to the disease. Considering the increasing demand of patients diagnosed with advanced cancer, or of those who evolve to progressive and irreversible disease during treatment, considerable investment in the area of palliative care is necessary, principally in relation to human resources (multi-professional teams, volunteers, etc.), and materials (such as access to pain killers, mainly opioids).

Wright *et al.* (2006), in a study aiming at evaluating the level of palliative care development in the world, has proved that nearly half of the 234 researched countries do not make accessible palliative care services available to their population. In the rest of them, this kind of service needs structure adjustments and many times is restricted to dedicated places, which make them inaccessible to the majority of the population and individuals with no integration to the existing health services. They have observed that there is a direct relation between palliative care services on offer and these countries' human development level. For instance, in the United Kingdom there is around 1 palliative care service for each 40 thousand inhabitants. However, in Pakistan there is only 1 palliative care service for 158 million inhabitants. Brazil has palliative care services in the proportion of 1 for each 13 million inhabitants. The researchers have concluded that the challenges related to the programme of palliative care implementation in the world include, among many aspects: political, economic and social instability; low level of population awareness; care of people with life-threatening diseases not seen as a priority; lack of appropriate government regulations; lack or incorrect use of opioids; palliative care being considered as a low-prestige subject; absence of content related to palliative care in the health professionals' courses and curriculum; current demands resulting from the need of a multi-professional team; insufficient number of interested professionals in this area; cultural differences, including death related taboos and diagnosis revelations.

10.3   Bioethics and palliative care

Caring for the dying tends to create a strong feeling of impotence in the professional. This impression of 'defeat' can make the professional reticent when dealing with terminal patients. Care for the terminally ill patients reminds us of the challenge of accepting our own human finitude.

It is important to point out that cancer treatment does not finish when possibilities of cure appear exhausted. This moment requires a change of focus, from cure to care searching for palliation. Palliative care provision is society's appropriate answer to the concern with care and comfort at the end of life, making the patients' autonomy stronger. Palliative therapeutics focus on symptomatic control, without healing function, aiming at preserving quality of life towards its end. Quality of life can be considerably improved with the implementation of a relatively small amount of resources. According to the WHO, palliative care is a recommended option when a patient's disease is incurable and aggressive treatments to make life longer may produce exaggerated morbidity and high personal cost with little benefit. This recommendation is based not only on moral and scientific elements but also on ethical principles.

The ethics of palliative care aim to identify the specific needs that emerge in the end-of-life context. Medical action always produces an effect to the patient, and it must be evaluated whether medical intervention will have a beneficial or detrimental effect. Often, during treatment, it is difficult to establish clearly a line between useful and futile. In cases of terminal patients, the therapeutic plan must have some aspects in sight, such as whether the proposed treatment may improve, maintain or restore quality of life, benefit the patient in terms of comfort, well-being or general appearance aspects, or, perhaps, relieve symptoms and suffering. In case these objectives cannot be met, medical treatment can be considered futile and results in extending agony and suffering. This action is considered 'therapeutic obstination', or 'disthanasia', that is 'the use of therapeutic processes whose effect is more harmful than the effects of the illness, or useless because cure is impossible and the expected benefit is less than foreseen inconvenience' (Pessini, 2001).

The principles of beneficence, autonomy and justice need to be analysed under the scope of palliative care. In the curable phase of a disease, beneficence must prevail. The main goal in this phase is the preservation of life, and the introduction of extraordinary measures is justifiable. Yet, in the phase of unavoidable death, where cure is no longer possible, efforts must be concentrated on non-maleficence (not institution of measures considered to be futile). The principle of autonomy refers to the patient's rights of taking part in the decision making process with regards to their situation. If the patient is unable to make decisions, the principle of autonomy will be exercised by family or legal representatives. The principle of justice refers to adequate evaluation of resources that will be used on a patient, considering the other principles discussed as well as the benefits and cost for the patient, also its effectiveness in promoting adequate symptom control, avoiding disproportional measures that may extend suffering but could benefit other patients. Additionally, there are other ethical principles to be considered in the praxis of palliative care and will be described below.

The principle of veracity refers to the trust that is fundamental in interpersonal relations. It consists of communicating the truth to patients and their families, which represents a benefit for both (beneficence) and enables active participation in decision-making processes (autonomy). In communication of bad news, a certain care with *what, how, how much (many), when, who and whom to inform*, should be taken. 'Silence conspiracy', a mechanism often present in these situations, can only be responsible for new forms of patient suffering.

The proportionality principle consists of the moral obligation of implementing all therapeutic measures that are relative to the proportion between means employed and foreseen result, in which the usefulness and uselessness of the action must be judged, as well as other alternatives considering risks and benefits, prognosis with or without the measure, and costs of physical, psychological, moral or economic nature, imposed to the patient, family and team.

The double effect principle marks the conditions that must be observed, so that performing a two-effect act – a good one and a bad one – is legal. This principle must be observed, for instance, in the case of sedation of a patient in extreme suffering for the difficulty of controlling the advanced disease symptoms. This intention of promoting relief through sedation (beneficence) surpasses the undesirable effect that may occur, respiratory depression (maleficence).

The prevention principle is concerned with the awareness of preventing the most frequent symptoms, the most possible complications related to disease evolution itself, and the needed implementation measures for its prevention, aiming at avoiding unnecessary suffering and decision-making which would lead to disproportionate interventions.

Finally, the principle of not-abandoning and pain treatment refers to assisted care up to the end of life and to pain control, as much as possible; receiving necessary care and not being abandoned, so that the patient may die with dignity, that is, with their symptoms adequately under control.

10.4 Basic principles in palliative care

Patient care at the end of life phase demands, in addition to technical and scientific knowledge, high humanistic sense, so that patients can be assured of their right of dying with dignity. Comfort and quality of life for cancer patients in palliative care are related to having family, friends and health team support, provided with an adequate care structure that allows patients to be into a family environment and obtain adequate control of cancer progression secondary symptoms. These results meet palliative care premises of promoting comfort and quality life to cancer patients at the end of their lives. It is necessary that patients are cared for by a multi-professional team, have psychosocial support and adequate control of the secondary symptoms of cancer progression.

An interdisciplinary approach and family and patient attention are fundamental to the palliative care exercise. Accordingly, the existence of a multi-professional team is necessary and must include nurses, social workers, psychologists, physiotherapists, religious representatives, volunteers, occupational therapists and physicians, in order to allow for a broader consideration of the patient's needs. Professional intervention must be based on communication and information as therapeutic tools. Among the existing barriers to communication, socio-cultural and family questions and professionals' fears with possible consequences of the act of communicating bad news are highlighted. When receiving news of cancer diagnosis, patient and family often feel sentenced to death. Many euphemisms are used to talk about this disease. Their main metaphors refer to topography ('scatter'; 'disseminates') and the biggest fear, even overcoming fear of death, is that of mutilation and pain.

Prejudice from some disease fear, considered as taboos, constitute a huge obstacle to a patient adequate approach. Difficulties in freely talking about patient diagnosis/prognosis may take professionals to a paternalist attitude or distancing attitudes which lead to an increase in patient and family suffering.

Communication is currently viewed as a fundamental element in professional–patient relationship, and many protocols currently offering suggestions and strategies on how to inform patients about their disease and/or death have been elaborated. Many barriers linked to the socio-cultural environment, where denial of death itself is evident, favour what is called a 'conspiracy of silence'. This consists in excluding nature and disease development as situation analysis elements to establish professionals' specific actions.

The vast majority of patients express the desire that their physician be realistic and provide opportunities for patients to ask questions, as well as a wish that they should be seen as an individual during prognosis discussion. The physicians' behaviour during this process is particularly important, appearing optimistic when providing data about the best available treatment, showing knowledge about the pathology and cancer patient care, and confirming that pain should be controlled. On the other hand, most patients feel that during prognostic discussion, physicians often demonstrate discomfort and nervousness, discuss issues with the families before talking to the patient, use euphemisms, avoid talking about cancer and only discussing the treatment itself. This behaviour can generate discouragement and hopelessness.

Some steps can be observed to make professional–patient communication easy: guaranteeing privacy, start the conversation at a calm place, no demonstration of hurry, avoiding interruptions; the presence of the patient's relative or close friend, chosen by the patient themselves, is recommended; information must be provided observing what the patient already knows and to what extent they would like to know; not imposing information on the patient; stopping when the patient shows they would not like to continue talking; always having the facts at hand in order to eliminate any shadow of doubt in relation to diagnosis and/or prognosis; providing clear and simple explanations; avoiding technical terms and euphemisms (e.g. 'ulcer' to designate 'cancer'); verifying patients comprehension; allowing patients' to express fear, negation, rage and to demonstrate hearing availability.

In palliative care, the family is also considered to be a care unit because it suffers with its relative's illness and death. In some countries, mainly in developing countries, it is observed that in cases of incapacitating diseases, which imply a high level of dependence, care has been provided by an informal support system that includes family care givers, friends, neighbours or community members whose activities are, in general, performed voluntarily, with no wage. Family and friends are the first source of care.

Assistance to the family, as health care unit, implies knowing how each family cares and identifies their strength, difficulties and efforts to share responsibility. Professional work with the families and/or care givers must contemplate information and reflection, and it is necessary to instruct family on care praxis as well as observing their emerging feelings towards the patient. Family care givers receive a physical and emotional overload, owing to their responsibility and care activities, continuous living with suffering and loss feelings and what it represents in their future life. Many times, the care givers face ruptures to their emotional ties, have their life deteriorate, have no vacations and low social participation. The care giver's activity is almost a lonely, restless, tiring, with non-stop daily repeating one and, many times, invisible. However, despite negative aspects, positive transformations are reported by care givers who have their lives changed, giving them a meaning that had never existed before, with interior experience of growing and transformation.

Another important aspect in palliative care is the place where these procedures are carried out/conducted. Hospitalization, which implies costs for the health system, drives the patient into an unknown environment with little flexible time and restrictions on visitors' numbers and time. On the other hand, home stay contributes to raising the patient's quality of life, allowing the patient's family and friends' home life, with an environment which is familiar to them, flexibility of hygiene, feeding and leisure time. Nevertheless, for home stay to foster comfort and avoid the patient's feeling abandoned by their health team due to having an incurable disease, it is necessary that a support structure is put in place that allows for professional assistance and access to necessary drugs for adequate control of symptoms and family support.

In developed countries, home care is a practice that has shown to be effective both to cost reduction and to foster the well-being that staying at home provides. This can be an important strategy for implementation of palliative care programmes in developing countries, which need to balance costs to the health system with problems related to poverty and social inequality, as infectious parasitic diseases and malnutrition are known to raise chronic diseases such as cancer.

10.5 Symptom control in oncology palliative care

The presence of pain and other signs and symptoms related to cancer progression in advanced cancer patients is very common. A person in cancer palliative care has special needs as do their family and care givers. A study by Higginson (1998) about the prevalence of the main problems that cancer people present at the end of life has shown the following results: pain (84 per cent), anorexia (71 per cent), nausea and vomits (51 per cent), insomnia (51 per cent), respiratory problems (47 per cent), constipation (47 per cent), wounds (47 per cent), depression (38 per cent), urinary control loss (37 per cent), mental confusion (33 per cent), intestinal control loss (25 per cent), anxiety and severe worry (25 per cent), disagreeable odour (19 per cent). Many of these problems may be associated directly with the disease, or be the result of intensive therapeutic interventions. Thus, cancer patients have needs that go far beyond physical comfort, which is why the importance of a differentiated care for them and their families has been highlighted. For the appropriate handling of these signals and symptoms and many other physical, emotional, social and spiritual factors, the health professional who acts in palliative care must consider some key aspects, such as evaluation, planning, and care implementation, therapeutic relationship development and outcomes evaluation.

Palliative care professionals must have the knowledge of the principles of anatomy and physiology for all organic systems; pharmacology of principal groups of drugs used in oncology palliative care; technological procedures that help in cancer diagnosis and treatment; and knowledge of psychiatric and physical aspects of the disease in its advanced phase as well as the related complications with the evolution of the disease itself and the side effects of the several procedures to which the patient has been submitted during the treatment. Such preparation is needed so that they are able to provide appropriate care at an opportune time in order to promote maximum comfort and quality of life for the patients.

10.5.1 Pain relief in cancer

Pain is an awkward and subjective sensorial and emotional experience, which is described according to previous individual experiences. Acute and chronic pain are frequent in advanced oncological disease, and may be caused by a primary tumour, metastasis, treatment or not-related conditions to oncologic disease. Pain prevalence increases with cancer progression and occurs in a moderate or intense way in 30 per cent of advanced cancer patients receiving treatment, and a total of 60 per cent to 90 per cent of advanced cancer patients.

However, this symptom can be relieved in about 90 per cent of the cases and maintained within acceptable levels in the rest, if it is appropriately evaluated and suitable therapeutics are instituted. Although there have been great pharmacological advances in last few years, pain control still represents an important challenge. One important aspect is the difficulty of diagnosis and pain evaluation by health professionals, due to insufficient knowledge of its symptoms and causes and the subjective nature of pain, which varies according to age, culture and psychological condition of the patient, as well as the generalized prejudice among patients and health professionals with regards to analgesic therapy, chiefly in relation to use of opioids.

Pain relief in cancer, considering this symptom has a significant effect on several aspects of the patients' lives, must be one of the main aims of professionals who work in oncology. In implementing an effective programme of pain control, some aspects must be observed: existence of a national policy for pain control, enforced through education and provision of access to appropriate analgesics; health professional education through inclusion of the subject into health professionals' curricula; and efficient policies not only for analgesic drug availability but also prescription, dispensing and adequate administration.

In palliative care, the concept of 'total pain' is used to indicate a consideration of the physical, social, psychological and spiritual aspects for its approach, resulting in the need for a multidisciplinary approach for the effective control of the symptom, as many factors including fear, anxiety, depression, hopelessness and fatigue can influence pain perception. Thus, for more effective pain control, it is necessary to consider the emotional, cultural and psychological aspects together with the physiopathological characteristics related to the illness.

It is crucial for the health professional to seriously consider the patient's complaint, evaluate it appropriately, relate it to the actual treatment methods to which the patient has been subjected, and use pharmacological and non-pharmacological resources to obtain the most effective control of this symptom in order to provide suffering relief and improve quality of life. Complementary methods of pain control could include care coordination, massage, relaxation, positions that diminish pain, immobilization, helping relations' and patient's family therapeutic adherence. On the other hand, avoiding self-medication practices through client education and their care giver with regards to pharmacological and not-pharmacological treatments is crucial to avoid damage.

The health professional must register pain evaluation clearly and precisely, detailing its location, intensity, pain start, duration and painful episode periodicity, quality of sensibility, evolution pattern, pain aggravating and attenuating factors and other associated symptoms. Many tools are used for pain evaluation. These tools must be chosen whilst taking into consideration the patient comprehension easiness and most used are the numerical scales and verbal descriptors.

Numerical scales are graded 1 to 10, where zero means pain absence and 10, the worst imaginable pain. Another much-used resource is the verbal scale, with simple terminology, where the patient must describe pain intensity using four terms: absent, light, moderate and intense pain. There are other scales, such as faces, bodies, etc., which may also be useful in cases where patients present difficulty in understanding the numerical scale. Furthermore, scales and diagrams of the body, such as the dermatome diagram where patients point to the region of the body with the most intense pain on a drawing, are used for the assessment of pain.

Various principles must be observed in the administration of analgesic drugs, according to the WHO, 'by the mouth, by the clock, by the stairs, individualization and attention to the detail'. The choice administration is the oral one and intravenous or muscle injectable drugs should be avoided for their technical difficulty, especially concerning self-care, and discomfort related to the procedure. Rectal administration should be considered as an alternative for patients with oral access restrictions as dysphagia or uncontrollable vomiting. Another alternative is transdermic administration for analgesics like fentanyl. However, the high cost of the particular drug limits its use in developing countries and it is reserved only for situations where patients present intolerance to morphine or are incapable of oral ingestion due to illness progression.

Subcutaneous administration can be an important alternative for patients who cannot medicate orally. It has the advantage of being available for home use due to its

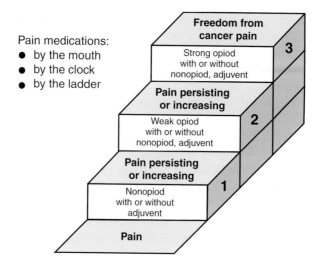

Pain medications:
- by the mouth
- by the clock
- by the ladder

Figure 10.1 WHO pain ladder

easy handling, particularly as care givers receive adequate training by professionals. However, subcutaneous administration is not indicated for generalized oedema, fragile peripheral circulation and in the cases where repetitive infections in puncture area of the patients occur.

Analgesic administration at regular times is another basic principle in controlling pain in cancer, as it ensures that the drug's plasma concentration remains within prescribed levels and the patient does not experience periods of pain. Besides administration of painkillers at regular times, additional doses may be necessary in case of intermittent or sudden pain. These additional doses must be calculated from the proposed therapeutic scheme, the patient must be orientated in relation to their use, and such incidents should be registered and used for a later principal scheme adjustment. The therapeutic scheme for pain control must be individualized, according to patient needs. Attention to detail is an important aspect for treatment success, and care in relation to dose, interval, prescription elaboration clarity and patient and family advice with regards to the use of the drug and its side effects, both concerning adverse reactions identification and dealing with predictable effects, such as constipation in patients who use of opioids, must be observed.

The WHO has developed a strategy to guide pain treatment in a sequential manner, the three-step 'ladder' for cancer pain relief (Figure 10.1), using its intensity as parameter:

1. Mild cancer pain; the indicated therapeutics in this case are non-opioid pain killers combined with adjuvant analgesic (drugs that are initially not indicated for pain treatment but provide this effect in certain situations, e.g., antidepressants, anticonvulsants, corticosteroids, neuroleptics, bisphosphonates, etc.).

2. Moderate to intense pain that did not have relieved symptom in the prior scheme. The therapeutics consists of the addition of weak opioid analgesics (codeine, tramadol) to the previous scheme.

3. Intense pain (intensity referred by patient or no effective relief from the previous scheme); the drug treatment, in this case, consists of substituting the weak opioid for a strong one (morphine, fentanyl, methadone), maintaining the administration of non-hormonal anti-inflammatory analgesics and adjuvant analgesics.

The treatment goal is relieving discomfort caused by pain, mainly when performing daily life activities. To achieve this goal, it is necessary to continuously evaluate the established analgesic therapy. Besides drugs therapeutics, other treatment modalities for pain control may be instituted, such as radiotherapy that may be used for neuropathic pain.

10.6   Advanced cancer: related symptoms and interventions

10.6.1   Fatigue

Fatigue is one of the most prevalent symptoms in oncologic palliative care and constitutes a complex and subjective phenomenon. Its intensity varies from patient to patient and it is necessary that its real scale is accessed by the healthcare professional who evaluates the patient. Its presence and consequent chronic effect in advanced cancer patients contributes to its status and favour the manifestation of other characteristic signals and symptoms, such as depression.

Fatigue, according to Carpenito (2002) 'is the self-recognized status in which the individual presents a sustained and dominated sensation of exhaustion and decrease of mental and physical capacity, not relieved by rest'. In advanced cancer patients, fatigue can be related to biochemical factors that arise from the presence of actively growing tumour. This can result in important loss of the organism's protein reserves, which constitutes an alteration in the anorexia–cachexia syndrome (CAS) present in advanced cancer. Other factors that contribute to fatigue are anaemia, loss of appetite, pain, sleep alterations, infections, hypoxia, fever, diabetes, intestinal constipation and anxiety, as a result of the tumour or as side effects of the therapeutic regime.

Apart from the physical causes, fatigue can also be related to cognitive, emotional, spiritual and social aspects. This multi-factorial characteristic makes fatigue an enduring symptom in advanced cancer patients. However, pharmacological and non-pharmacological measures may be implemented to maintain patient functional capacity, promoting quality of life and minimizing unnecessary energy losses, always aiming for a beneficial effect to the patient.

Pharmacological examples for controlling fatigue include: anti-depressants, non-opioid and opioid analgesics attempting to achieve pain control, corticosteroids, antibiotics (in the case of infections), etc. Besides, one can also exploit hydration with electrolytic replacement and blood transfusions as this treatment can also be effective in dealing with fatigue.

Non-pharmacological fatigue care includes allowed physical exercises according to location and extension of disease, clinical indication and treatment regimes. Planning and prioritization of activities need to be developed day by day; sleeping time organization, avoiding the change of day for night often observed in this kind of patient, particularly those who are in bed. Although there is lack of direct evidence for the effectiveness of these measures, as mentioned before, their implementation is easy and often results in perceived improvement.

10.6.2 Dyspnoea

Dyspnoea is another frequent symptom in advanced cancer patients and causes intense discomfort, fear and anxiety, and, for most patients, it also represents proximity of death, thus worsening the performance status and consequently affects prognosis.

Dyspnoea is also a subjective sensation that constitutes the disagreeable perception of difficulty of breath or effort needed to breathe. Thus, only the patient is able to provide data on its characteristics and intensity. Dyspnoea follows many clinical conditions in palliative care, even when primary or metastatic disease is not pulmonary in nature. Therefore, it must be fastidiously investigated before therapeutic intervention is warranted and determined. In general, dyspnoea in oncology patients occurs in situations of metabolic exhaustion that is present in anorexia–cachexia syndrome, grave ascites, recurrent pleural flood, gasometric alterations, visceromegaly, pulmonary system primary or metastatic cancer itself, neuromuscular diseases and emotional unbalance. Other co-morbidities that may cooperate in its graveness include congestive heart failure, asthma, chronic obstructive pulmonary disease and renal failure.

Healthcare professionals must be attentive to the presence of dyspnoea, noting and assessing its graveness, aggravating factors and respiratory cycle frequency, as well as, contribute to the determination and verification of effectiveness of therapeutic regimes, in close interaction with the oncology multi-disciplinary team.

Severe dyspnoea can result in brain hypoxia, causing cognitive disturbances, with movement agitation pictures. In some cases, the situation can become so grave that the best procedure is terminal sedation, reducing the patient's and family's, as well as the health team's, suffering. This measure is considered when the prognosis indicates rapid deterioration in the condition of the patient, as often is the case in primary lung advanced cancer and respiratory system metastasis. Any medical decisions must be discussed with patient and family and approval should be sought. Furthermore, the health team must respect all decisions of the patient, or family, when they are unable to talk for themselves, even if this does not constitute the most appropriate medical choice of action.

The most commonly used pharmacological therapies in oncologic palliative care for the control of dyspnoea are corticosteroids, diuretics and antibiotics. Diuretics must be used with caution due to the risk of dehydration. A number of alternative procedures can also be used, including thoracocentesis, tracheotomy, pleurodesis, blood transfusion, paracentesis, and sodium restriction in the diet.

For the immediate control of dyspnoea, the following resources are available: anticholinergics and anti-histaminics, which reduce secretion; bronchodilators; anxiolytics to reduce anxiety; anti-coughing opioids, which reduce coughing, reduce secretion and venous return and decrease pre-charge; moist oxygen administration using a nasal catheter or mask; superior airways aspiration; raised bed-head maintenance and provision of a calm environment.

The use of oxygen is indicated for cases where dyspnoea is related to hypoxia, in some acute dyspnoea cases and in situations where patient and family psychologically depend on it. However, use of oxygen may cause discomfort, due to the use of a mask, and may lead patients to dependency and anxiety for its use, greatly limiting their quality of life. That is why it is indicated only for cases in which dyspnoea is related to hypoxia, for cases of acute dyspnoea and situations in which both patient and family present psychological dependence to it.

10.6.3 Cognitive aspects

Another important aspect in the care of advanced cancer patients is concerned with potential cognitive alterations, mainly present in elderly patients, resulting from the presence of an incurable disease, as well as undesirable effects of drugs used in the therapeutic control of chronic pain. Cognitive aspects include consciousness, attention, perception and memory. Any disturbance in one of these criteria indicates presence of cognitive alteration. The main observations of cognitive alteration in palliative care cancer patients are delirium, dementia, anxiety and depression.

The patient's cognitive status must be carefully evaluated in order to ensure early identification of any kind of alteration or aggravation of pre-existing alterations that may disturb their coherence and clarity. Such aspects must be evaluated, as they can contribute to non-compliance to the efficacious therapeutic regime, thus hampering other indications and advanced cancer symptom control. Besides, alterations in cognition directly influence in self-care capacity and it may thus be necessary to relieve the care giver, bringing the patient to the hospital once more, to avoid potential delays in intervention.

Very often, cognitive alterations are treated in an inadequate way or under treated, which is why there is need of early identification and correlation with other factors, such as: brain hypoxia due to dyspnoea, systemic processes such as acid–base disturbance, nutritional deficit, metabolic encephalopathy, polypharmacy, and the disease itself compromising the central nervous system may cause cognitive alterations.

As usual in oncological palliative care, prevalence of cognitive alterations increases with proximity of death. Depression indications often rise when the patient is hospitalized. Furthermore, this is often associated with increased anxiety and it can result in increased perception of physical symptoms such as pain, thus further worsening quality of life. Clinical conditions and patient prognosis must be accurately evaluated before implementing pharmacological measures against depression as there is a temporal window until their anti-depressant effect appears efficacious. In situations where a poor diagnosis is involved, it is worth administering psycho-stimulants that improve appetite, reduce fatigue and promote general well being.

10.6.4 Constipation

Constipation is another very frequent symptom in oncological palliative care. Nearly 50–80 per cent of patients in palliative care present constipation. Constipation may be related to many factors, such as, reduction of liquid and fibre ingestion, reduction of general physical activity, and lack of privacy, principally during hospitalization. Furthermore, changes in vital organs due to advanced cancer presence can result in constipation, especially when these compromise abdominal organs that are capable of causing intestinal compression and consequent intestinal sub-occlusion. Finally, constipation could be caused by the direct effect of cancer on the gastrointestinal tract, metabolic changes, drug adverse effects, or medullary. The important thing in this case is to be attentive to the patient's intestinal habits, as well as evaluate the abdominal region during physical examination, auscultating peristaltic movements regularly and promoting new adaptations daily. Often the use of laxatives, suppositories and enemas, in addition to the use of mineral oil orally, laxative diets and increased of fluid intake when there is no counter-indication, is needed. Such a measure must be initiated by the time of opioid pharmacological therapy begins, to ensure intestinal constipation prevention.

Constipation creates further loss of appetite, fatigue, and concern with proximity of death and social isolation. The latter is related to the invasive procedures used in attempting to resolve the problem, which compromises the patient's privacy, alters their mood and causes irritability. Considering these factors, it is concluded that constipation contributes to reduction in quality of life and is one of the issues that need to be addressed within the remit of palliative care.

10.6.5 Anorexia

As many other symptoms in oncological palliative care, anorexia is multi-factorial. The bad nutrition and loss of appetite is directly related to cachexia resulting from the CAS, which is one of the greatest challenges for a multi-professional team. Anorexia can be related to taste and smell alterations, as well as alterations on the hypothalamus hunger regulator centre, caused by the disease or as a result of side effects from the therapy. As mentioned before, constipation and intestinal obstruction are also able to cause loss of appetite. Besides, digestion and food absorption related disturbances might severely contribute to CAS.

All these factors contribute to significant weight loss in advanced cancer patients, promoting important alterations in their well being, in their performance status, in their prognosis and, consequently, their quality of life.

The presence of a tumour in progression determines a minor availability of energy to the patient so that they may perform their daily life activities. The tumour promotes a significant depletion to protein reserves and adipose tissue loss, leading to progressive malnutrition and dehydration. This process is expedited when the tumour location compromises the digestive system. Not eating or not wanting to eat during the end-of-life process brings important social, symbolic, nutritional and psychological implications to the patient and principally to their family. Eating and drinking are elementary actions of daily life, and thus, the process of providing appropriate care is closely related to the offer of food and liquids. When the care givers find themselves unable to perform this basic activity, a pathological condition prevails, making advanced phase disease implications stronger. Not achieving feeding of the body abundantly and promoting pleasure means absence of protection and defence against disease – as if feeding was the only connection to life.

Interventions against CAS primarily focus on the evaluation of conditions associated with pain, modified taste, bad mouth conditions, oral cavity tumour lesions, halitosis, bleeding, xerostomia, mucositis, constipation, nausea and vomiting, dysphagy, alterations in self-care and cognitive functions and their appropriate management.

In dealing with CAS, the following procedures are indicated: fractionation of diet, increased flexibility of time according to the patient's desires; mild diets that are much more tolerable; amount of food adequate and to the patient's desire, not forcing them to ingest bigger volumes of food than they are supposed to tolerate; choice of foods that the patient prefers, not insisting in high calorie or high protein contents, neither specific diets that the patient may not tolerate. Attention to food presentation must be paid and appropriate amount of food and size of plate are aspects that may contribute to a better acceptance of diet. The use of nasogastric catheters or other invasive feeding forms must be limited to situations where there is some high obstruction by the tumour (pharynx, oesophagus) that implies difficulty in oral feeding. Use of invasive methods for feeding, in the case of CAS patients have not demonstrated effectiveness in improving their clinical status, although they contribute to increase of suffering, and are thus not indicated in CAS management.

10.6.6   Nausea and vomiting

Nausea and vomiting represent a significant problem for advanced cancer patients, affecting their quality of life directly. For efficient control of these symptoms it is necessary to recognize their aetiology. They may happen because of chemotherapy or radiotherapy side effects, as a result of advanced disease or medication side effects from controlling other signs and symptoms. With regards to measures for controlling nausea and vomiting, the fractionation of diet and reduction in portion volume; provision of cold and attractive food; therapeutic environment; use of anti-emetic drugs as rescue drugs in severe cases; and establishment of appropriate oral hygiene are highlighted.

Frequently, nausea is more difficult to control than vomiting. It may be associated with gastric stasis and peristaltic movement alterations. Nausea and vomiting are common in hyperkalaemia, aggravating dehydration and worsening prognosis and is very common in bone metastasis. As therapeutic measures for hyperkalaemia expansion with saline solution, which reduces dehydration, and use of intravenous biphosphate are highlighted. These control hyperkalaemia by blocking osteoclastic osteolysis and reduce bone metastasis. However, the possibility that these may result in renal failure, coma and death must also be recognized.

10.6.7 Ulcerated lesions

Another problem related to cancer progression is the presence of tumoral ulcerated lesions, which, often compromise patients' quality of life due to their size and leaky nature, and in some cases cause pain, bleeding, and a fetid odour. Pain control, exudation and maintenance of externally clean and dry dressings as well as promotion of a therapeutic and confident environment are essential measures to promote patient comfort.

10.7 Psycho-spiritual aspects in oncology palliative care

In today's society, death is often a taboo, synonym of loss, injustice and something that is not natural. This reason results in constant negation of death and search for immortality. Patients under oncology palliative care face the reality of being finite, and many times fear does not reside only in death itself but also in everything that surround them, disease situation, fear of suffering and being left alone.

When facing the fact of having an incurable, terminal disease, attitudes of anger, negation, bargain and depression are common (see also Chapter 12) until the patients accept for themselves the irreversibility of the disease process and imminent death. To deal with that patients need to find meaning in life and live their last moments thoroughly with all the support they need, whether professional, family-based, social and/or spiritual, to understand this process.

In advanced cancer patients, quality of life is related to both *physical* integrity, manifested in the need to control symptoms, and *non-physical* integrity that can be experienced even when the body already presents signs of decline. The patient has the need to resolve dependencies, to feel in peace, and often finds the necessary support in faith and religious beliefs when dealing with proximity of death. These aspects must be valued and the multi-professional team's presence is important to enable the patient's access to the resources they need to feel comfortable despite the adverse situations they are experiencing.

Spirituality seems to be important to help the patient in facing disease processes. It is important to mention that spirituality is not necessarily related to religiosity and it is important that healthcare professionals and other members (religious personnel, volunteers, etc.) who play a role in palliative care must be attentive to enable patients to exercise their faith, belief or rituals, observing what is the patients' wish, without imposing on them personal, team, friend or family's beliefs.

10.8   Conclusion

The increase in cancer cases diagnosed and the continuous improvements in the diagnostic and therapeutic interventions available, resulting in an increase survival time with the disease, imply an increased need for adequate care to cope with patients' demands.

Palliative care services and pain control policies still remain a world challenge, particularly in the poorest countries. The fight for a more equitable world also implies a fight for all people to have access to health services and receive adequate treatment whenever and at whatever stage they need it, not only aiming to increase life expectancy, but also to die with dignity, painlessly, with other uncomfortable symptoms under control and as much as possible in their own home.

Providing pain and suffering relief for patients who are under your care is every healthcare professional's duty, independently of their specialty and available resources. The healthcare professional is entitled to make the best use of available resources, keeping in mind the highest benefit and least damage to the patient, so that the impact of their actions improve patients' quality of life.

To provide appropriate care for people at the end of their life it is necessary to recognize the limit where treatment can assist with control of the disease before it becomes damaging to the patient. Professionals should be technically competent and sensitive to the needs of the patient and the provision of palliative care at the right time, enabling improved comfort and quality of life. Control of symptoms like pain, constipation, nausea and vomiting, cachexia and anorexia are important for patient relief, particularly in end-of-life care, to ensure that patients maintain their dignity. The ability of the patient to remain at home and maintain some of their basic functions are crucial during this process and both pharmacological and non-pharmacological approaches are available to relieve such symptoms. As we have seen in the previous chapter, a number of therapeutic regimes are now administered with palliative care agents, such as antiemetics, to reduce suffering, whilst prolonging life. However, value of life, allowing dignity, respect and autonomy for the terminally ill, are equally important factors to be considered by the carer.

10.9   Self-assessment questions

A 65-year-old patient with breast cancer with bone metastasis (metastatic implants in sternum, ribs, lumbar spine, pubis and left femur, liver and lung), after presenting disease progression during chemotherapy treatment, has been sent to the palliative care team. During team evaluation, she showed nervousness and signs of knowing that her disease had not responded to the chemotherapy treatment. She presented weakness (asthenia) and generalized bone pain that limited her in her daily activities. She referred to irregular use of Dipyrone, without effective pain control. Furthermore, she complained of absence of appetite and difficulty in sleeping due to the pain. She appeared to be worried about her family's attitude that appeared reticent as to her actual clinical condition and felt the need of talking about her disease, but had no opportunity of doing so. Based on this story, address the following points as requested:

Question: What are the relevant aspects (problems) to be considered by the team in order to implement appropriate palliative care?

Answer: Many problems are relevant in this case and deserve special attention: the pain, which is not being effectively controlled, limiting her daily activities and making sleep difficult; the asthenia, the anorexia and the need to talk about her clinical condition with her family.

Question: Indicate which principles should be observed in pain management?

Answer: Initially, detailed evaluation of pain should be performed: initiation, characteristics (burning, stinging), location, intensity, developing factors, improving factors, worsening factors, impact on daily activities and in quality of life. It is also important to identify other factors that may interfere in pain perception, e.g. anxiety, depression etc. It is important to know her previous history, ability of comprehension and self-care, available resources for it, level of support, and family involvement. With regards to the treatment, concerning pharmacological intervention, WHO principles must be observed: preferably use orally administered medication, use of medication in regular intervals, use of pain scale to determine the drugs of choice. Pain must be approached in an individual way and details in relation to factors that may influence treatment compliance must be considered. Yet, non-pharmacological measures for pain control as psychotherapy and physiotherapy must also be considered.

Question: With regards to asthenia, indicate the procedures relevant to its evaluation and management.

Answer: Identify which factors are related to asthenia and how they can be reversed, e.g. anaemia, pain, loss of appetite, depression, etc. Employ pharmacological measures if they can be effective. Non-pharmacological management of fatigue includes allowed physical exercises according to the location and stage of disease and clinical status; inform about the importance of planning and prioritization of activities on a daily basis; organize sleeping time, avoiding day–night changes.

Question: Describe the approach to be adopted by team members in face of patient's desire to talk about their illness and the family attitude of not talking about it.

Answer: Discuss the subject with relatives, reporting the patient's desire, allowing them to express their feelings about the situation they are living. Promote dialogue between patient and relatives, granting privacy, starting talk at a quiet place with no interruptions; allowing the patient to choose which relative or relatives should be present; and expressing her feelings in relation to their disease and proximity to death. Provide every support available to patient and family, e.g. psychotherapy and spiritual support etc.

Question: Describe the role of the multi-professional team in supporting the family who is experiencing this process.

Answer: Remember that, in palliative care, the family is a health care unit, which implies the need to know how each one cares and to identify their difficulties and efforts to share responsibility. It is necessary to instruct relatives in care practice, allowing expression of feelings that emerge in relation to the patient, to the moment they are living, to loss and what it represents for their future life, about death and mourning. Remind relatives and care givers that, although it is a difficult moment, positive aspects such as the possibility of internal growth from this experience can be found.

10.10   Further reading and resources

Adderley U and Smith R. Topical agents and dressings for fungating wounds (Protocol for a Cochrane Review). In: *The Cochrane Library*, Issue 2, 2005. Update Software, Oxford.

American Cancer Society. *Cancer facts & figures 2005*. American Cancer Society, Atlanta GA, 2005.

Baile WF, Buckman R, Lenzi R, Glober G, Beale EA and Kudelka P. Spikes – a six-step protocol for delivering bad news: application to the patient with cancer. *Oncologist* 2000, **5**, 302–311.

Barreto SS. Associação entre qualidade de vida e conforto de pessoas com câncer em cuidados paliativos no domicilio. [Dissertação de Mestrado em Enfermagem]. Faculdade de Enfermagem da Universidade Estadual do Rio de Janeiro, Rio de Janeiro, 2005.

Bauer C, Gerlach MA and Doughty D. Care of metastatic skin lesions. *J Wound Ostomy Continence Nurs* 2000, **27**, 247–251.

Bertolino M. Estreñimento/constipacíon. In: Bruera E and Lima E (eds). *Cuidados paliativos: guia para el manejo clínico*. Organizacion Panamericana de Salud & International Association for Hospice and Palliative Care, Washington DC, 2004, pp. 55–60.

Breaking bad news. Preparing to break bad news. Available from: www.breakingbadneuws.co.uk [accessed 28 Jan 2007]

Bruera E and Driver L. Astenía/fatiga. In: Bruera E and Lima E (eds). *Cuidados paliativos: guia para el manejo clínico*. Organizacion Panamericana de Salud & International Association for Hospice and Palliative Care, Washington DC, 2004, pp. 75–78.

Campbell T and Hately J. The management of nausea and vomiting in advanced cancer. *Int J Palliat Nurs* 2000, **6**(1), 18–23.

Caponero R. A evolução do movimento hospice. In: Pimenta CAM, Mota DDCF and Cruz DALM (eds). *Dor e cuidados paliativos – enfermagem, medicina e psicologia*. Manole, São Paulo, 2006, pp. 1–28.

Carpenito LJ. *Diagnósticos de enfermagem – aplicação à prática clínica*, eighth edition. Artmed, Porto Alegre, 2002.

Chaves LD. Dor pós-operatória: aspectos clínicos e assistência de enfermagem. In: Leão ER and Chaves LD (eds). *Dor – 5° sinal vital: reflexões e intervenções de enfermagem*. Editora Maio, Curitiba, 2004, pp. 151–168.

Davies J and McVicar A. Issues in effective pain control 1: assessment and education. *Int J Palliat Nurs* 2000, **6**(2), 58–65.

Doyle D, Geofrey H and Macdonald N. Introduction. In: Doyle, D; Geofrey H and Macdonald N (eds). *Oxford Textbook of Palliative Medicine*, second edition. Oxford University Press, Oxford, 2003, p. 3–8.

Elsayem A, Driver L and Bruera E. *The M.D. Anderson Symptom Control and Palliative Care Handbook*. The University of Texas Health Science Center at Houston, Houston TX, 2003.

Elsayem A, Driver L, Walker P, Fisch M, Sivesin D and Bruera E. Other problems in patients with cancer. In: Bruera E, Lima L, Wenk R and Farr W (eds). *Palliative Care in the Developing World: Principles and Practice*. International Association for Hospice and Palliative Care, Houston TX, 2004, pp. 125–142.

Farias MLF. A hipercalcemia nas malignidades: aspectos clínicos, diagnósticos e terapêuticos. *Arq Bras Endocrinol Metab* 2005, **49**(5), 816–824.

Ferrel BR. The impact of pain on quality of life: a decade of research. *Nurs Clin North Am* 1995, **30**(4), 609–624.

Fihser ES and Silva MJP. Reações emocionais da enfermeira no atendimento ao paciente fora de possibilidades terapêuticas. *Rev Nursing* 2003, **66**(6), 25–30.

Firmino F. Lutas Simbólicas das Enfermeiras no Processo de Implantação do Centro de Suporte Terapêutico Oncológico (CSTO) do Instituto Nacional de Câncer. [Dissertação de Mestrado em Enfermagem]. Escola de Enfermagem Anna Nery da Universidade Federal do Rio de Janeiro, Rio de Janeiro, 2004.

Floriani A and Schramm FR. Atendimento domiciliar ao idoso: problema ou solução? *Cad Saúde Pública* 2004, **20**(4), 986-994.

Foucault M. *O Nascimento da Clínica*, sixth edition. Forense Universitária, Rio de Janeiro, 1982.

Franco M. La comunicación con el paciente terminal y su familia. In: Bruera E and Lima E (eds). *Cuidados paliativos: guia para el manejo clínico*. Organizacion Panamericana de Salud & International Association for Hospice and Palliative Care, Washington DC, 2004, pp. 15–20.

Friedrichsen M and Erichsen E. The lived experience of constipation in cancer patients in palliative hospital-based home care. *Int J Palliat Nurs* 2004, **10**(7), 321–325.

Fukuda C. Controle da constipação intestinal. In: Pimenta CAM, Mota DDCF and Cruz DALM (eds). *Dor e cuidados paliativos – enfermagem, medicina e psicologia*. Manole, São Paulo, 2006, pp. 219–239.

Garcia-Calvente MM, Mateo-Rodrigues I and Maroto-Navarro G. El impacto de cuidar en la salud y la calidad de vida de las mujeres. *Gac Sanit* 2004, **18**(suppl 2), 83–92.

Gutierrez PR and Oberdiek HI. Concepções sobre a saúde e a doença. In: ANDRADE, SM et al. Bases da Saúde Coletiva. Rio de Janeiro (RJ): EDUEL/ABRASCO/NESCO; 2001.

Hagerty RG, Butow PN, Ellis PM *et al.* Communicating with realism and hope: incurable cancer patient's views on the disclosure of prognosis. *J Clin Oncol* 2005, **23**(6), 1278–1288.

Higginson I. Needs assessment and audit in palliative care. In: Faull C, Carter Y and Woof R (eds). *Handbook of Palliative Care.* Blackwell Science, London, 1998, pp. 44–54.

International Association for Study of Pain. Consensus development conference statement: the integrated approach to the management of pain. *J Accid Emerg Med* 1994, **6**(3), 291–292.

Johnston B. Overview of nursing developments in palliative care. In Lugton J and Kindlen M (eds). *Palliative Care: The Nursing Role.* Churchill Livingstone, Edinburgh, 1999, pp. 1–26.

Kovács MJ. Bioética nas questões da vida e da morte. *Psicol Univ São Paulo* 2003, **14**(2), 115–167.

Kübler-Ross E. *Sobre a morte e o morrer.* Martins Fontes, São Paulo, 2002.

Lavor MFS. Cuidados Paliativos na Atenção Básica: visão dos enfermeiros do Programa Saúde da Família. [Dissertação de Mestrado em Enfermagem]. Escola de Enfermagem Anna Nery – Universidade Federal do Rio de Janeiro, Rio de Janeiro, 2006.

Lobb EA, Butow PN, Kenny DT and Tattersall MHN. Communicating prognosis in early breast cancer: do women understand the language used? *Med JAust* 1999, **171**(6), 290–294.

Maguire P. Breaking bad news: explaining cancer diagnosis and prognosis. *Med J Aust* 1999, **171**(6), 288–289.

Manfro G, Dias FL, Lima RA and Reis T. Relação entre idade, sexo, tratamento realizado e estágio da doença com a sobrevida em pacientes terminais com carcinoma epidermóide de laringe. *Rev Brasileira Cancerologia* 2006, **52**(1), 17–24.

Márquez BC. Valoración del dolor por cáncer. In: Bruera E and Lima E (eds). *Cuidados paliativos: guia para el manejo clínico.* Organizacion Panamericana de Salud & International Association for Hospice and Palliative Care, Washington DC, 2004, pp. 27–30.

Mcmillan SC and Weitzner M. How problematic are various aspects of quality of life in patients with cancer at the end of life? *Oncol Nurs Forum* 2000, **27**(5), 817–823.

Menezes MFB and Camargo TC. A fadiga relacionada ao câncer como temática na enfermagem oncológica. *Rev Latino-am Enfermagem* 2006, **14**(3), 442–447.

Ministério da Saúde (BR). Instituto Nacional de Câncer. Alívio da dor no câncer. INCA, Rio de Janeiro, 1997.

Ministério da Saúde (BR). Instituto Nacional de Câncer. Cuidados paliativos oncológicos – controle de dor. INCA, Rio de Janeiro, 2001.

Ministério da Saúde (BR). Instituto Nacional de Câncer. Ações de enfermagem para o controle do câncer. INCA, Rio de Janeiro, 2002.

Montejo G and Delírio. In: Bruera E and Lima E (eds). *Cuidados paliativos: guia para el manejo clínico.* Organizacion Panamericana de Salud & International Association for Hospice and Palliative Care, Washington DC, 2004.

Moraes TM. Atuação do enfermeiro na dor oncológica. In: Leão ER and Chaves LD (eds). *Dor – 5° sinal vital: reflexões e intervenções de enfermagem.* Editora Maio, Curitiba, 2004, pp. 170–179.

Mota, AR and Mota DDCF. Alterações cognitivas em cuidados paliativos. In: Pimenta CAM, Mota DDCF and Cruz, DALM. *Dor e cuidados paliativos – enfermagem, medicina e psicologia.* Manole, São Paulo, 2006, p. 279–300.

National Comprehensive Cancer Network. *NCCN Clinical Practice Guidelines in Oncology. Adult cancer pain.* National Comprehensive Cancer Network, Philadelphia, 2006.

National Comprehensive Cancer Network. *NCCN Clinical Practice Guidelines in Oncology. Palliative care.* National Comprehensive Cancer Network, Philadelphia, 2006.

Oliveira VZ, Oliveira MZ, Gomes WB and Gasperin C. Communication of the diagnostic: implications on threatening adolescents with chronic illness. *Psicol estud* 2004, **9**(1), 9–17.

Organização Pan-Americana de Saúde. Doenças crônico-degenerativas e obesidade: estratégia mundial sobre alimentação saudável, atividade física e saúde. Organização Pan-Americana de Saúde, Brasília, 2003.

Pessini L. *Distanásia, Até quando prolongar a vida?* Editora do Centro Universitário São Camilo & Loyola, São Paulo, 2001.

Pessini L. A filosofia dos cuidados paliativos. In: Pessini L and Bertachini L (eds). *Humanização e cuidados paliativos*, third edition. Centro Universitário São Camilo: Loyola, São Paulo, 2004. p. 181–208.

Pimenta CAM and Ferreira KASL. Dor no doente com câncer. In: Pimenta CAM, Mota DDCF and Cruz DAL (eds). *Dor e cuidados paliativos – enfermagem, medicina e psicologia*. Manole, São Paulo, 2006, pp. 124–166.

Pimenta CAM and Mota DDCF. Fadiga em pacientes com câncer avançado: conceito, avaliação e intervenção. *Rev Brasileira Cancerologia* 2002, **48**(4), 577–583.

Pimenta CAM and Mota DDCF. Controle da fadiga. In: Pimenta CAM, Mota DDCF and Cruz DALM. *Dor e cuidados paliativos – enfermagem, medicina e psicologia*. Manole, São Paulo, 2006, pp. 193–218.

Piva, JP and Carvalho, PRA. Considerações éticas nos cuidados médicos ao paciente terminal. *Bioética* 1993, **1**(2), 129–138.

Plancarte R, Guillén MR, Guajardo J and Mayer F. Ascitis em los pacientes oncológicos. Fisiopatogenia y opciones de tratamiento. *Rev Soc Esp Dolor* 2004, **11**, 156–162.

Portenoy RK, Sibirceva U, Smout R, *et al.* Opioid use and survival at the end of life: a survey of a hospice population. *J Pain Sympt Manag* 2006, **32**(6), 532–540.

Rincon HG, Gomez JE and Lima L. Depresion e ansiedad em pacientes terminales. In: Bruera E and Lima E (eds). *Cuidados paliativos: guia para el manejo clínico*. Organizacion Panamericana de Salud & International Association for Hospice and Palliative Care, Washington DC, 2004, pp. 85–90.

Rodrigues R. Náusea crónica y vómito en el paciente com cancer. In: Bruera E and Lima E (eds). *Cuidados paliativos: guia para el manejo clínico*. Organizacion Panamericana de Salud & International Association for Hospice and Palliative Care, Washington DC, 2004, pp. 41–48.

Rodriguez CJ. *O Tabu da Morte*. Achiamé, Rio de Janeiro, 1983.

Rodríguez EDG. Sintomas respiratorios I: dispnea e HIPO. In: Sancho MG (ed.). *Cuidados paliativos: atención integral a enfermos terminales*. Instituto Canario de Estúdios y promoción social y sanitária, Spain, 1998, pp. 549–558.

Rosario MAB and Fraile AA. La comunicación con el paciente con enfermedad en fase terminal. *Atención Primaria* 2002, **30**(7), 463–466.

Saunders C. Foreword. In: Doyle D, Geofrey H and Macdonald N. *Oxford Textbook of Palliative Medicine*, second edition. Oxford University Press, Oxford, 2003, p. v–xi.

Saunders C. Prefácio. In: Sociedade Francesa De Cuidados Paliativos & Colégio De Cuidados De Enfermagem. *Desafios de Enfermagem em Cuidados Paliativos: Cuidar: ética e práticas*. Lusociência, Lisbon, 2000, pp. 9–10.

Schramm RF. Morte e finitude em nossa sociedade: implicações no ensino de cuidados paliativos. *Rev Brasileira Cancerologia* 2002, **48**(1), 17–20.

Silva CHD. A moralidade dos cuidados paliativos. *Rev Brasileira Cancerologia* 2004, **50**(4), 330–333.

Silva YB and Silva J. Controle da dispnéia. In: Pimenta CAM, Mota DDCF and Cruz DALM. *Dor e cuidados paliativos – enfermagem, medicina e psicologia*. Manole, São Paulo, 2006.

Simone GG. El final de la vida: Situaciones clinicas y cuestionamentos éticos. *Acta Biomédica* 2001, **VI** (1), 49–62.

Sociedad Española de Cuidados Paliativos. Guia de Cuidados Paliativos. [on line] España: SECPAL. Available from: http://www.secpal.com/guiacp/ [accessed Jan 31 2007]

Sontag S. *A doença como metáfora*. Edições Graal, Rio de Janeiro, 1984.

Souter J. Using a model for structure reflection on palliative care nursing: exploring the challenges raised. *Int J Palliat Nurs* 2003, **9**(1), 6–12.

Souza FAEF and Hortense P. Mensuração da dor. In: Leão ER and Chaves LD. *Dor – 5° sinal vital: reflexões e intervenções de enfermagem. Editora Maio, Curitiba*, 2004, pp. 151–168.

Taboada P. Princípios éticos relevantes em medicina paliativa. In: Bruera E and Lima E (eds). *Cuidados paliativos: guia para el manejo clínico*. Organizacion Panamericana de Salud & International Association for Hospice and Palliative Care, Washington DC, 2004, p. 9–14.

Taboada, P. Ethical issues in palliative care. In: Bruera E, Lima L, Wenk R and Farr W (eds). *Palliative Care in the Developing World: Principles and Practice*. International Association for Hospice & Palliative Care, Houston TX, 2004, pp. 39–51.

Tapiero AA. La sedación terminal. Aspectos éticos. *Med Interna Madrid* 2003, **12**(20), 645–649.

Teixeira MJ. Dor no doente com câncer. In: Teixeira MJ(ed.) *Dor: contexto interdisciplinar*. Maio, Curitiba, 2003, pp. 327–341.

Teng CT, Humes EC and Demetrio FN. Depressão e comorbidades clínicas. *Rev Psiq Clín* 2005, **32**(3), 149–159.

Thoroddsen A. Applicability of the Nursing Interventions Classification to describe nursing. *J Caring Sci* 2005, **19**(2), 128–139.

Twycross R. *Palliative Care*. Climepsi, Lisbon, 2001.

Twycross RG and Lack AS. *Terapêutica em câncer terminal*. Artemed, Porto-Alegre, 1991.

Valera JP and Aubry R. Morphine – doctor's belief and the myths. *Eur J Palliat Care* 2000, **7**(5), 178–182.

World Health Organization & UICC – Unión Internacional Contra el Cáncer. Accíon mundial contra el cáncer. Versión Rev. WHO, Geneva, 2005.

World Health Organization. Collaborating Centre for Palliative Care. Looking forward to cancer pain relief. International consensus on the management of cancer pain. CBC, Oxford, 1997.

World Health Organization. Consejo Ejecutivo. *Control del cáncer*. Informe de la Secretária. WHO, Geneva, 2004.

World Health Organization. *WHO definiton of Palliative Care*. WHO, Geneva, 2005. [cited 2005 Aug 22]. Available from: http://who.int/cancer/palliative/definition/en/

Wright M, Wood J, Lynch T and Clark D. Mapping levels of palliative care development: a global view. International Observatory on End of Life Care, Lancaster University, UK, 2006. [accessed Jan 21 2007]. Available from: http://www.nhpco.org/files/public/palliativecare/World_map_report_ final-0107.pdf

Younes RN and Noguchi Y. Pathophysiology of cancer cachexia. *Rev Hosp Clín Fac Med S Paulo* 2000, **55**(5), 181–193.

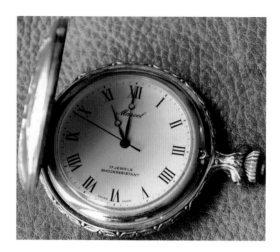

Following the chapters about diagnosis, imaging and treatment of cancer, we are now looking at the last hours of this book. The patient by this stage would have been diagnosed with cancer, undergone surgery, assisted by imaging techniques, and would have either chemotherapy or radiotherapy, or both. At this stage, the patient would (i) be struggling to rejoin normal life, through the side effects of the treatment, (ii) be under treatment, such as hormone therapy, having passed in the stage of living with a chronic disease, or (iii) be at a terminal stage and try to have the best quality of life possible during this very difficult last stage of life.

In this chapter we will see how physiotherapy, as well as other disciplines allied to medicine, can assist the patient recover from the side effects of surgery, chemotherapy or radiotherapy. The nature and use of physiotherapy has changed during the last years and the multidisciplinary nature of dealing with cancer is discussed during this chapter. Improved therapeutic approaches can extend the life of the patients, but they often leave them with severe and debilitating side effects and impairments. Physiotherapy can improve the physical condition of the patients and assist their rehabilitation. As we will see in this chapter, physiotherapy can provide a number of services, specialized to the various form of cancer and the individual needs of the patient, and assist in their quick return to the society and their regaining of functions that were affected from disease or treatment.

11

Physiotherapy in cancer patients

Mario Bernardo-Filho[1], Anke Bergmann[2] and Ângela Tavares[3]

1. *Universidade do Estado do Rio de Janeiro and Instituto Nacional de Câncer, Brasil*
2. *Physioterapy Department, Hospital do Câncer III, Instituto Nacional de Câncer, Brasil*
3. *Faculdade de Fisioterapia, Fundação Oswaldo Aranha, Brasil*

11.1 Physiotherapy and oncology

Physiotherapy has a relevant role in the healthcare of people of all ages and with different kinds of clinical conditions, including in the treatment and the prevention of diseases or complications. Physiotherapists use physical agents, such as therapeutic exercises, electrotherapy and manipulative therapy to provide a holistic approach to the prevention, diagnosis and therapeutic management of disorders. Involving the movements of the body and the optimization of the functions of the tissues, they aim to enhance the health, welfare and quality of life of people throughout their lifespan.

Physiotherapy is a profession defined by great diversity in areas of clinical practice with the purpose of developing, maintaining and restoring the maximum movement and functional ability of each person, considering the specific limitations of the individual. Moreover, increasing complexity and breadth in physiotherapy has led to the development of specialized areas to provide patient care with respect to prevention of diseases, decrease of recovery time and risk of recurrence, appropriate management of the condition and improvement of the quality of the life of the patient. Physiotherapy includes the provision of procedures in circumstances where movement and function are threatened by the process of ageing or that of injury or disease.

The role of the physiotherapist within the interdisciplinary clinical group (physician, nurse, nutritionist, occupational therapy, social worker, psychologist, speech therapist) has also changed. There is increased responsibility for interpreting information and

The Cancer Clock   Edited by Sotiris Missailidis
© 2007 John Wiley & Sons Ltd

advising other health professionals on appropriate patient management. Developments in the complexity and the use of physiotherapy clinical equipment, such as real-time ultrasound, non-invasive ventilators and electrotherapy, adjuncts to the treatment of several clinical conditions and have increased the level of knowledge and responsibility required by physiotherapists. Furthermore, advances in the understanding of the mechanisms of manipulative techniques support the actions of the physiotherapist. Finally, the increase in scientific information about the mechanism of action of acupuncture has permitted the use of this technique as an important tool in the clinical practice of the physiotherapist.

Oncology is the study of tumours or neoplasms. Cancer is the common term for all malignant tumours. Advances in medical procedures (early diagnosis, improved chemotherapy and radiotherapy) and surgical techniques, as well as in the field of oncology, have strongly influenced the practice of physiotherapy. People are living longer with their cancers as a result of early detection and advances in treatment options. Thus, physiotherapists need greater knowledge of the clinical conditions and require greater skill in managing of patients with cancer, before, during and after the specific medical procedures (surgery, radiotherapy, chemotherapy). They also have the responsibility of managing and treating patients during the pre- and postoperative periods with the provision of the best physiotherapeutic interventions to each patient. Besides this knowledge about clinical interventions, the physiotherapist needs to be in contact with the scientific literature in general. In oncology, for example, there is increasing evidence, initially only from epidemiological studies but increasingly from studies in individuals, that risk to some cancers, particularly cancers of the colon and rectum, breast, prostate and non-Hodgkin's lymphoma may be reduced in people living in areas of high ambient solar radiation or with high sun exposure than in those where the converse is the case. Of course, it is also known that sunlight is the primary causative agent in the pathogenesis of several types of cancer involving the skin. In these cases the physiotherapist can intervene and inform about sun protection. It is also necessary that the physiotherapist working with oncology patients needs to have a range of knowledge that encompasses the oncology specialty itself as well as other clinical areas such as neurology and the musculoskeletal and cardiopulmonary systems.

11.2 The importance of studies about cancer and physiotherapy

Cancer is considered a national health priority area in several countries because of the burden it places on the individual, families and the community. Cancer control is a public approach aimed at reducing causes and consequences of cancer. The World Health Organization works towards the prevention, research, education and control of cancer. Important medical developments have permitted that people with cancer can survive with their disease and with the side effects of their disease and treatment for longer. The high relevance of the cancer can also be demonstrated by the number of scientific research identified in the database system PubMed (a service of the National

Library of Medicine and the National Institutes of Health). It is possible to identify using the word 'cancer' approximately 2 000 000 full papers. Physiotherapists have had to keep up with these developments as well as change practice to meet health policy initiatives of keeping people at home for longer and returning them home sooner after a hospital stay. As a result, physiotherapists working with people with cancer that have undergone a clinical intervention can be found in acute care facilities, in rehabilitation facilities, in hospices, in the community and in home-based care, providing services along the entire spectrum of patient care. There is also a considerable role for physiotherapists in the evaluation of the clinical conditions and management of the patients, as well as in assisting people's return to work and normal life, as it is often the fatigue and weakness caused by the disease and the treatment that delays this return or limits some actions of the specific individual (see Figure 11.1).

Surgery is being seen as the optimal early intervention to remove many localized cancers, due to new imaging techniques, such as positron emission tomography (PET) with fluorine-18 fluorodeoxyglucose (18FDG; see Chapter 7), providing better tumour definition. It is essential that physiotherapists working with cancer patients have a clear and comprehensive understanding of the individual cancers and their staging and development, as well as the techniques that are being used in the diagnosis and treatment

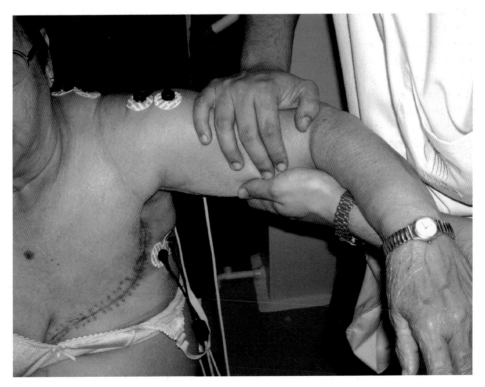

Figure 11.1 Physiotherapeutic evaluation and management of a patient who has undergone a modified radical mastectomy

of a determined disease. The physiotherapist needs to have knowledge of the consequences and complications of clinical procedures, as chemotherapy and radiotherapy, and their potential side effects (such as neuropathies and cardiomyopathies). Radiotherapy is a cancer treatment that uses high-energy X-rays or other types of ionizing radiation to try to kill the cancer cells in various organs/tissues. There are mainly two types of radiotherapy: (i) external radiotherapy that uses a source of radiation that is outside the body and (ii) internal radiotherapy that uses a radioactive substance sealed in needles, seeds, wires, or catheters that are placed directly into or near the cancer (brachytherapy; see also Chapter 7). Various severe complications following radiotherapy can be found and these complications depend on the type of the radiotherapy technique. The physiotherapist needs to know how these medical procedures can affect the physiotherapeutic interventions and to select the best procedure for each patient.

The physiotherapist also needs to know more about individual medications as patients can survive longer using new cancer treatments, often with much more severe side effects, due to improved medical care, but they get much weaker and sicker during the process. Hormonal therapy, for example, has an important effect on the muscle mass. The decrease in muscle mass, leading to muscle weakness and general debility, can be minimized by specific exercise programmes. These exercises are established and implemented by physiotherapists considering the specific capabilities and limitations of each patient. Stem cell transplantation is another example that allows survival from very intensive chemotherapy, where recovery can be enhanced and length of hospital stay reduced by physiotherapy.

11.3   Possible interventions of the physiotherapist in specific types of cancer

11.3.1   Breast cancer

Carcinoma is the most common malignancy of the breast, and breast cancer is the most common non-skin malignancy in women. Carcinoma arising in the male breast is a rare occurrence, with a frequency ratio to breast cancer in the female less than 1:100 or a lifetime risk of 0.11 per cent compared to about 13 per cent in women. Breast cancer is the most commonly detected cancer in women and the cancer causing most death in females in several countries. There have been many advances made in the management of breast cancer in the last decades. The increasing 5-year survival rate places an emphasis on the need for an excellent functional outcome to improve long-term quality of life and return to pre-surgical activities. The modified radical mastectomy and the development of the surgical technique of axillary node dissection and breast conservation rather than radical mastectomy have had a relevant importance. This new technique comes with new complications of nerve and shoulder joint injury. The patients that have undergone axillary lymphadenectomy have a 30 per cent lifetime risk of lymphoedema as a complication. To try and minimize the surgical complications, sentinel node biopsy (SNB) was developed. In SNB, the first axillary node receiving the lymphatic drainage from the breast is removed. As early discharge is a priority in several clinical situations, the length of hospital stay has been reduced to 1 day in most cases. This has meant that the physiotherapists working in oncology, managing patients postoperatively, have had to develop more complex and efficient discharge education programmes for these women. Because of the understanding of the great benefits of early mobilization, it is expected that patients can be out of bed moving around very shortly after treatment.

It is the role of the physiotherapist to get people with mobilization difficulties out of bed and assist with their return to normal mobility function. Physiotherapists have had to keep up with particular postoperative management of more individual interventions to ensure that the person can commence rehabilitation early, with no detrimental outcome. Manual lymphatic drainage is a procedure that the physiotherapist can use to try to avoid lymphoedema (see Figure 11.2 and Box 11.1).

The physiotherapist can also help the patient in the pre-surgical period, during which the exercises that will be done in the post-surgical period can be learned early by the patient. Furthermore, physiotherapeutic evaluation in the pre-surgical phase can aid in the identification of factors that can contribute to the appearance of complications due to the surgical procedure. This is of great significance for women both from the perspective of continuing the activities of daily life and also from the perspective of needing a good range of movement of their shoulders to assume the position required to undergo radiation therapy. When the prescribed exercise programmes and specific interventions are well established, they can assist the recovery from surgery, self-esteem

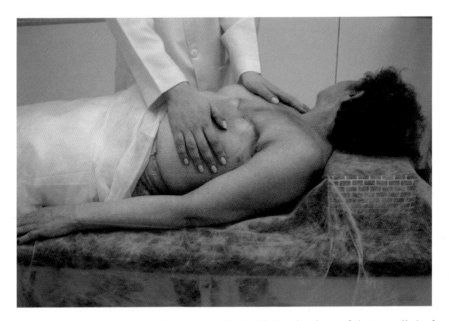

Figure 11.2 Manual lymphatic dreinage in a patient with lymphoedema of the upper limb after a modified radical mastectomy

and control of some of the side effects of chemotherapy and radiotherapy or another modality of treatment.

Box 11.1   Lymphoedema and breast cancer

Lymphoedema is one of the complications normally found in the ipsilateral arm of patients with breast cancer that have undergone surgery and/or radiotherapy. Lymphoedema is a high-protein swelling resulting from a dysfunction of the lymphatic system. The complications of lymphoedema include fibrosis, limb dysfunction, increased risk of cellulitis with subsequent infection and psychological distress. The management of lymphoedema in breast cancer patients has been based on results from case studies, clinical experience, anecdotal information, and only a few randomized trials. Several therapeutic interventions exist to treat this potentially distressing and disabling condition. Complex physical therapy (CPT) is the most accepted method for managing lymphoedema after breast cancer treatment. It is a four-fold approach which includes manual lymphatic drainage, compression therapy with garments or bandages, skin care and exercises, and is performed in phases. The goals of the first, also known as the intensive or decongestive phase, are to mobilize the protein-rich fluid and minimize the fibrosclerotic tissue. In the second phase, the goal is to maintain the results of the first phase, when the maximum level of decongestion was achieved. The effectiveness of CPT has been reported in a number of papers, but no consensus has been reached as to what constitutes optimal or definitive treatment of lymphoedema. Because of these doubts, the role of the physiotherapist is relevant in identifying the best management of the patient with lymphoedema. Specialist lymphoedema physiotherapists play a significant role in managing all of these complications by controlling lymphoedema itself and providing education for patients to self-manage their condition. The management of lymphoedema is of critical importance for patients because of fibrosis that leads to decrease in the function in the affected limb. The limitation of limb movement can lead to both poor functional outcomes and other related disorders like hip and back pain as other parts of the body take on extra loads. Cellulitis and infection is both painful and costly to the individual and the community.

11.3.2 Gynaecological cancers

The role of the physiotherapist is also highly relevant in the pre- and post-surgical period for patients with gynaecological cancers. Diseases of the female genital tract are extremely common and include complications of pregnancy, inflammation, tumours, and hormonally induced effects. The main problem in patients with ovarian cancer is early detection and the accurate and adequate staging of the disease before beginning treatment. Tumours of the vulva are the most important lesions to affect this region. The vagina is a portion of the female tract that is remarkably free from primary disease. The major serious primary lesion of this structure is the uncommon primary carcinoma. The cervix is both a sentinel for potentially serious upper genital tract infections and a target for viral and other carcinogens, which may lead to invasive carcinoma. The uterus is subject to a variety of disorders, the most common of which result from endocrine imbalances, complications of pregnancy and neoplastic proliferation. Rehabilitation of gynaecological cancer patients, after extensive and complex surgery and/or radiotherapy, requires knowledge and new approaches are necessary to improve the best clinical conditions for the patient. Some complications after the surgery and/or radiotherapy have been reported. Vaginal fibrosis, a side effect in some of these patients, means that vaginal dilation is required to allow examination, specimen collection and normal sexual functioning. The appropriate procedures to permit this dilation are conducted by a physiotherapist. Therapeutic intervention for the treatment of pain and sensitivity in vestibulitis has been undertaken and acupuncture has been an option. The presence of scar can limit the movements of some muscles and the manipulation of these scars is necessary. The pelvic girdle instability rehabilitation, to assist pelvic floor function, continence (urinary and/or faecal) and low back pain, has advanced and several scientific studies have demonstrated its importance and efficiency. Lymphoedema management in patients with gynaecological cancers has also been carried out and the early intervention in lymphoedema, as in many other areas, has been shown to minimize dysfunction and expedite eventual discharge. This management also limits the extent of fibrotic effects, decreases the risk of infection and improves the quality of life of the patient.

11.3.3 Prostate cancer

Only three pathological processes affect the prostate gland with sufficient frequency to merit discussion; inflammation, benign enlargement and cancer. Adenocarcinoma of the prostate is the most common form of cancer in men and the second leading cause of cancer death. The early-stage detection of prostate cancer with improved male health screening and the development and widespread use of prostate-specific antigen (PSA) testing (see Chapter 6) has somewhat improved the outcome for prostate cancer. Surgery is advised for non-benign and some benign presentations of this disease, with the resection of the groin lymph nodes in some cases. Radical prostatectomy is the appropriate therapy for any patient whose tumour is clinically confined to the prostate, has a life expectancy of 10 years or more, and has no serious co-morbid conditions that would contraindicate surgery. Improved knowledge of pelvic anatomy has resulted in major improvements in the surgical technique of radical retropubic prostatectomy (RRP). One of the most bothersome complications of this operation is urinary incontinence (UI), with a prevalence ranging from 5 to 60 per cent. UI after RRP has a major impact on the quality of life and it is therefore of utmost importance to minimize its prevalence after this kind of surgery. Physiotherapy assists with postoperative respiratory recovery, early mobilization, lymphoedema prevention education and garments if required, as well as the later management of pelvic floor re-education, continence advice and lymphoedema treatment if necessary. Moreover, the physiotherapist can also help the patient in the pre-surgical period in which the exercises for the pelvic floor and for the respiration that will be done in the post-surgical period can be learned early by the patient. Authors have demonstrated beneficial effects of pre- and postoperative pelvic floor re-education, since both the duration and degree of IU after RRP decreased. Physiotherapy has responded to the improved outcomes and patient demand for quality of life improvements by instituting new treatments and education, such as informing about the possible impor-tance of the sunlight in the prevention of the prostate cancer and as to protect against the harmful effects of the ultraviolet radiation, or about the options of physiotherapy for rehabilitation and re-integration to normal life.

11.3.4   Head and neck cancers

Most head and neck tumours are squamous cell carcinomas or a variant, including lymphoepithelioma, spindle cell carcinoma, verrucous carcinoma, and undifferentiated carcinoma. The possible usefulness of PET with 18 FDG for predicting tumour aggres-siveness and response to intra-arterial chemotherapy and radiotherapy in head and neck carcinomas has been evaluated. The uptake of this radiopharmaceutical in the tumour might reflect tumour aggressiveness, which is closely related to the proliferative activity and cellularity. Pre-treatment PET with 18 FDG is useful in predicting the response to treatment, and post-treatment PET with 18 FDG is of value in predicting residual viable tumours. This procedure has a profound impact on the treatment strategy for head and neck carcinomas. Intra-arterial chemotherapy using high dose cisplatin, combined with systemic neutralization in patients with head and neck cancer is used to reduce the tumour volume preoperatively. The physiotherapists need to know about the possibi-lities of these examinations to present suggestions and to work with the interdisciplinary group to improve the conditions of the patient.

Significant post-treatment morbidity can occur in patients treated for head and neck cancer. Co-morbid problems are common in these patients, like alcohol abuse, poor nutritional status, and cardiopulmonary diseases. Because of the extensive surgical and radiotherapeutic treatment, visible and functional deficits can occur, and may interfere with socialization and employment.

The physiotherapy must be preventive and may begin prior and continue throughout oncological intervention and treatment. The patient who receives radiotherapy, chemo-therapy or surgery needs oral exercises to maintain movement of the lips, tongue and jaw.

11.3.5   Melanoma and non-melanocytic skin cancers

Malignant melanoma is a relatively common neoplasm that not long ago was considered almost uniformly deadly. The great preponderance of melanomas arises in the skin, whereas other sites of origin include the oral and anogenital mucosal surfaces, oesophagus, meninges, and, notably, the eye. Malignant melanoma of the skin is usually asymptomatic, although itching may be an early manifestation and the importance of the physiotherapist in these cancers is mainly in the early detection and in the education in primary care to prevent this kind of cancer. Physiotherapists will very often need to treat a person with their outer clothing removed and thus are very likely to be in a position to recognize a skin lesion, for example on the back or neck of a patient. With skin cancer rates increasing and awareness programmes publicized, this is a role that the physiotherapist has developed in the last decades. Early detection is vital to the management of melanoma, so this important role cannot be underestimated. Again the physiotherapist is involved with post-surgical recovery, especially if tissue grafting is done, as well as in the advanced stage of the disease, particularly where lymph node was removed and subsequent swelling occurs. Moreover, the harmful effects of the ultraviolet radiation of the sun are indisputable, with much research showing that the sunlight is the primary causative agent in the pathogenesis of basal cell carcinoma, squamous cell carcinoma and malignant melanoma. In these cases the physiotherapist can act in the primary intervention, informing about sun protection in the form of sun avoidance, sun-protective clothing and sunscreens. Peak times for ultraviolet radiation exposure are between 10 am and 4 pm, and sun avoidance should be encouraged during this time.

11.3.6 Colorectal cancer

Carcinoma of the colon is curable, if discovered early. Surgery is the primary treatment for colorectal tumours and recurrences. In inoperable patients, radiotherapy or chemotherapy, or both, provides palliation. The early treatment of bowel cancer involves surgical resection and post operative mobilization is complicated by pain, respiratory compromise and many attachments such as drains, i.v. lines and oxygen delivery devices. As with other surgical procedures, the length of hospitalization is now much reduced, and the benefits of early mobilization are well documented. Physiotherapists have changed their practice to facilitate these changes with new services, education and outpatient clinics.

Rehabilitation includes exercise programmes to expedite cardiorespiratory recovery, abdominal muscle rehabilitation, pelvic floor muscle functional recovery, continence programmes for bladder and bowel function and earlier return to previous activities. Education for coping with functional activities that increase intra-abdominal pressure and place strain on surgical sites and the bladder and bowel has also advanced considerably to prevent complications of these procedures.

11.3.7 Lung cancer

Lung cancer is currently the most frequently diagnosed major cancer in the world and the most common cause of cancer mortality worldwide. In men, malignancy of the lung had been rising steadily but has plateaued in the last years, and is expected to decline in the future. Unfortunately, as more and more women are smoking, it has become the most common malignancy in women in several countries, surpassing even breast cancer (see also Chapter 1). The survival time for people with small cell lung cancer and mesothelioma has been enhanced by new chemotherapy and radiotherapy regimes. Radical surgery is an option for mesothelioma patients. Longer survival is accompanied by the opportunity for these cancers to metastasize to other areas. The role of physiotherapy in assisting symptom control and functional ability is now to support these people in their survival.

As stated previously, the benefits of maintaining aerobic fitness is now seen as a life-enhancing strategy for these people, to help them function better and also to assist their coping with the rigour of their treatment, improve their quality of life and limit complications of the disease and its treatment. Strength training helps preserve lean muscle mass, limiting fatigue and assisting with upper limb functional activities since muscle training is recognized as being muscle specific. In the more advanced cases, there is more complex input required from the physiotherapist to determine what respiratory equipment is needed to assist the patients in returning home. This is done by way of using physiotherapy rehabilitation data to determine home oxygen prescription. Additionally, physiotherapy functional assessments are used to assist with planning discharge. A greater focus on carer education has also developed in order to expedite discharge home and to assist with decreasing readmission rates. Depending on the severity of the type of the cancer, the physiotherapist can help the patient as palliative treatment or in improving the quality of life.

11.3.8 Non-Hodgkin's lymphoma

Non-Hodgkin's lymphoma differs from Hodgkin's disease and is characterized by the presence of malignant cells in any area of the lymphoid system, including lymph nodes, bone marrow, spleen, gastrointestinal tract, and skin. There are two histological types, the follicular and the diffuse. The increasing presentation of the non-Hodgkin's lymphoma, despite newer and more potent treatments such as peripheral blood stem cell transplants and allogenic transplants, has placed research and learning demands on physiotherapists. As with so many other cancers, survival is longer with a better quality of life. There is much research on the benefits of exercise to cope with treatment and return to a better performance status sooner. Related diseases, such as some of the leukaemias and multiple myeloma, have shown similar responses in fatigue levels and return to work. The choice of treatments depends on the stage of the disease and histology, and cures are rare in patients with follicular lymphomas. Physiotherapy care in the palliative phase has progressed as in the other cancer presentations. Surgical interventions for spleen removal and bowel obstruction, often with platelet support, low haemoglobin and neutrophil counts, place increased demands on our knowledge of physiology and pharmacology.

The presentation and increased survival with oncology emergencies, such as neutropenic sepsis and tumour lysis syndrome, require the knowledge to manage much more unstable patients. Knowledge of respiratory care regarding positioning, oxygen therapy and management of the patient is necessary and can be vital in several situations. The increased treatment for achieving remission, or survival, places a greater demand on the intensive care required for these patients in crisis. The skills and knowledge required for this care, together with new techniques and equipment for monitoring, artificial ventilation and rehabilitation after much longer periods of having been paralysed and ventilated, significantly increases the demands on physiotherapists treating such patients.

11.4 Physiotherapy, exercise prescription and technology advances

The most prevalent symptom in cancer is fatigue. Fatigue has overtaken pain as the most common distressing symptom in cancer, since pain management has improved. There is much evidence to suggest that appropriately prescribed exercises play a significant role in the decrease of cancer fatigue and the improvement of the quality of life of the patient. The reduction of cancer fatigue is highly relevant and desirable, and very important in a number of ways, which include: (i) the ability to continue functioning at work; (ii) the conditions to develop daily activities at home; and (iii) participation in social activities. Some scientific works have shown that exercises protect the organism against the protein turnover that contributes to loss of body weight. People with primary lung cancer or with cardiopulmonary side effects from their particular cancer or medical intervention (medication and/or radiotherapy) have shown decreased physical capacity. Lung resection for primary lung cancer or mesothelioma requires physical rehabilitation in addition to physiotherapy management in the early postoperative recovery stage. The physiotherapist uses an oximeter to help in the evaluation of the clinical condition of the patient, to assess the lung capacity of the patient and to determine the appropriate exercise and functional levels, as well as using it for assessing the patient for home oxygen requirements. Physiotherapy skills in providing respiratory rehabilitation have progressed with time and the physiotherapists need to be able to know to select, to read and to understand the available and convenient postoperative monitoring devices used in recovery, intensive care and on the wards. The respiratory care of these patients requires an understanding of the oxygen delivery systems available, and the humidification devices that are commonly used. Telemetry, which monitors heart function, is another tool that can be used by the physiotherapists to assist the patient with his/her specific exercise regime.

11.5 Physiotherapy and palliative care in oncology

In the final stages of cancer, the palliative care aim of treatment becomes paramount. This conduct, due to the natural history of each type of cancer, is very variable, and this stage may last a few days or several months. Physiotherapy in palliative care is used for pain, lymphoedema, dyspnoea and other symptom assessment and treatment, as well as for the education on safe transfer and mobility management of the patient. Constipation, nausea, sleep disturbance (insomnia), fatigue, dyspnoea, pain scores and appetite are all improved or prevented by physiotherapy intervention. The lymphoedema management in the terminally ill has developed more effectively in recent years with evidence supporting complex physiotherapy treatment and the integration with other professionals.

The beneficial effects of the pelvic floor exercises instituted prior to RRP are well defined. The evaluation of the consequences of the early pelvic floor re-education on the degree and duration of IU after RRP has identified that the time period toward continence after RRP can be shortened relevantly if pelvic floor re-education is started directly after catheter removal. The complications of advanced disease and its treatment, for example, bone metastasis (coping with functioning, bone pain, fractures and the consequent repair surgery, and at times spinal cord compression and paralysis); lung disease and subsequent breathlessness and infection, loss of airway potency and functional ability, and also brain metastasis, are all areas of significant physiotherapy development. The drugs used to treat the problem of metastases can cause neuropathies that partially respond to rehabilitation.

In advanced colorectal cancer and in inoperable patients, physiotherapists assist with the symptoms of metastatic disease such as lymphoedema, the breathlessness associated with ascites, the fatigue and loss of function seen with liver disease. The frequency of colorectal liver metastases is very high. Moreover, the postoperative intervention can be complicated with surgery for bowel obstruction in very weak patients, who can now survive this intervention, and the participation of the physiotherapists in the management of these patients is highly relevant.

The mobilization of the scars (see Figure 11.3) to avoid adherence and important alterations in the posture of the patient is highly relevant and contributes to improve the quality of life of the patient in the future.

The discharge destination is more likely to be to home, rather than to another institution, and from social perspectives this conduct has very positive impacts on the patients and their families. In consequence, this has meant more responsibility and complexity for the discharging by the physiotherapist and has increased the responsibility for the physiotherapists providing care in the home of the patient. The interdisciplinary interventions, when provided at the correct time, delay the onset of disability and maximize function for as long as possible. Intervention may help to correct lean tissue loss, muscle atrophy and deterioration in functional capacity, thus restoring self-efficacy, correcting disruption in social, sexual and family relationships and enhancing overall quality of life. It is also recommended that, just as early identification and treatment of cancer is crucial, early allied health professional assessment and intervention is also essential, rather than waiting for functional disabilities to develop. The physiotherapists need also work in this model, receiving early outpatient referrals from the palliative care team, and reviewing all the needs of the inpatients. It is important that the physiotherapists develop new skills of appropriate goal setting and work more closely with carers, patients and other palliative care specialists, in an

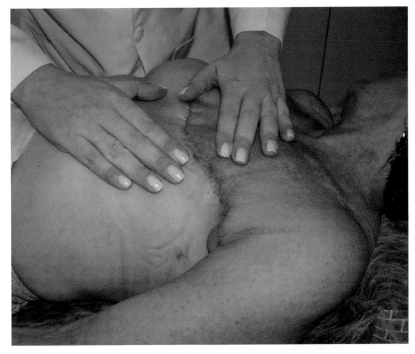

Figure 11.3 Scar mobilization in a patient with tissue adherence, after a modified radical mastectomy

interdisciplinary environment, to provide optimal supportive care for the level of function and stage of disease for each patient. The discharge timing and destination is now planned with a large input from physiotherapists and other allied health professionals.

With the aim of aiding the patient and their family, it is also crucial that physiotherapists understand the process of overcoming grief in a patient with a life-threatening or terminal disease and know how to seek resources in the hospital, in the community or in other centres that have patients in similar conditions.

The complications of lymphoedema in several post-surgical conditions include fibrosis, limb dysfunction, increased risk of cellulitis and subsequent infection and psychological trauma. The knowledge of the varied disease processes and stages, possible complications and symptoms, to allow effective optimal outcome for the patient and the family is essential. What equipment is now available and where to source it is a valuable aid to stressed and weary patients and carers, as is assessing when visiting outpatient facilities is no longer in the patients' best interests so that new home services can be instituted or physiotherapy treatment withdrawn.

Concerning palliative care, the physiotherapist is often asked to advise when their intervention for airway maintenance is no longer achieving a helpful symptom management outcome, or to suggest ways of maintaining a patient's airway, or to indicate more appropriate equipment. The increased knowledge of the benefits of positioning, respiratory physiology and the availability of nasopharyngeal airways, non-invasive ventilation and mini-tracheotomies and new oxygen delivery devices and the benefits of humidification has increased the possibilities of the physiotherapists' aid to a patient in the final stages of cancer, improving, at least, the quality of life of the patient. Primary or secondary bone cancer can be treated with more complicated resection and recon-struction surgery. The knowledge of the surgical approach, technique and patient's physiological healing capacity in the setting of the complexities of cancer and other co-morbidities is essential to a safe and effective rehabilitation in the case of bone allografts, autografts and prosthetic implants.

11.6 Physiotherapy in the actions, community expectations and quality of life in oncology

Various complications following the treatment of the various types of cancer have been reported. Perhaps more than in most other areas of health, meeting community expectations in managing oncology patients has grown in complexity. Many phy-siotherapists practise in a specialized area and it is important that the profession promotes specialization. Physiotherapy plays an important role in the prevention, reduction, and alleviation of adverse effects from the cancer treatment. The importance of a new career structure for the physiotherapy profession, the need for recognition of general specialization process, as in oncology, within this structure has been highlighted. The relevance of specialization in the health sciences for the advancement of clinical skills, approaches, research, and organization as well as training supervision and teach-ing has been recognized. Cancer has gained much publicity in the media, with new developments in its detection and management publicized regularly, and more infor-mation about this disease is available. Information can assist in the early detection and effective treatments of a further one-third of cases of cancer in the world. The various programmes and actions to aid in the prevention, research, education and control of cancer have been supported by governmental, national and international institutions and private organizations. Cancer is also a very emotive subject (see Chapter 12) with its status as a potentially terminal disease adding great fear to its diagnosis. In consequence, the physiotherapists and other medically allied professionals have had to develop new approaches to deal not only with the patient and their presenting condition, but also with the quality of information that the patient has obtained via the internet and the media in general. The film *Calendar Girls* shows the meaning of the interactive process of co-operation when it touches public opinion for humanitarian causes. Moreover, this film shows the relevance of a simple and creative action to obtain money to help in the research about cancer. The implementation of the physiotherapy routine for patients with cancer undergoing cancer treatment aims to prevent complications through homecare measures and orientation, as well as diagnosis and intervention, seeking to improve quality of life and to reduce personal and hospital costs. In depth knowledge of the clinical area, based on the best available evidence, is critical for physiotherapists to assist the patient come to terms with the diagnosis and likely prognosis. Moreover, the physiotherapist will also play a role in the formation of a database bank on risk factors, incidence and complications, evaluation of various approaches, and service plans.

Clinical actions have undergone constant changes aiming to improve the techniques used in health sciences, as well as the availability of competent professionals and material resources of appropriate quality and quantity. Moreover, clinical specialization will help to analyse, evaluate, and improve physiotherapy, and will promote greater expertise and intelligent use of the scientific evidence. While advances have made it possible for patients to have better outcomes and survival rates from cancer, they are, as mentioned previously, also often living longer with more complex complications of the disease. These complications may significantly affect the quality of life of a person and the contribution by other professionals, including the physiotherapist, in various cancer services is highly desired.

Specialization will help to drive research and the development of new ideas within the physiotherapy practice. Such developments in physiotherapy management in the area of oncology have made relevant contributions to patient care, including: (i) decreasing length of stay in acute facilities (early discharge planning, outpatient follow up and education, involvement in palliative care facilities and physiotherapy services in the home); (ii) improving functional capacity (early mobilization, management of complications of surgery, convenient manipulations of the areas submitted to radio-therapy and other treatments, treating lymphoedema) (see Figure 11.4); (iii) improving

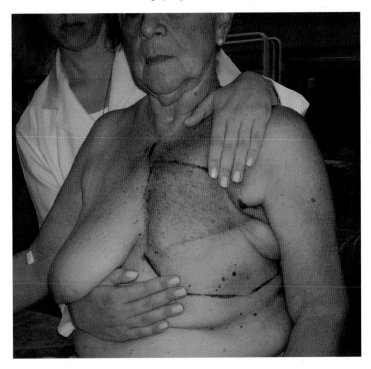

Figure 11.4 Tissue mobilization of a patient submitted to a modified radical mastectomy that is under adjuvant radiotherapy.

lymphoedema management that have lead to decreased hospital admissions for cellulitis (a feature of poorly controlled lymphoedema) and decreased need for costly and at times uncomfortable pressure garments; (iv) improving exercise capacity (prevention of loss of body weight and managing the side effects of the disease, medication and surgery); (v) shortening the period of time of UI after prostatectomy; and (vi) affecting quality of life factors for all cancer sufferers and their carers and families.

These all provide examples where physiotherapy intervention contributes considerably to health care provision and demonstrate how the various disciplines allied to medicine are working together either bring the now healthy individual back to normal life and re-integration to the society, or improve the quality of life of patients that have to live with cancer as a chronic disorder and those that are in the terminal stages of the disease and life.

11.7   Self-assessment questions

Question:	In general practice, which physiotherapeutic agents are used in oncology?
Answer:	Physiotherapists use physical agents, such as therapeutic exercises, electrotherapy, non-invasive ventilators, acupuncture and manipulative therapy.
Question:	In the past, the main purpose of physiotherapy was just in the rehabilitation of physical and functional sequelae. Today, with the progress of science and the knowledge of physiopathology, physiotherapy has a much wider role in the field of health sciences. Which are the current objectives of the physiotherapy in oncology patients?
Answer:	Treatment and prevention of diseases or complications; prevention, diagnosis and therapeutic management of disorders involving the movements of the body; optimization of the function of the tissues to enhance health; development, maintenance and restoration of maximum movement and functional ability of each human being considering the specific limitations of each one; prevention of diseases, recovery time and risk of recurrence; improvement of the quality of the life; interpreting information and advising other health professionals on appropriate patient management; assisting people returning to work; minimizing consequences and complications of clinical procedures, such as chemotherapy, surgery, hormonal therapy and radiotherapy and their potential side effects and complications.

Question: Lymphoedema is one of the main complications following breast cancer surgery, and severely affects the quality of life of these patients. The management of lymphoedema in breast cancer patients requires a specialist lymphoedema physiotherapist. Which is the most accepted method for management of lymphoedema of the upper limb?

Answer: The most accepted method for managing lymphoedema after breast cancer treatment is the complex physical therapy (CPT). It is a four-fold approach which includes manual lymphatic drainage, compression therapy with garments or bandages, skin care and exercises, and is performed in phases. The goals of the first, also known as the intensive or decongestive phase, are to mobilize the protein-rich fluid and minimize the fibrosclerotic tissue. In the second phase, the goal is to maintain the results of the first phase, when the maximum level of decongestion was achieved.

Question: The role of the physiotherapist is highly relevant in patients with gynaecological cancer. Which are the main complications that can be anticipated or minimized through physical therapy intervention?

Answer: Vaginal fibrosis, pain and sensitivity, movement restriction, alteration of the scar, incontinence (urinary and/or faecal), lymphoedema.

Question: Prostate cancer is the most common form of cancer in men and the second leading cause of cancer death. Radical prostatectomy has co-morbid conditions that can be treated by precocious physiotherapy. In which ways can physiotherapy assist in the alleviation of symptoms following the treatment of such patients?

Answer: Physiotherapy assists with pre- and postoperative pelvic floor and respiratory exercises, early mobilization, lymphoedema prevention, education and treatment, management of pelvic floor re-education, continence advice.

Question: Fatigue is a common distress symptom after cancer treatment. How can exercises decrease this symptom?

Answer: The reduction of cancer fatigue is highly relevant and desirable, and it will be very important in a number of ways which include: (i) the ability to continue functioning at work; (ii) the conditions to develop daily activities at home; and (iii) participation in social activities.

Some scientific studies have shown that exercises protect the organism against protein turnover that contributes to loss of body weight.

Question: In palliative care, the physiotherapist can be useful to relieve pain, lymphoedema, dyspnoea, constipation, nausea, sleep disturbance (insomnia), fatigue and appetite. Taking into account the breathing alterations, which would be the aim of the intervention of physiotherapy?

Answer: The physiotherapist is often asked to advise when their interventions for airway maintenance are no longer achieving a helpful symptom management outcome, or to suggest ways of maintaining a patent airway, or to indicate the most appropriate equipment. The increased knowledge of the benefits of positioning, respiratory physiology and the availability of nasopharyngeal airways, non-invasive ventilation and mini-tracheotomies, as well as new oxygen delivery devices and the benefits of humidification, has increased the possibilities for the physiotherapists to aid a patient in the final stages of cancer, improving, at least, the quality of life of the patient.

11.8 Further reading and resources

Baum M and Schipper H. *Fast Facts, Breast Cancer*. Health Press, Oxford, 2005.

Bennett CJ and Grant MJ. Specialisation in physiotherapy: a mark of maturity. *Aust J Physiother* 2004, **50**, 3–5.

Bergmann A, Ribeiro MJ and Maia A. Breast cancer physiotherapy: results of a preventive routine. Proceedings, 13th International Congress on senology of the Senology Society in cooperation with all the senology Societies and the FLAM, p. 230, 2004.

Bergmann A, Ribeiro MJ, Pedrosa E, Nogueira EA and Oliveira ACG. Physical therapy in breast cancer: clinical protocol at the Cancer Hospital III / INCA. *Rev Brasil Cancerologia* 2006, **52**, 97–109.

Bernardo RM, Oliveira E, Mendonça FAP and Bernardo-Filho M. Cancer, Prevention, Research and the 'Calendar Girls'. IV International Symposium on Extracellular Matrix, Búzios, Rio de Janeiro, Brasil, p:136, 2006.

Consensus document of the International Society of Lymphology. *Lymphology* 2003, **36**, 84–91.

Cornel EB, de Wit R and Witjes JA. Evaluation of early pelvic floor physiotherapy on the duration and degree of urinary incontinence after radical retropubic prostatectomy in a non-teaching hospital. *World J Urol* 2005, **23**, 353–355.

Gerber LH. Cancer rehabilitation into the future. *Cancer* 2001, **Suppl 92**, 975–979.

Kaplan RJ. Cancer and rehabilitation. E-medicine. Available in http://www.emedicine.com/pmr/topic226.htm. [Accessed January 29 2007]

Kricker A and Armstrong B. Does sunlight have a benefificial influence on certain cancers? *Progr Biophys Molec Biol* 2006, **92**, 132–139.

Kumar V, Abbas AK and Fausto N. *Robbins and Cotran Pathologic Basis of Disease*. Elsevier Saunders, seventh edition, China, 2005.

Moon SJ, Fryer AA and Strange RC. Ultraviolet radiation, vitamin D and risk of prostate cancer and other diseases. *Photochem Photobiol* 2005, **81,** 1252–1260.

Santiago-Palma J and Payne R. Palliative care and rehabilitation. *Cancer* 2001, **Suppl 92,** 1049–1052.

Wilke LG, McCall LM, Posther KE, *et al.* Surgical complications associated with sentinel lymph node biopsy: results from a prospective international cooperative group trial. *Ann Surg Oncol* 2006, **13,** 491–500.

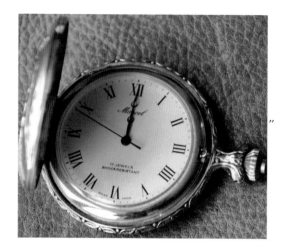

Cancer is associated with emotional responses at all stages, from the moment one takes a diagnostic assay and is diagnosed with the disease, through all stages of treatment and side effects associated with it, to their passing in the last stages of the disease, living with cancer as a chronic disorder, or returning to normal life. It would be perhaps prudent to have this chapter as individual sections in all chapters throughout the book. However, psychosocial oncology is now recognized as a discipline of its own and the professionals are part of the multidisciplinary team that deals with oncology patients. As we saw in the previous chapters with oncology nursing and physiotherapy, a whole range of disciplines are working together to provide the best care and improve therapeutic output or quality of life for cancer patients. This can be to ease their passing at the last stages of their life, or to provide them the necessary support to cope with the disease and ideally return to fully functional members of the society that can enjoy life to the full. Various feelings can be experienced by cancer patients, ranging from anxiety and anger, to fear and uncertainty, coping strategies for pain, side effects such as weight and hair loss, changes in physical appearance from surgery, or fear of potential recurrent disease. Many of these issues as well as the role of the social environment and the appropriate strategies assumed by the professional to provide the best patient care possible are discussed in this chapter.

12
Psychosocial oncology

Ian J. McCubbin and Craig A. White

West of Scotland Cancer Network, Ayrshire Central Hospital, UK

12.1 Introduction

There are many different known types of cancer, each with a different aetiology, treatment regime and prognosis and, as such, a vast array of factors that will influence the psychological concerns or problems experienced by people who have cancer. As with all physical illnesses, the psychological variability between patients with very similar illness characteristics and experiences can be significant. For example, a patient who has experienced breast cancer in the context of adequate personal and supportive care resources, a good understanding of treatment, and has no major problems relating to treatment side effects, will experience an entirely different set of thoughts and feelings to a patient with head and neck cancer who has few supportive relationships and a past history of alcohol abuse. Although both patients' lives are influenced by cancer, there are significant differences in how patterns of adjustment occur. Such differences in psychological experiences are further accentuated when one considers that the latter patient had also experienced a range of disfiguring surgical treatments and has been told that their overall treatment is no longer curative. In addition to cancer type, prognosis and treatment regime, aspects such as a patient's life history and current personal and social resources are also very likely to have a bearing upon the precise interaction between cancer and the person with cancer.

The Cancer Clock   Edited by Sotiris Missailidis
© 2007 John Wiley & Sons Ltd

12.2 Cancer and psychological distress

The concept of cancer-related distress has become a useful way of thinking about the range of ways in which people experience cancer. It has been defined as:

'...an unpleasant emotional experience of a psychological, social, or spiritual nature that may interfere with a patient's ability to cope with cancer and its treatment. Distress extends along a continuum, ranging from common normal feelings of vulnerability, sadness, and fear, to problems that can become disabling, such as depression, anxiety, panic, social isolation, and spiritual crisis'. (National Comprehensive Cancer Network, 1999)

Though often dismissed as 'understandable', distress is a treatable cause of reduced quality of life and poorer clinical outcome. It is increasingly recognized that a substantial proportion of patients experience psychological problems that have a significant negative impact on functioning and quality of life. Comprehensive cancer care should aim to identify patients at risk of these higher levels of distress, identify problems when they occur and then provide evidence-based care and, when indicated, appropriate interventions. Distressing thoughts can have a significant impact on patient's lives, although practical or financial problems sometimes give rise to the biggest emotional distress. For some people a cancer diagnosis results in a range of 'positive' psychological responses (e.g. enhanced meaning in life, greater investment in personal relationships) but many patients will experience 'negative' psychological responses (e.g. depression and hopelessness, withdrawal from personal relationships). Good psychological care occurs when positive and negative psychological reactions to cancer are identified and discussed as an integral part of an overall care plan. This is particularly important when one considers that many of the unmet needs reported by patients relate to psychological adjustment. Homsi et al. (2006) reported that the median number of symptoms reported by patients on systematic assessment was ten fold higher than those volunteered. Interestingly, 79 per cent of the most distressing symptoms were not spontaneously reported.

Increasing medical advances have meant that more people are living with cancer than ever before. These changing circumstances mean cancer is increasingly being conceptualized as a chronic illness. Almost everyone who is told that they have cancer will experience a period of shock and psychological distress. For the majority of patients, this will be a self-limiting experience, one that does not cause any lasting psychological problems and that can be understood as part of a normal adjustment reaction. Some people will experience more severe distress. Currently available estimates suggest that this severity of distress will apply to around 25 per cent of people who have cancer, though there are some cancer sites where this figure is higher. Patients with this level of distress are more likely to be experiencing psychological problems that significantly interfere with their quality of life and ability to function on a day-to-day basis. Those patients who experience severe psychological problems are likely to have one or more of the more common risk factors for higher levels of distress.

A cancer patient is at greater risk of developing severe psychological distress if they

- Are younger;

- Are single by virtue of separation, divorce or being widowed;

- Live alone;

- Have children aged under 21 years old;

- Are experiencing economic adversity;

- Have a perceived lack of social support;

- Have poor marital or family functioning;

- Have a history of psychiatric problems;

- Have cumulative stressful life events;

- Have a history of alcohol or other substance abuse.

More severe distress is more likely at the time of diagnosis or recurrence, at advanced stages of cancer, in the presence of a poorer prognosis and when someone is experiencing more treatment side effects. The presence of symptoms such as lymphoedema, pain or fatigue also increases the risk of such distress.

Many patients have to face treatment regimes that are difficult to tolerate, that require frequent hospital visits and levels of motivation that can be difficult to generate or sustain. Some patients will experience anxiety, depression or trauma symptoms that, although not experienced at sufficient severity to warrant a diagnosis, can cause problems. Indeed, non-physical treatment side effects such as anger, anxiety or apprehension are often rated by patients as being more severe than physical side effects such as nausea or hair loss. Some patients may even drop out of chemotherapy because of psychological problems. Some treatment procedures (e.g. bone marrow transplantation) result in psychological problems because of the particular demands that they involve (e.g. prolonged exposure to isolation). Chemotherapy is more challenging for patients with fears of needles and radiotherapy can be distressing for people that have fears of enclosed places. Advances in drug therapies have resulted in a reduction in the incidences of nausea and vomiting associated with chemotherapy. However, conditioned nausea and vomiting do still occur (particularly among those with an anxious disposition) and aversions to food can also develop. Even after the end of treatment, patients' lives may be affected throughout the follow up period, as they attend appointments to determine whether the cancer has returned. The need to better appreciate the experience of cancer survivors and the concept of survivorship is also being recognized.

Progress in cancer genetics has resulted in increased awareness of the possibility of negative psychological reactions to increased genetic predisposition for cancer. Researchers have examined the way in which patients manage uncertainty about this, make decisions about treatment (e.g. prophylactic mastectomy) and how, in some cases, beliefs about genetic risk of cancer can precipitate or mediate psychological problems. Although people who have had cancer may feel relieved that their active treatment has ended, they may experience fear and anxiety about the uncertainty associated with the future. Fear of recurrence is thought to be almost universally present, though it is more likely to be experienced on a continuum as with other fears and anxiety. There are also undoubtedly some patients that have to address this more directly as a result of the initial pathological staging of their tumour and/or by virtue of knowledge about increased genetic risk. Beliefs about the likelihood of cancer recurrence are thought to be influenced very significantly by exposure to information within the popular press and media.

Treatments can also have an impact on sexual functioning (e.g. hormonal therapies or surgically induced damage to pelvic autonomic nerves). Quality of relationship is an important correlate of sexual functioning. Radiotherapy and chemotherapy can be associated with reduced sexual desire, related particularly to the occurrence of physical side effects such as fatigue, constipation or weight changes that reduce the extent to which an individual feels 'sexual'. Fatigue is one of the most common unrelieved symptoms in cancer patients and is a major factor affecting quality of life, both during and following treatment. Fatigue associated with cancer is generally more severe and persistent than 'everyday' fatigue and tends to persist even in the presence of adequate amounts of sleep and rest. For some cancer survivors, fatigue does not decline to premorbid levels following treatment and can become chronic. In an attempt to standardize the definition for, and improve the recognition of cancer related fatigue, diagnostic criteria for cancer-related fatigue (CRF) have been proposed. Studies that have used these criteria have reported prevalence estimates of 17–21 per cent. Fatigue is often associated with psychological morbidity, sleep problems and reduced activity levels.

Given the many psychological consequences of cancer and cancer treatment, it is not surprising that clinical psychologists are regarded as essential core members of the multidisciplinary team in cancer and palliative medicine teams. Clinical psychology can be applied to the assessment, formulation and intervention elements of clinic work. However, it is also being recognized that clinical and other applied psychologists can make a valuable contribution teaching psychological care skills to colleagues (e.g. communication skills training).

12.3 Assessment process

Many patients will not have had the opportunity to talk to staff about their cancer experiences (sometimes referred to as their 'cancer story'), from the time that they presented with symptoms to the point at which they are being psychologically assessed. For these patients, the process of psychological assessment can, in itself, be therapeutic.

Meaning is a concept that has relevance from a number of perspectives in understanding the psychology of cancer. Cancer challenges people's views of the world as meaningful, purposeful and coherent – 'what it all means' is a common focus of thinking. Coward (1997) has suggested that the experiences associated with cancer result in 'severe spiritual dis-equilibrium' and that process of searching for meaning is a response to this state. Thus, Lepore and Helgeson (1998) suggested that 'integrating the cancer experience into (their) pre-existing mental models should promote psychological adjustment'. O'Connor *et al.* (1990) defined the process of searching for meaning as '. . . questions about the personal significance of a life circumstance, such as cancer, in order to give the experience purpose and to place it in the context of a total life pattern . . .' Sometimes cancer leads to changes in the way people think about what they want from life and how they will approach each day.

While there are some patients who are able to retain feelings of self-control and worth throughout their cancer experiences, there is a substantial minority of others where loss of control becomes a significant issue influencing adjustment. Cancer, like many other physical illnesses, has an impact on the nature of the relationships that the person with cancer has with others in their lives. The social and family support that is experienced by some patients can act as a significant personal resource and for others the lack of such support leads to feelings of isolation and loneliness.

Most patients want to be fully informed about their care and treatment. Satisfaction with information is a very significant determinant of overall psychosocial adjustment, particularly during the early stages of cancer care and treatment. Ensuring that patients are asked about their current level of understanding of their cancer and treatment can reveal misconceptions and informational needs that then become a key factor in subsequent intervention.

In most cases, families act as a helpful resource to support and assist a family member with cancer. Indeed, families are often very involved with decision making about treatment and tend to provide emotional support throughout the duration of a physical illness affecting a family member. There are usually some members of the family who have more frequent contact with the person being assessed, who demonstrate greater empathy and understanding, who offer more practical support and in whom the patient will find it easier to confide.

When screening suggests that there may be family issues influencing presentation, family members' experiences of cancer need to be assessed. A patient who has had the experience of both of their parents, siblings and a brother-in-law die as a result of cancer will have a very different understanding of the impact of cancer than someone who has not had any previous experience of cancer. It is of course also possible that someone will have been exposed to illnesses other than cancer and that this experience within their family unit will have some bearing upon understanding their and the family's psychological experience of cancer within the family. Families may express their thoughts about the most appropriate way in which to meet the needs of family members who have cancer ('We don't think that you should tell him that it has spread to his liver') and clinical colleagues will often look to clinical psychologists for advice on how best to manage these situations.

12.3.1   Integrating sources of information

Psychological assessments aim to incorporate a range of sources of information on the content areas that have been referred to. Questioning within a consulting room or at the bedside is complemented by review of medical and nursing notes, interview of clinical colleagues, observations, the completion of self-report questionnaires and also of diaries. As with clinical psychology practice in general, there are many self report measures that have been developed for use with people who have cancer:

The Mental Adjustment to Cancer Scale (MACS) takes approximately 10 minutes to complete and comprises five subscales:

- Fighting spirit;

- Helplessness/hopelessness;

- Anxious preoccupation;

- Fatalistic;

- Avoidance.

The Cancer Behaviour Inventory assesses self-efficacy for coping with cancer. The brief version has 12 items and the longer version has 36. Respondents rate the degree to which they feel confident in their ability to accomplish the behaviour asked about.

The Cancer Coping Questionnaire is a 21-item measure that consists of 14 individual items and an additional 7 items that can be completed to assess the coping responses as they relate to close relationships of patients.

All these measures have good data on validity and reliability. These measures can be used with a standard assessment and may lead to follow-on assessment questions, or repeat administration can be used to determine whether interventions had the desired affect.

12.3.2   Using diaries for assessment

Assessment using diaries and written records to collect information for review in the out patient department (see Schumacher *et al.*, 2002 for experiences with a cancer pain diary) can be particularly useful when there is uncertainty about the potential links between two or more variables than have been identified elsewhere within an assessment. Patients are encouraged to note the intensity of a symptom like pain on a 0–100 scale and, at the same time, monitor other factors such as distress, also on a 0–100 scale. Diary assessment can be helpful when there is a need to help a patient become more aware of the links between variables that have been discussed during interview or on the basis of information that has been obtained from other assessment sources (e.g. ward-based staff). The inclusion of an element of assessment that involves writing in greater detail about thoughts and feelings can also be therapeutic in itself and/or lead to greater clarity on the part of patients about what precisely they have been most concerned about.

12.4 Formulation

Following the assessment, all the information that has been obtained is incorporated into the patient's case formulation. A formulation is an explanation of the psychological factors and processes that are thought to account for the onset, maintenance and expression of the psychosocial problems.

Faulkner and Maguire (1994) have suggested that psychosocial adjustment to cancer is associated with six hurdles: managing uncertainty about the future; searching for meaning; dealing with a loss of control; having a need for openness; needs for emotional support; and needs for medical support. They suggest that a failure to deal with these results in psychosocial problems. It can be a useful starting point to think in terms of the extent to which they have been successfully surmounted and whether they are helpful in constructing the formulation. A case formulation should offer an account (using information from the assessment) about why some hurdles are more of a challenge than others and the processes that contribute to this observation.

A patient's perception of the severity and course of their cancer has a crucial role in determining their psychological responses. In most cases, patient perceptions are accurate and reflect what they have been told by their oncologists. However, there are some patients who have unrealistic perceptions (e.g. an overoptimistic viewpoint or in some instances it may be inappropriately pessimistic) regarding their illness and its treatment. This can mediate problems, particularly when it becomes clear that their perception of their cancer is at odds with information from other sources (e.g. when they develop problems with functional abilities due to spread of their cancer). Expectations tend to influence emotional reactions in response to new events. Patients who experience a recurrence of their cancer that is unexpected tend to be more distressed than those who had a certain level of expectation that the recurrence might happen. Patients with a greater perception of discrepancies between actual experiences and ideal aspects of their self concept tend to be more depressed.

The stage of an individual patient's 'cancer journey' will be important, as the type of psychological problems experienced will depend upon this. Patients (particularly those with higher risks toward vulnerability) are more at risk when the illness is diagnosed, during the early months of treatment, when all treatment has ended or when a recurrence or spread of the cancer is discovered. Patients within the first few weeks of their chemotherapy are likely to have formulations that include the presence of physical side effects, personal experiences of coping with treatment demands and emotions relating to considering whether the treatment is working. The concept of problematic re-entry to a pre-morbid lifestyle can be used to conceptualize obstacles for patients who have psychological problems after treatment has ended.

All relevant aspects of the patients' current and past life experiences in relation to their cancer (e.g. how cancer related problems link with events such as prior abuse or current problems with social isolation) are taken into account and included (provided this adds explanatory value). These experiences need not be events that have been experienced personally but can be experiences that have been observed. The presence or absence of adequate levels of social support often moderates the expression or severity of a psychological problem. The predominant coping pattern preferred by the patient should be outlined in the formulation, as it may be that there is a restricted pattern of coping where patients rely on one strategy for all problems, as opposed to varying strategies depending upon the demands of the situation. Escape-avoidance coping has been consistently shown to be associated with distress, whereas emotionally expressive coping has been shown to have benefits. Although literature in this area tends to give the impression that coping style is consistent across time and with different problem domains, this is not the case.

12.5 Psychological interventions

Once an assessment of the problems and processes that are relevant in understanding an individual patient's experience of cancer has been described in a formulation that accounts for the onset, maintenance and manifestation of presenting problems, clinical psychologists can begin to plan an intervention. There are a range of psychological models and constructs that can be used to intervene in psychosocial oncology. There is some evidence to support the application of a range of interventions, though future work needs to address methodological weaknesses in this areas of research in order to maximize the chance of a more compelling case being made for the effectiveness of these across the range of problems and patient experiences. Many of these target similar psychological processes, though they may do so using different strategies and in a way that emphasizes different processes of change. The following section will be divided into two. First, the range of processes that are commonly influenced by psychological therapy in cancer care settings will be outlined. Second, the main schools of psychological therapy will be outlined, with information on how they can be used to address psychological problems in cancer care.

In practice, most clinicians will tailor their application of psychotherapy with people with cancer to take account of the presenting problems and implement elements of educational, supportive, expressive or existential emphasis. In this respect, psychotherapy with cancer patients illustrates the way in which differing therapeutic modalities can be tailored to the presenting problems and issues facing the person who is physically ill. Barraclough (1999) and Burton and Watson (1998) provide helpful overviews of how psychological interventions can be applied in cancer settings.

12.5.1   Processes targeted in psychological interventions

Tackling avoidant behaviour and thinking

As with many presentations in clinical psychology practice, avoidance is often a significant maintaining factor for many cancer related psychological problems. It may involve avoidance of people, situations or appointments and frequently extends to the avoidance of talking about cancer within sessions. Interventions should therefore target both the nature of the fears and thoughts about coping ability. All psychological interventions target avoidance, though they differ in the extent to which they explicitly emphasize this. Psychodynamically focused therapeutic sessions might reverse avoidance by focusing on emotionally charged material on transference and counter-transference and tackle avoidance by making interpretations relating to defence mechanisms, thus enabling patients to gain insight into this. Cognitive psychotherapy would tend to be more explicit about the role of avoidance and may set up behavioural experiments that are aimed to enable patients to consider how this might operate to reinforce their symptoms and to gain evidence that can be used to develop alternatives.

Avoidance is usually mediated by intermediate beliefs about the predicted consequences of not avoiding ('If I talk about cancer then I will be overwhelmed'). Patients are often very reluctant to give up their avoidance behaviour and often need to be offered an explanation of why avoidance should be addressed ('You seem to be reluctant to spend any time at the Day Hospice as you have been thinking that everyone will start to speak to you about death'). This may involve exploring advantages and disadvantages of the strategy and testing out the effects of dropping avoidance for a period of time.

Box 12.1   Dialogue between therapist (T) and patient (P)

T: This is certainly a common experience of many of my patients – they would rather avoid everything to do with cancer than have the unpleasant feelings associated with facing up to whatever it is that they are avoiding.

P: My view is; why feel bad if you can avoid it?

T: I would agree with you. Avoidance certainly makes you feel better at the time. Some people find that avoidance does not work in the long run or that it gets more and more difficult to avoid unpleasant feelings.

P: It seems to work for me.

T: It may be that there is no downside to your avoidance in which case this may have nothing to do with the agitation and unpleasant thoughts you were telling me about. On the other hand it may be that it is this which is making things more difficult and we may need to work on helping you to reverse the avoidance.

P: I can see that it might be a problem.

T: Do you find that there is any change in how often you have to push the thoughts out of your mind or how often you have to make an effort to avoid reminders of cancer?

P: I am not sure.

T: Given the fact that your avoidance could be crucial in keeping your problems going, would you consider monitoring this for a week to see when and how often you have to do this?

P: If you can show me how to do that and you think it might help me.

This patient (see Box 12.1) returned to the next session having discovered that she was having to engage in significant effort to avoid reminders of cancer. This was used for discussion of the advantages and disadvantages of avoidance and as a way of trying out alternative strategies to address her urge to avoid unpleasant reminders. Modification of intermediate beliefs ('If I get frightening memories then I should block them from my mind') about avoidance can be combined with behavioural experiments designed to evaluate the emotional, cognitive and behavioural consequences of engagement with cancer stimuli. Patients should be advised to keep note of the advantages of reversing cognitive and behavioural avoidance. Reversal of cognitive avoidance is essential for patients who are experiencing problems related to intrusive memories, flashbacks and nightmares. Patients often find it easier to consider this if intrusive phenomena are normalized. Therapists may need to help patients address problematic metacognitions, which influence cognitive and behavioural avoidance. Avoidance is often reinforced by the avoidance behaviours displayed by cancer care staff – who may themselves promote avoidance in their interactions with patients and have problems that relate to their own exposure to distress.

Facilitating control

Many psychological problems associated with cancer can be minimized if people can control the impact of the disease and treatment on their lives. The very process of engagement within psychological therapy provides patients with experience of exerting control over the problems that have resulted in their presentation for help. Group psychotherapeutic approaches also enable participants to learn more about the ways in which others have developed control over their problems.

The use of Weekly Activity Schedules can be implemented during assessment and linked with intervention in this regard. Forward planning can be used to enable people to pre-empt problems associated with treatment by scheduling activities around treatment days. There may be occasions when a patient has to be in isolation – because of an immunocompromised state or because of radioactivity (in the case of brachytherapy). The use of an activity schedule can be helpful and provide the patient with structure to buffer the negative emotions which exposure to these scenarios can cause. Patients can be encouraged to keep written records of their fatigue and daily activity levels. These can be used to plan responses to fatigue and to schedule appropriate amounts of rest. The Multidimensional Fatigue Inventory can be used to monitor outcome. Patients may have difficulty accepting the need for rest and the limitations which accompany a diagnosis. This can often be addressed by enabling them to set more achievable goals and changing the thoughts which make activity more difficult at times of diminished energy.

The extract in Box 12.2 outlines how planning activities was discussed with a patient with metastatic ovarian cancer who was struggling to cope with weakness during a course of chemotherapy:

Box 12.2 Dialogue between therapist (T) and patient (P)

T: You feel that there is nothing you can do – the chemotherapy takes control over your routine.

P: It seems to get in the way of anything I try to do.

T: Do you remember using the activity diary when we first met?

P: The thing on the grid.

T: Yes.

P: Yes.

T: I wondered if we could use it again – this time, to try to work round the chemotherapy. You know when you have to come for it and now that you have been in twice we could probably work out when you were feeling at your worst and work around it.

P: I see . . . keeping a note of what I do again.

T: The main thing will be to make a plan – keeping a note of what you do will be a good idea though as you can check out how the plan goes.

P: Right.

T: When do you get the chemotherapy again?

P: I come in on Friday morning.

T: What do you think then about beginning to make the plan from Saturday to Thursday? We can meet up again next Friday to see how you got on.

P: Just the idea of doing something to try to break the monotony helps.

T: Good. Let's start with Saturday morning and what you usually like to do on a Saturday?

P: I usually try to get out to Tesco for 8.30 – for its opening, to miss the rush.

T: When was the last time that you did that?

P: A month ago.

T: How realistic is it, based on the past two chemo visits, that you will be able to do that on Saturday?

P: Mmm, I would like to be able to get it done . . . but I need to sleep

T: That's what this planning will be about . . . being realistic about what you can achieve. This way you can feel that you have achieved something. Before you were getting down because you did not achieve anything – mainly because your plan was not sensitive to the temporary changes in your life.

P: I see.

T: Is there another shop that you could go to? or could you go at another time? or day?

Enhancing social, partner and family support

Given the pivotal role of social, partner and family support, the formulation for some patients will outline the central negative influence of a lack of a social network or adequate social, partner or family support. Here the therapist's role is to facilitate changes within the patient's environment and in the case of more prolonged therapeutic contacts, the psychologist themselves becomes part of a supportive framework. Patients must first be helped to determine the main reasons why there is diminished social support. This could relate to hopelessness, anxiety, procrastination or a lack of opportunity to socialize. Diminished support may relate to individual family members feeling threatened as a result of the cancer diagnosis and/or having developed psychological problems which require intervention in their own right. Friends and relatives may avoid patients, resulting in less social support being available. When relatives are uncertain about how best to help the patient, therapists can arrange to provide advice on practical strategies and how to overcome some of the obstacles to providing support. Significant others may need help to evaluate beliefs about the consequences of expressing any negative emotions ('If I talk to her about her cancer then I will make things worse'). The management of communication problems that have been triggered by the cancer is generally easier than scenarios in which communication problems are a long-standing feature of the patient's life and cancer just another example of how it can become manifest.

Patients may have held beliefs about the support that they thought that they would have received from friends and family and become depressed when this does not materialize. Support may be withdrawn prematurely and/or be provided when it is not needed. Patients who are making predictions about the unrewarding nature of social interaction can be encouraged to identify and evaluate these thoughts and, if appropriate, evaluate them using a behavioural experiment. Some patients find that they have no idea what they will say to other people who ask about their cancer and may need assistance, both in evaluating their predictions about this and in developing skills to confidently manage their interactions with others (Box 12.3).

Box 12.3   Dialogue between therapist (T) and patient (P)

T: So you have very few contacts with other people at the moment?

P: I suppose so. That's why they want me to go to the day centre.

T: Has that always been the case – that you don't tend to see too many people during the week?

P: No, I used to fill my week without a problem.

T: What sorts of things filled your week that you don't have happening now?

P: I had my visits to the church lunches on a Tuesday, my sister visited on a Wednesday, I did some voluntary work on a Friday and Saturday was always my day for seeing the family.

T: When was the last time that your week had this normal pattern for you?

P: Let me see, must have been about 2 weeks before the surgery – yes, that would be the last time I had a 'normal' week for me.

T: What would you see as being the main things that have interfered with you being in touch with other people like you used to be?

P: I don't know.

T: Let's look at it another way – what would need to happen for you to have a week which was more like the ones that you used to have?

P: It would need to be 2 months time – that's how long the doctor said it would be before I had fully recovered.

T: That's certainly one way of looking at it. Can you think of any disadvantages of relying on the passage of time alone?

P: I get very low with no-one around.

T: That's what I was thinking too – your depression does seem to relate to having few contacts at the moment. Is there any way that you could have contact with the people from your normal week but not have to go out and about to see them all?

P: I couldn't ask them to all come and seem me.

T: Could you ask some of, or even one of them, if they would like to come for a visit?

P: Yes, maybe they are waiting to be asked.

Handling uncertainty

The uncertainty associated with a cancer diagnosis triggers powerful emotional responses. All psychological therapies focus upon enabling patients to articulate and express these, although they differ slightly in the ways in which they might address this process. Psychodynamic and supportive–expressive psychological therapies help patients express and tolerate the powerful emotions linked with uncertainty. In some circumstances the main vehicle of therapeutic change relates to the support and nurturance that the psychologist provides in enabling patients to 'stay with' this powerful emotion (contrasted with the pervasive avoidance that is often reflected in the responses of society and significant others). There is a huge variability in the psychosocial correlates of uncertainty – some patients interpret this as a positive reason to 'live for the moment' and others tend to respond to uncertainty with hopelessness and fear. Some patients can accept the uncertainty associated with the course of their disease. They interpret this as an inevitability which cannot be avoided and are able to keep their thinking focused upon what is known to them, without becoming preoccupied with 'what ifs'.

The way in which cancer services are delivered can worsen problems with uncertainty. Waiting for test results, appointment scheduling arrangements and the way in which information is provided to patients (as 'indirect' psychological intervention components) can all be modified with good results to minimize the problems of those struggling with uncertainty. Therapists should consider environmental and situational strategies as first line intervention strategies.

Cognitive intervention strategies for uncertainty begin by enabling patients to understand that it is not the uncertainty which is mediating their problems, but that it is their thoughts and beliefs about uncertainty which are causing difficulty. Life is always full of uncertainties – it is just that most of the time we choose to avoid thinking about this. The following extract (Box 12.4) illustrates how cognitive interventions can be used to enable patients to build a new way of viewing the uncertainties associated with cancer:

Box 12.4 Dialogue between therapist (T) and patient (P)

T: The last panic attack was in the clinic?

P: Yes.

T: That was the time that you were having thoughts that you were going to go mad and end up in Gartnavel? (Note: a local psychiatric hospital in Scotland).

P: I couldn't stand not knowing – the uncertainty was unbearable.

T: This is perhaps something else that we could work on by looking at your thoughts ... your thoughts about uncertainty and your ability to deal with it.

P: I need certainty.

T: What would you like to have certainty about?

P: That the cancer will not come back.

T: You want to be told for certain that the cancer will never return?

P: I know, I know I can't have that ... that would solve the panic though.

T: What is it about knowing it wouldn't come back that would help you feel less panicky?

P: I would know that I could control things again.

T: What sort of things?

P: Well, I could still work, could still see my children and have some sort of life.

T: Is it that you think that this is not going to happen? – being with your children and having some sort of life.

P: When I feel panicky, yes.

T: So, you think about the fact that you cannot be certain about the cancer coming back, this then leads you to feel panicky?

P: I just think. . . ... I can't deal with the uncertainty, it is going to drive me mad. It will all come back, I know it will.

T: So your awareness of the uncertainty leads you to think things will go out of control – that the cancer will come back. Feeling more in control you think might help you to feel less panicked about it?

P: Yes.

T: Perhaps we could also put together an action plan of all of the things you could do if the cancer were to come back – this might mean that you have less need to keep going over this possibility in my mind.

P: Not just yet, if I can feel more in control then I think I could just about face this.

T: I agree, let's spend our next session on that topic – helping you to feel more in control and able to deal with the certainties in life.

12.5.2 Specific treatment modalities

Cognitive behavioural and problem solving approaches
Cognitive behavioural interventions and therapies have been shown to be effective when applied to the psychosocial issues and problems experienced by cancer patients. Moorey *et al.* (2003) have published guidance on the application of cognitive behavioural psychotherapy with people who have cancer. Cognitive behaviour-based interventions, such as adjuvant psychological therapy, have been shown to improve anxiety and depressive symptoms and be superior to supportive counselling. Problem-solving

therapy has been shown to be effective in reducing cancer related distress and improving quality of life. Some interventions, although not strictly cognitive behavioural therapy, incorporate cognitive and behavioural strategies as part of a package of psychoeducation. There is good evidence of their application to depression and pain in cancer. Most cognitive behavioural approaches to psychosocial morbidity in cancer are characterized by short term approaches, consisting of time limited interventions that enable patients to acquire strategies to regulate their feelings and behaviour in relation to cancer and its impact on their lives. They aim to enhance confidence with ability to cope with the hurdles which cancer can present and successfully manage the practical aspects of living with cancer.

In some circumstances, it may be necessary to devote more therapy time to the coverage of existential themes, particularly when working with those patients who have advanced disease. Kissane *et al.* (1997) outline details of this in an approach that they called cognitive existential therapy. Concentrating on emotional expression as a therapeutic component is important part of cognitive behaviour therapy, especially with regard to 'realistic' thoughts and in the presence of avoidant coping. Cognitive behavioural therapies can also be delivered in a group format for cancer patients. Supportive expressive psychotherapy has traditionally been delivered in this format and will be considered next.

Supportive expressive psychotherapy

Supportive expressive therapy has been traditionally delivered in a group and in the context of work to evaluate the impact of participation in such groups on survival. One of the major goals of this modality is to enable individuals to express all emotions (negative and positive). Based on the premise that most people tend to avoid the fear and anxiety associated with the possibility of death, supportive expressive therapy enables someone to express and tolerate the affect associated with thoughts of death and dying. This has been referred to as 'detoxifying death'. It has been suggested that therapy with this focus may be more appropriate for patients with advanced cancer. The therapy consists of the building of bonds between participants, facilitating emotional expression, assisting with the redefinition of life priorities, enabling increased access to the support of family and friends, improving doctor–patient relationships and improving coping skills.

Interventions that focus on family dynamics

Family therapy has traditionally been applied to the psychosocial needs of families with a physically ill child, with problems seen with children and adolescents and usually with mental health problems, though this has been changing over the past two decades. In psychosocial oncology, most family-oriented interventions seek to enhance communication and facilitate relationships that are sensitive to the emotional and psychological dimensions, their being a member of the family who has cancer. Treatment goals often involve enabling patients to tackle avoidance of communication, particularly on emotionally charged topics such as death. Therapeutic work may focus upon enabling families to ensure that cancer does not become a dominant feature in influencing all relationships and responses to everyday events. Families often find it useful to focus on the identification of shared assets and to engage in a process whereby they begin to prioritize the problems that face them or consider how they might have untapped resources that could be used to address problems. The majority of families are able to maintain a degree of stability, ensuring that the non-medical needs of the family are addressed. However, therapeutic time may need to be devoted to reinforcing the non-medical needs of the index patient (and possibly those of key family members, especially those of young children). This is particularly the case when a conceptualization reveals that families have been neglecting well-being as individuals and within a family.

Interventions with a psychodynamic focus

In psychodynamic therapies the major goal is to enable the patient to experience and express distressing emotions within a non-judgemental, supportive relationship. The therapist also helps the patient to explore underlying conflicts, and understand their expression within current relationships. The aims, when using a psychodynamic approach to psychological therapy with people who have had cancer, is to move patients from rigid, limiting defences to proactive, positive coping efforts. As with all psychodynamically based interventions in general adult practice, the therapeutic relationship with the person who has cancer is key to the process. The clinical psychologist working within this framework works toward enabling a patient to have deep trust within the therapeutic relationship, feeling able to let defences down and to open up and allow emotional exploration. Psychodynamic psychotherapy highlights unresolved childhood conflicts. This can help patients understand the role that these conflicts play in current relationships. This way the patient can gather and experience appropriate support and re-establish a sense of personal control. Patients may transfer old feelings and ways of relating that were established with parents, causing distortions and conflict. Cancer (like any physical illness) can often foster dependency on the therapist. Patients can idealize their clinical psychologist as the 'only one who understands'. Patients may become extremely angry when the nurturance they seek is not provided and will often resist the therapist's efforts to guide or explore their psychological experience of cancer, particularly when there are unresolved authority issues.

Some patients project the anger that they have about the diagnosis and course of their cancer on the therapist. The opportunity to work through these issues, to accept mature relationship boundaries, to face dependency needs or work with, not against, an authority figure can provide significant opportunities for emotional growth. Therapists also develop counter-transference feelings, i.e. emotional responses to the patient that may be rooted in the therapist's own needs and conflicts. The therapist may feel out of control and helpless to impact the illness. He/she may be uncomfortable in relation to signs of medical illness (e.g. scars and disfigurement). He/she may fear loss and sadness if the patient dies. He/she may struggle with a need to nurture the patient and foster an unhealthy dependency. A psychologist may use his/her own defences to cope with these feelings, which will then influence the therapeutic relationship. The therapist pays attention to the patient's deepest unexpressed feelings, to help him/her understand and process those feelings. When the patient does not need to expend emotional energy defending against feelings he/she is better able to cope with illness-related distress.

12.6   Does psychological intervention influence survival?

In the context of a growing interest in the effects of psychosocial factors on health and illness over the past two decades, there have been various attempts to examine the influence of psychosocial factors on mortality and the potential benefits of psychological intervention on survival.

The well-known work of David Speigel found significantly longer survival time in metastatic breast cancer group members and led to a great deal of interest in the effect of group social support on morbidity and mortality. However, studies of the effect of group interventions on survival are inconsistent with some showing longer survival time and immunological response for cancer group members but others failing to demonstrate such a connection. Higher helplessness/hopelessness scores on the Mental Adjustment to Cancer Scale are associated with a moderately detrimental effect on survival. It is possible that psychotherapy targeted at helplessness/hopelessness might produce survival benefits.

12.7   Summary

This chapter has aimed to provide a brief overview of some of the work carried out in psychosocial oncology and discuss the various ways in which psychological theory has been applied to the treatment of individuals who have a cancer diagnosis.

An individual's psychological adjustment to their cancer journey can vary according to a wide range of different factors. These factors can include: the specific type of cancer the individual has been diagnosed with, the particulars of their treatment, the range of support that is available to them and their own individual characteristics.

Psychological distress is increasingly recognized in oncology as a treatable feature of an individual's reduced quality of life. Psychologists can assess individuals who may be suffering from psychological distress, formulate a treatment plan, specific to that individual, and provide targeted psychological interventions. There are a number of different psychological approaches which have been shown to be effective at targeting some of the key processes that can negatively influence an individual's adjustment to their diagnosis and treatment. Trained clinicians can apply these approaches (e.g. cognitive behavioural therapy or psychodynamic therapy) to address the different processes (e.g. targeting avoidant thinking or handling uncertainty) that are involved in an individual's psychological distress. Also, there is a significant body of research that suggests that interventions targeted at reducing psychological distress can improve the clinical outcomes of patients, as well as improving their quality of life.

12.8   Self-assessment questions

Question: What are the risk factors associated with developing severe psychological distress?

Answer: Patients who: are younger, are single by virtue of separation, are divorced or widowed, live alone, have children aged under 21 years old, are experiencing economic adversity, have a perceived lack of social support, have poor marital or family functioning, have a history of psychiatric problems, have cumulative stressful life events, have a history of alcohol or other substance abuse.

Question: What is a formulation?

Answer: A formulation is an explanation of the psychological factors and processes that are thought to account for the onset, maintenance and expression of the psychosocial problems.

Question: At what times in a patient's cancer journey is the greatest risk of developing psychological problems?

Answer: Patients (particularly those with higher risks toward vulnerability) are more at risk when the illness is diagnosed, during the early months of treatment, when all treatment has ended or when a recurrence or spread of the cancer is discovered.

Question: What are examples of some of the processes described in this chapter that can be targeted or facilitated by psychological interventions in oncology?

Answer: Avoidant behaviour and thinking, facilitation of control, enhancing social, partner and family support, and handling uncertainty.

Question: What patient group has it been suggested that supportive expressive psychotherapy may be most appropriate for?

Answer: Patients with advanced cancer.

12.9 Further reading and resources

Andersen BL, Cyranowski JM and Espindle D. Men's sexual self-schema. *J Pers Soc Psychol* 1999, **76**, 645–661.

Andersen BL, Woods XA and Copeland LJ. Sexual self schema and sexual morbidity among gynaecologic cancer survivors. *J Consult Clin Psychol* 1997, **65**, 221–229.

Arai Y, Kawakita M, Hida S, Terachi T, Okada Y and Yoshida O. Psychological aspects in long term survivors of testicular cancer. *J Urol* 1996, **155**, 574–578.

Barraclough J. *Cancer and Emotion. A Practical Guide to Psycho-oncology*, third edition. John Wiley, Chichester, 1999.

Barsevick AM, Sweeney C, Haney E and Chung E. A systematic qualitative analysis of psychoeducational interventions for depression in patients with cancer. *Oncol Nurs Forum* 2002, **29**, 73–87.

Bottomley A. Group cognitive behavioural therapy: an intervention for cancer patients. *Int J Palliat Nurs* 1996, **2**, 131–137.

Brennan J. Adjustment to cancer – coping or personal transition? *Psycho-Oncology* 2001, **10**, 1–18.

Brewin C, Watson M, McCarthy S, Hyman P and Dayson D. Memory processes and the course of anxiety and depression in cancer patients. *Psychol Med* 1998, **28**, 219–224.

Burton M and Watson M. *Counselling People with Cancer*. John Wiley, Chichester, 1998.

Cameron LD, Leventhal H and Love RR. Trait anxiety, symptom perceptions, and illness-related responses among women with breast cancer in remission during a tamoxifen clinical trial. *Health Psychol* 1998, **17**, 459–469.

Cella D, Davis K, Breitbart W and Curt G. Cancer-related fatigue: prevalence of proposed diagnostic criteria in a united states sample of cancer survivors. *J Clin Oncol* 2001, **19**(14), 3385–3391.

Cella DF and Tross S. Psychological adjustment to survival from Hodgkin's disease. *J Consult Clin Psychol* 1986, **54**, 616–622.

Coates A, Abraham S, Kaye SB, Sowerbutts T, Frewin C, Rox RM and Tattersal MHN. On the receiving end - patient perception of the side effects of cancer chemotherapy. *Eur J Cancer Clin Oncol* 1983, **19**, 203–208.

Cottrell D and Boston P. Practitioner review: the effectiveness of systemic family therapy for children and adolescents. *J Child Psychol Psychiatry* 2002, **43**(5), 573–586.

Coward DD. Constructing meaning from the experience of cancer. *Semin Oncol Nurs* 1997, **13**, 248–251.

Cull A, Anderson EDC, Campbell S, Mackay J, Smyth E and Steel M. The impact of genetic counselling about breast cancer risk on women's risk perceptions and levels of distress. *Br J Cancer* 1999, **79**(3/4), 501–508.

Cunningham AJ and Edmonds C. Group psychosocial support in metastatic breast cancer (letter). *N Engl J Med* 2002, **346**(16), 1247–1248.

Cunningham AJ, Edmonds CVI, Jenkins GP, Pollack H, Lockwood GA and Warr D. A randomized controlled trial of the effects of group psychological therapy on survival in women with metastatic breast cancer. *Psycho-Oncology* 1998, **7**, 508–517.

Deimling GT, Kahana B, Bowman KF and Schaefer ML. Cancer survivorship and psychological distress in later life. *Psycho-Oncology* 2002, **11**(6), 479–494.

D'Errico GM, Galassi JP, Schanberg R and Ware WB. Development and validation of the Cancer Worries Inventory: a measure of illness-related cognitions. *J Psychosoc Oncol* 1999, **17**, 119–137.

Derogatis LR, Morrow GR, Fetting J, *et al.* The prevalence of psychiatric disorders among cancer patients. *JAMA* 1983, **249**, 751–757.

Devine EC. Meta-analysis of the effect of psychoeducational interventions of pain in adults with cancer. *Oncol Nurs Forum* 2003, **30**, 75–89.

Dunkel-Schetter C, Feinstein LG, Taylor SE and Falke RL. Patterns of coping with cancer. *Health Psychol* 1992, **11**(2), 79–87.

Edelman S, Lemon J, Bell DR and Kidman AD. Effects of group CBP on the survival time of patients with metastatic breast cancer. *Psycho-Oncology* 1999, **8**, 474–481.

Fallowfield L, Jenkins V, Farewell V, Saul J, Duffy A and Eves R. Efficacy of a Cancer Research UK communication skills training model for oncologists: a randomized controlled trial. *Lancet* 2002, **359**, 650–656.

Faulkner A and Maguire P. *Talking to Cancer Patients and Their Relatives*, Chapter 2. Oxford University Press, Oxford, 1994.

Fawzy FI. Psychosocial interventions for patients with cancer: what works and what doesn't. *Eur J Cancer* 1999, **35**, 1559–1564.

Fawzy FI, Fawzy NW, Arndt LA and Pasnau RO. Critical review of psychosocial interventions in cancer care. *Arch Gen Psychiatry* 1995, **52**, 100–113.

Finney JW and Bonner MJ. The influence of behavioural family intervention on the health of chronically ill children. *Behaviour Change* 1993, **9**, 157–170.

Gilbar O and De-Nour K. Adjustment to illness and dropout of chemotherapy. *J Psychosomatic Res* 1989, **33**, 1–5.

Goodwin PJ, Leszcz M, Ennis M, *et al.* The effect of group psychosocial support on survival in metastatic breast cancer. *N Engl J Med* 2001, **345**(24), 1719–1726.

Greer S and Moorey S. Adjuvant psychological therapy for cancer patients. *Palliat Med* 1997 **11**, 240–244.

Greer S, Moorey S, Baruch JD, *et al.* Adjuvant psychological therapy for patients with cancer: a prospective randomised trial. *Br Med J* 1992, **304**, 675–680.

Homsi J, Walsh D, Rivera N, *et al.* Symptom evaluation in palliative medicine: patient report vs systematic assessment. *Support Care Cancer* 2006, **14**, 444–453.

Hopwood P. Psychological issues in cancer genetics: Current research and future priorities. *Patient Educ Couns* 1997, **32**, 19–31.

Jenkins V, Fallowfield L and Saul J. Information needs of patients with cancer: results from a large study in UK cancer centers. *Br J Cancer* 2001, **84**, 48–51.

Kangas M, Henry JL and Bryant RA. Posttraumatic stress disorder following cancer. A conceptual and empirical review. *Clin Psychol Rev* 2002, **22**, 499–524.

Katz MR, Rodin G and Devins D. Self esteem and cancer. *Can J Psychiatry* 1995, **40**, 608–615.

Kissane DW, Bloch WI *et al.* (1994). Psychological morbidity in the families of patients with cancer. *Psycho-Oncology* **3**, 47–56.

Kissane DW, Bloch S, Miach P, Smith GC, Seddon A and Keks N. Cognitive-existential group therapy for patients with primary breast cancer-techniques and themes. *Psycho-oncology* 1997, **6**, 25–33.

Lee-Jones C, Humphris G, Dixon R and Bebbington Hatcher M. Fear of cancer recurrence – a literature review and proposed cognitive formulation to explain exacerbation of recurrence fears. *Psycho-Oncology* 1997, **6**, 95–105.

Lepore SJ and Coyne JC. Psychological interventions for distress in cancer patients: a review of reviews. *Ann Behav Med* 2006, **32**(2), 85–92.

Lepore SJ and Helgeson VS. Social constraints, intrusive thoughts and mental health after prostate cancer. *J Soc Clin Psychol* 1998, **17**, 89–106.

Manne SL. Intrusive thoughts and psychological distress among cancer patients: the role of spouse avoidance and criticism. *J Consult Clin Psychol* 1999, **67**, 539–546.

Merluzzi TV and Sanchez MAM. Assessment of self efficacy and coping with cancer: development and validation of the cancer behaviour inventory. *Health Psychol* 1997a, **16**, 163–170.

Merluzzi TV and Sanchez MAM. Factor structure of the psychosocial adjustment to illness scale (self-report) for persons with cancer. *Psychol Assess* 1997b, **9**, 269–276.

Moorey S, Frampton M and Greer S. The Cancer Coping Questionnaire: a self-rating scale for measuring the impact of adjuvant psychological therapy on coping behaviour. *Psycho-Oncology* 2003, **12**, 331–344.

National Breast Cancer Centre and National Cancer Control Initiative. Clinical practice guidelines for the psychosocial care of people with cancer. National Breast Cancer Centre, Camperdown, NSW, 2003.

National Comprehensive Cancer Network. NCCN practice guidelines for the management of psychosocial distress. *Oncology* 1999, **13**, 113–147.

O'Connor AP, Wicker CA and Germino BB. Understanding the cancer patient's search for meaning. *Cancer Nurs* 1990, **13**, 167–175.

Osborne RH, Elsworth GR, Kissane DW, Burke SA and Hopper JL. The Mental Adjustment to Cancer (MAC) Scale: replication and refinement in 632 breast cancer patients. *Psychol Med* 1999, **29**, 1335–1345.

Osowiecki D and Compas BE. Psychological adjustment to cancer: control beliefs and coping in adult cancer patients. *Cogn Ther Res* 1998, **22**, 483–499.

Ryan H, Schofield P, Cockburn J, *et al*. How to recognise and manage psychological distress in cancer patients. *Eur J Cancer Care* 2005, **14**, 7–15.

Sadler IJ, Jacobsen PB, Booth-Jones M, Belanger H, Weitzner MA and Field KK. Preliminary evaluation of a clinical syndrome approach to assessing cancer-related fatigue. *J Pain Symptom Manage* 2002, **23**(5), 406–416.

Sanson-Fisher R, Girgis A, Boyes A, *et al*. The unmet supportive care needs of patients with cancer. *Cancer* 2000, **88**, 226–237.

Schumacher KL, Koresawa S, West C, Dodd M, Paul SM, Tripathy D, Koo P and Miaskowski C. The usefulness of a daily pain management diary for outpatients with cancer-related pain. *Oncol Nurs Forum* 2002, **29**, 1304–1313.

Speice J, Harkness J, Laneri H, *et al*. Involving family members in cancer care: focus group considerations of patients and oncological providers. *Psycho-Oncology* 2000, **9**, 101–112.

Sprangers MAG, Cull A, Groenvold K, Bjordal K, Blazeby J and Aaronson NK. The European Organisation for Research and Treatment of Cancer approach to developing questionnaire modules: an update and overview. *Quality of Life Research* 1998, **7**, 291–300.

Sprangers MAG, te Velde A and Aaronson NK. The Construction and Testing of the EORTC Colorectal Cancer-specific Quality of Life Questionnaire Module (QLQ-CR38). *Eur J Cancer* 1999, **35**, 238–247.

Stanton AL, Danoff-Burg S, Sworowski LA, Collins CA, Branstetter AD, Rodriguez-Hanley A, Kirk SB and Austenfeld JL. Randomized, controlled trial of written emotional expression and benefit finding in breast cancer patients. *J Clin Oncol* 2002, **20**, 4160–4168.

Stanton AL, Danoff-Burg S, Cameron CL, *et al*. Emotionally expressive coping predicts psychological and physical adjustment to breast cancer. *J Consult Clin Psychol* 2000, **68**, 875–882.

Thornton AA. Perceiving benefits in the cancer experience. *J Clin Psychol Med Settings* 2002, **9**, 153–165.

Veach TA and Nicholas DR. Understanding families of adults with cancer: combining the clinical course of cancer and stages of family development. *J Couns Develop* 1998, **76**, 144–156.

Vickberg SMJ, Bovbjerg DH, DuHamel KN, Currie V and Redd WH. Intrusive thoughts and psychological distress among breast cancer survivors: global meaning as a possible protective factor. *Behavi Med* 2000, **25**, 152–160.

Walker LG, Walker MB, *et al*. Psychological, clinical and pathological effects of relaxation training and guided imagery during primary chemotherapy. *Br J Cancer* 1999, **80**, 262–268.

Walker LG, Ratcliffe MA and Dawson AA. Relaxation and hypnotherapy: long term effects on the survival of patients with lymphoma. *Psycho-Oncology* 2000, **9**, 355–356.

Watson M. What to do when a depressed or anxious cancer patient refuses further treatment. *Drug Benefit Trends* 2000, **12**, 5–9.

White CA and Macleod U. Cancer. In: *ABC of Psychological Medicine*. BMJ Books, London, 2002.

White CA. The measurement of meaning in psychosocial oncology. *Psycho-Oncology* 2004, **13**, 468–481.

Yurek D, Farrar W and Andersen BL. Breast cancer surgery: comparing surgical groups and determining individual differences in post operative sexuality and body change stress. *J Consult Clin Psychol* 2000, **68**, 697–709.

Index